PIONEERING DISCOVERIES IN

NANOTECHNOLOGY

FOR HEALTH AND WELLBEING

Other Titles by the Editors

Tissue Engineering and Nanotheranostics
ISBN: 978-981-314-918-2

The World Scientific Encyclopedia of Nanomedicine and Bioengineering I: Nanotechnology for Translational Medicine: Tissue Engineering, Biological Sensing, Medical Imaging, and Therapeutics
(A 4-Volume Set)
Volume 1: Noble Metal Nanoparticles for Biomedical Applications
Volume 2: Application of Nano-structured Materials and Devices in Chemical and Biological Sensing
Volume 3: Nanotechnology in Gene Delivery
Volume 4: Nano Imaging: From Fundamental Principles to Translational Medical Applications
ISBN: 978-981-4667-65-4 (Set)
ISBN: 978-981-4667-61-6 (Vol. 1)
ISBN: 978-981-4667-71-5 (Vol. 2)
ISBN: 978-981-4667-70-8 (Vol. 3)
ISBN: 978-981-4667-63-0 (Vol. 4)

The World Scientific Encyclopedia of Nanomedicine and Bioengineering II: Bioimplants, Regenerative Medicine, and Nano-Cancer Diagnosis and Phototherapy
(A 3-Volume Set)
Volume 1: Biomaterial Implants for Tissue Regeneration and Engineering
Volume 2: Graphene Quantum Dots for Biomedical Applications
Volume 3: Advanced Nanomaterials for Bioimaging and Cancer Therapy
ISBN: 978-981-4667-58-6 (Set)
ISBN: 978-981-4667-64-7 (Vol. 1)
ISBN: 978-981-4667-62-3 (Vol. 2)
ISBN: 978-981-4667-69-2 (Vol. 3)

Bio-Inspired Nanomaterials and Applications: Nano Detection, Drug/Gene Delivery, Medical Diagnosis and Therapy
ISBN: 978-981-4616-91-1

Bioengineering in Wound Healing: A Systems Approach
ISBN: 978-981-314-457-6

PIONEERING DISCOVERIES IN NANOTECHNOLOGY FOR HEALTH AND WELLBEING

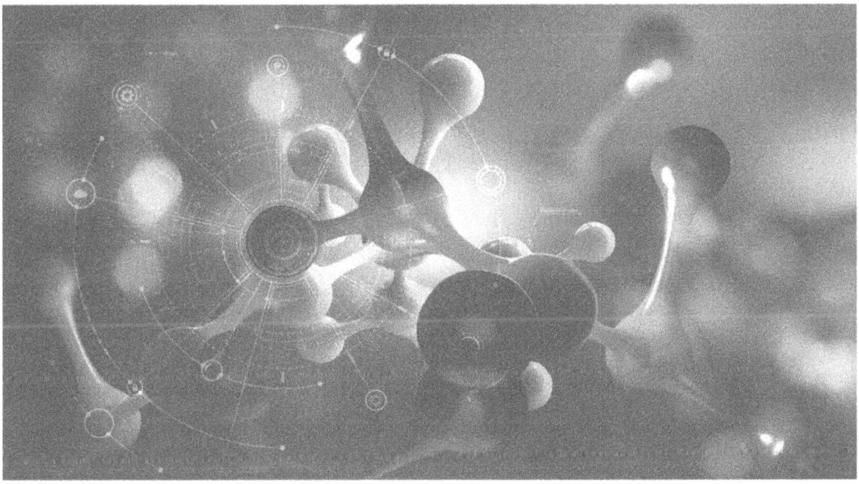

EDITED BY

DONGLU SHI

University of Cincinnati, USA

MARTIN L YARMUSH

Rutgers University, USA

World Scientific

NEW JERSEY • LONDON • SINGAPORE • GENEVA • BEIJING • SHANGHAI • TAIPEI • CHENNAI

Published by

World Scientific Publishing Co. Pte. Ltd.
5 Toh Tuck Link, Singapore 596224
USA office: 27 Warren Street, Suite 401-402, Hackensack, NJ 07601
UK office: 57 Shelton Street, Covent Garden, London WC2H 9HE

Library of Congress Control Number: 2024060704

British Library Cataloguing-in-Publication Data
A catalogue record for this book is available from the British Library.

PIONEERING DISCOVERIES IN NANOTECHNOLOGY FOR HEALTH AND WELLBEING

ISBN 978-981-98-0901-1 (hardcover)
ISBN 978-981-98-0902-8 (ebook for institutions)
ISBN 978-981-98-0903-5 (ebook for individuals)

For any available supplementary material, please visit
https://www.worldscientific.com/worldscibooks/10.1142/14206#t=suppl

Desk Editor: Brittney Phitojo

Typeset by Stallion Press
Email: enquiries@stallionpress.com

https://doi.org/10.1142/9789819809028_fmatter

Preface

Over the past decade, nanotechnology has transformed the landscape of health and wellbeing, offering innovative solutions to some of the most complex challenges in medicine, biology, and environmental health. By leveraging the unique properties of materials at the nanoscale, researchers have unlocked unprecedented opportunities for precision medicine, advanced diagnostics, and sustainable healthcare systems. This period has been marked by remarkable progress in areas such as nanomedicine, regenerative therapies, and pandemic management, highlighting the intersection of engineering, biology, and technology.

One of the most significant advancements has been in nanomedicine, where nanoparticles and nanoscale systems are now routinely employed to deliver therapeutics with pinpoint accuracy. This has enabled the treatment of diseases such as cancer, cardiovascular conditions, and neurodegenerative disorders with reduced side effects and improved efficacy. The development of multi-functional nanoparticles capable of simultaneous imaging, diagnosis, and therapy has further bridged the gap between treatment and monitoring, embodying the promise of personalized medicine.

Regenerative medicine has seen a paradigm shift through nanotechnology. Electrospinning and electrospraying techniques have revolutionized biomanufacturing by creating scaffolds and matrices that mimic the extracellular environment, facilitating tissue engineering and organ regeneration. Advances in nanostructured biomaterials have enabled precise control over cell behavior, opening new doors for repairing and regenerating damaged tissues.

The past decade also underscored the critical role of nanotechnology in addressing global health crises, such as the COVID-19 pandemic. Rapid diagnostic tools, including nanosensor-based testing, proved instrumental in early detection and disease management. Moreover, nanoscale vaccines and drug delivery systems accelerated the development and deployment of life-saving therapeutics. These breakthroughs underscored how nanotechnology can quickly adapt to emergent challenges and enhance public health infrastructure.

From a fundamental research perspective, new insights into the biophysical properties of cells and tissues have emerged through nanotechnology. For instance, studies exploring the unique electrical charges of cancer cell surfaces have provided novel therapeutic targets, linking nanotechnology with cellular metabolism and tumor biology. These discoveries not only improve our understanding of disease mechanisms but also inspire the design of innovative therapeutic interventions.

As we reflect on the past decade, it is clear that the convergence of nanotechnology with life sciences has redefined the possibilities for improving human health and wellbeing. This collection of groundbreaking studies from *Nano LIFE* exemplifies the field's progress and its potential for future breakthroughs. From addressing the challenges of precision medicine to contributing to global health security, nanotechnology continues to expand the horizons of what is achievable in science and healthcare.

This volume celebrates the ingenuity, resilience, and transformative impact of nanotechnology research. It serves as a testament to the progress made and an inspiration for the future, as we continue to explore the possibilities that lie at the intersection of the nanoscale and the complexities of life.

As we celebrate the 15th anniversary of *Nano LIFE*, we reflect on the journal's profound impact on advancing nanotechnology for health and wellbeing. Over the years, *Nano LIFE* has served as a premier platform for innovative research that bridges the gap between nanotechnology and life sciences. To honor this milestone, we have curated a collection of 16 groundbreaking articles that exemplify the journal's commitment to excellence in this transformative field. These selected works, spanning a range of critical topics, highlight the versatility and significance of nanotechnology in addressing pressing biomedical challenges.

The collection begins with **"Electrospinning and Electrospraying with Cells for Applications in Biomanufacturing"** by Qilong Zhao and Min Wang. This pioneering work explores the application of electrohydrodynamic processes in integrating living cells with nanostructures. It underscores how nanotechnology enables the scalable production of bioengineered constructs for tissue engineering and regenerative medicine, opening new avenues for biomanufacturing.

Francois Berthiaume, in **"COVID-19 Testing: Frequency Wins over Sensitivity in Control of Disease Transmission,"** presents a compelling argument for the strategic deployment of rapid, frequent testing. The study employs mathematical modeling to demonstrate how nanotechnology-enhanced testing methods can be instrumental in curbing disease outbreaks, particularly during pandemics like COVID-19.

In cancer research, Donglu Shi's **"Cancer Cell Surface Negative Charges: A Bio-Physical Manifestation of the Warburg Effect"** uncovers a novel connection between cancer cell metabolism and cell surface electrostatics. This biophysical analysis provides a new framework for designing therapies targeting the metabolic vulnerabilities of cancer cells, potentially leading to more effective treatment options.

The field of regenerative medicine is advanced by **"Therapeutic Delivery of Stromal Cell-Derived Factor-1 for Injury Repair"** by Agnes Yeboah, Martin L. Yarmush, and Francois Berthiaume. This paper highlights how nanotechnology facilitates the delivery of bioactive molecules to sites of injury, enhancing the body's natural healing mechanisms and providing a targeted approach to tissue repair and recovery.

Isabel Perez *et al.*'s **"Novel Brain-Derived Neurotrophic Factor Controlled-Release Formulation Promotes Neuroprotection *In Vitro*"** investigates the development of nanoparticles for the controlled release of neurotrophic factors. By enabling sustained delivery of these critical proteins, the study provides a promising strategy to combat neurodegenerative diseases and support neural regeneration.

Daniel Rui Chen, Megha Chitranshi, Mark Schulz, and Vesselin Shanov, in "**A Review of Three Major Factors Controlling Carbon Nanotubes Synthesis from the Floating Catalyst Chemical Vapor Deposition,**" delve into the intricate factors that dictate carbon nanotube growth. This comprehensive review explores catalyst design, reaction parameters, and carbon sources, offering essential insights for optimizing nanomaterial production processes.

The potential of nanoparticles in oncology is showcased in "**Gold Nanoparticles in Cancer Imaging and Therapeutics**" by Huang-Chiao Huang *et al.* This paper highlights the dual diagnostic and therapeutic functionalities of gold nanoparticles, illustrating their ability to improve imaging precision while simultaneously enabling targeted cancer therapies.

Andrew J. Giustini and colleagues' "**Magnetic Nanoparticle Hyperthermia in Cancer Treatment**" presents a groundbreaking approach to cancer therapy by leveraging magnetic nanoparticle-induced hyperthermia. The study explores how controlled heating of cancerous tissues using magnetic fields can selectively destroy tumor cells without harming surrounding healthy tissues.

Suneel Kumar *et al.*'s "**Sizes and Sufficient Quantities of MSC Microspheres for Intrathecal Injection to Modulate Inflammation in Spinal Cord Injury**" discusses the fabrication of mesenchymal stem cell (MSC) microspheres for spinal cord injury therapy. This innovative work reveals how nanotechnology can enhance the therapeutic potential of stem cells by enabling precise control over their delivery and dosage.

P. C. Pandey *et al.*'s "**Effect of the Organic Functionality on the Synthesis and Antimicrobial Activity of Silver Nanoparticles**" examines how surface functionalization influences the antimicrobial properties of silver nanoparticles. This study provides critical insights into designing nanoscale antimicrobials with enhanced efficacy and specificity.

Lennert Molenaar *et al.*'s "**Quantification of Magnetic Nanoparticles in *ex vivo* Colorectal Lymph Nodes**" introduces a novel methodology for quantifying magnetic nanoparticles in biomedical imaging applications. The work highlights the role of nanotechnology in improving the detection of cancer metastases through precise and non-invasive imaging techniques.

Chen-Hua Ma *et al.*'s "**Intratumoral Photosensitizer Delivery and Photodynamic Therapy**" combines nanotechnology and photodynamic therapy to achieve localized cancer treatment. By optimizing the delivery of photosensitizers, this study enhances therapeutic outcomes while minimizing off-target effects.

Rebecca J. Thomson *et al.*'s "**Nanoparticles in Joint Arthroplasties**" investigates the use of nanoparticles in enhancing the longevity and performance of orthopedic implants. This work paves the way for next-generation materials in joint replacement surgeries, addressing common challenges like wear and inflammation.

Tanya Nanda *et al.*'s "**Iron Oxide Nanoparticles for Tissue Repair and Regeneration**" highlights the role of magnetic nanoparticles in promoting tissue repair. The paper explores their application in guiding cellular activities and improving regenerative outcomes, particularly in musculoskeletal systems.

Fei He *et al.*'s "**Adverse Outcome Phenomena and Toxicity Mechanisms of Micro and Nanoplastics in Human Health**" addresses the emerging concerns of nanotoxicology. The study provides a detailed analysis of how micro- and nanoplastics impact human health, underscoring the importance of developing safer nanomaterials.

Scott R. Burge *et al.*'s "**Exploiting the Electrical Nature of Biofilms for Long-Term Monitoring of Quiescent Aquatic Environments via Open-Circuit Microbial Potentiometric Sensors: Evidence of Long-Distance Electrical Signaling**" presents innovative biosensing technologies using nanotechnology. The research offers solutions for real-time monitoring of environmental conditions, emphasizing the versatility of nanotechnology in addressing ecological challenges.

As editors, we extend our deepest gratitude to the authors, reviewers, and readers who have supported *Nano LIFE*. We hope this compilation serves as a vital resource for researchers, practitioners, and students, inspiring continued exploration and innovation in the transformative field of nanotechnology. These articles collectively represent the cutting-edge research published in *Nano LIFE* and reflect the ingenuity and dedication of researchers who harness nanotechnology to address complex biological and medical challenges.

Donglu Shi
University of Cincinnati, USA

Martin L. Yarmush
Rutgers University, USA

https://doi.org/10.1142/9789819809028_fmatter

About the Editors

Dr. Donglu Shi is a Professor of Materials Science and Engineering at the University of Cincinnati's College of Engineering. He served as the Chair and Graduate Director of the Materials Science and Engineering program from 2013 to 2023. Dr. Shi's research spans diverse fields, including nanoscience, energy materials, biomedical engineering, precision medicine, and condensed matter physics. His prolific work includes over 300 peer-reviewed journal publications, with many published in prestigious journals such as *Nature, Physical Review Letters, Advanced Materials, Biomaterials*, and *ACS Nano.* He has also authored 13 books on topics ranging from superconductivity and electronic materials to nanomedicine, magnetism, and biomaterials. Dr. Shi is the Editor-in-Chief of *Nano LIFE*, serves on the Editorial Board of *Biomaterials Advances*, and is an Associate Editor for the *Journal of Nanomaterials.* His contributions have been recognized with numerous awards, including the George Rieveschl Jr. Award for Distinguished Scientific Research, the Sarah Grant Barber Outstanding Faculty Advisor Award, the Neil Wandmacher Teaching Award, the Distinguished Engineering Researcher Award, and the Sigma Xi Research Recognition Award. A Fellow of ASM International and a Graduate College Fellow at the University of Cincinnati, Dr. Shi continues to make significant contributions to advancing materials science and engineering.

Professor Martin L. Yarmush is an internationally recognized bioengineer and translational scientist who has been a leader in the fields of tissue engineering and regenerative medicine, BioMEMS and nanotechnology, applied immunology and biotechnology, metabolic engineering, and medical device development. He currently serves as the Paul and Mary Monroe Endowed Chair and Distinguished Professor of Biomedical & Chemical Engineering at Rutgers University, and the Director of the Center for Engineering in Medicine and Surgery at the Massachusetts General Hospital (MGH). He has published over 580 refereed journal articles and over 60 patents & patent applications. He has also taught a spectrum of courses from molecular genetics, biochemistry, and immunology, thermodynamics and transport phenomena, to advanced biotechnology. Professor Yarmush is the recipient of over 30 local and national awards including Founding Fellow of AIMBE, Fellow of BMES, Fellow of the US National Academy of Inventors, and Fellow of the US National Academy of Engineering. He is also the founding editor-in-chief of the *Annual Review of Biomedical Engineering* and co-editor-in-chief of *Nano LIFE*. He has pioneered advancements in tissue engineering, stem cell therapies, bioartificial organs, organ storage methods for transplantation, and many more. Some of these innovations have led to patents and company formations, including Molecmo (later Novira), which developed novel antiviral drugs for Hepatitis B and was acquired by J&J in 2015 for $600M.

https://doi.org/10.1142/9789819809028_fmatter

Contents

https://doi.org/10.1142/9789819809028_0001

Chapter 1

Electrospinning and Electrospraying with Cells for Applications in Biomanufacturing*

Qilong Zhao†

Institute of Biomedical & Health Engineering
Shenzhen Institute of Advanced Technology
Chinese Academy of Sciences
Shenzhen 518035, P. R. China
ql.zhao@siat.ac.cn

Min Wang

Department of Mechanical Engineering
The University of Hong Kong
Pokfulam Road, Hong Kong, P. R. China
memwang@hku.hk

Biomanufacturing of cell-laden scaffolds with biomimetic cell-scaffold organizations resembling the structures and anatomy of human body tissues and organs holds great promise in tissue engineering and regenerative medicine. In human body tissues and organs, specific types of cells are supported by nanofibrous extracellular matrix (ECM) in well-defined three-dimensional (3D) manners. Electrospinning is a facile and effective technique for producing nanofibrous scaffolds, which exhibit high similarities in the structure compared to ECM that offers structural and mechanical supports to cells in the human body. The incorporation within the electrospun nanofibrous scaffolds has therefore been considered as a promising approach for biomanufacturing of cell-laden scaffolds with tissue-mimicking structures. However, limited by low controllability of conventional cell seeding

---

*To cite this article, please refer to its earlier version published in the *Nano LIFE*, Vol. 11, No. 4 (2021) 2141003 (19 pages), DOI: 10.1142/S1793984421410038

†Corresponding author.

strategies and small sizes of interconnected pores of normal electrospun scaffolds, it is highly difficult to incorporate living cells within electrospun scaffolds on demand and results in cell-laden scaffolds with desirable 3D cell-scaffold organization. With recent advances in electrospinning and electrospraying with cells, it is visible to directly incorporate living cells within scaffolds via cell microencapsulation approaches and therefore offer promising alternatives for biomanufacturing of cell-laden scaffolds with tissue-mimicking structures. In this review, we will summarize the applications and challenges of cell seeding strategies and cell microencapsulation technologies for incorporating cells within electrospun scaffolds. Some techniques with high potentials to be integrated with electrospinning for forming the cell-laden scaffolds in continuous and noncontact manners, including aerodynamic-assisted cell microencapsulation, hydrodynamic-assisted cell microencapsulation and electrohydrodynamic-assisted cell microencapsulation (i.e., cell electrospinning and cell electrospraying), are highlighted. In particular, the cell microencapsulation and the subsequent formation of cell-laden scaffolds directly by electrospinning and electrospraying with living cells are overviewed in a detailed manner. Finally, the perspective and challenges of electrospinning and electrospraying with cells for biomanufacturing of cell-laden scaffolds with tissue-mimicking structures are discussed.

Keywords: Electrospinning; electrospraying; tissue engineering; biomanufacturing; cell-laden scaffolds; cell microencapsulation.

1. Introduction

Tissue engineering and regenerative medicine aim to provide potential alternatives for treating the loss, damage or disease of human body tissues and organs by using multidisciplinary knowledges of life science, chemistry, engineering, etc.[1,2] In tissue engineering and regenerative medicine, scaffold-based strategies are commonly used, where the scaffolds with appropriate architectures, physicochemical and biological properties resemble the "natural" ones in human body tissues and organs, i.e., native extracellular matrix (ECM) is designed and developed.[3,4] In human body tissues and organs, ECM usually possesses porous and nanofibrous architectures, supporting specific types of cells by their structures to form well-defined cell-ECM organizations and guiding cell behaviors and functions by different bioactive molecules they contain.[5] Inspired by the architectures, properties and functions of ECM, a large variety of synthetic tissue engineering scaffolds possessing porous and three-dimensional (3D) structures allowing cell attachment and ingrowth and bioactivities enabling guiding the behaviors and functions of cells have been prepared by using various scaffold manufacturing techniques.[6–8] Among different scaffold manufacturing techniques, electrospinning exhibits multiple superiorities, including the ease to form ECM-like nanofibrous structures, the high versatility of forming scaffolds with varied and adjustable compositions ranging from various polymers to different composites, and the capability to deliver specific bioactive molecules such as growth factors, making electrospun scaffolds excellent candidates for tissue engineering and regenerative medicine applications.[9–12] Moreover, through cell incorporation by appropriate approaches such as post-electrospinning cell seeding, the resultant electrospun cell-laden scaffolds could mimic the native cell-ECM organizations of human body tissues and organs, which hold great promise in the field of biomanufacturing and have been investigated for regenerating/repairing human body tissues with relatively simple laminar anatomies.[13] However, since cell infiltration is usually limited through the small sized interconnected pores of normal electrospun nanofibrous scaffolds, the cells could only be located near the scaffold surface when incorporated via conventional post-electrospinning cell seeding methods.[14] The resultant cell-laden scaffolds therefore show significant limitations of presenting only two-dimensional (2D) cell-scaffold organization that differ from the 3D cell-ECM organizations of many tissues and organs with thick structures and complicated anatomies. Consequently, the biomanufacturing of cell-laden scaffolds for mimicking complex human body tissues and organs via electrospinning and post-electrospinning cell seeding procedures will be extremely difficult, if any likely. Developing and investigating new strategies for cell incorporation within electrospun nanofibrous scaffolds shall be of great significance for extending the scope in the applications of biomanufacturing.

Cell microencapsulation has been widely studied and verified effectively in building biocompatible microenvironments for cell preservation and cell delivery[15] which exhibit the possibilities to be used for incorporating cells within electrospun nanofibrous scaffolds on demand and biomanufacturing cell-laden scaffolds with tissue-mimicking structures. In a typical cell microencapsulation process, cells or cell cluster are enwrapped in a semi-permeable microstructure, which allows mass transfer for cell metabolism and protects the encapsulated cells from external environments.[16] Due to its high surface-area-to-volume ratio, spherical-shaped microsphere is preferred in cell microencapsulation owing to its optimized mass transfer efficiency.[16] Under suitable formulations, cell-encapsulated microspheres could be formulated into injectable cell-laden forms and delivered into specific sites of damaged or diseased tissues to act as bio-factories to secret specific bioactive molecules for specific therapeutic purposes.[17,18] It is also reasonable to envision that the integration of cell microencapsulation technologies with electrospinning can be used for delivering cells into designated sites of scaffold structures and resulting in tissue-mimicking cell-laden scaffolds.

With the assistances of some recent advanced technologies that are capable of producing cell-encapsulated structures in continuous and noncontact manners, including aerodynamic-assisted cell microencapsulation, hydrodynamic-assisted cell microencapsulation and electrohydrodynamic-assisted cell microencapsulation (i.e., cell electrospinning and cell electrospraying), the electrospinning and electrospraying with living cells for biomanufacturing tissue-mimicking constructs have become pratical.[19,20] In this review, we will overview the recent progresses in the field of electrospinning and electrospraying with cells, summarizing the incorporation of cells within electrospun tissue engineering scaffolds via both conventional cell seeding strategies and novel cell microencapsulation strategies. In particular, the cell microencapsulation and the subsequent formation of cell-laden scaffolds for both *in vitro* and *in vivo* applications directly by electrospinning and electrospraying with living cells are highlighted. The perspective and challenges of electrospinning and electrospraying with cells for applications in biomanufacturing are finally discussed.

2. Cell seeding for incorporating cells within electrospun scaffolds

Appropriate cell incorporation within porous structures of electrospun tissue engineering scaffolds is an important prerequisite for biomanufacturing of cell-laden scaffolds with tissue-mimicking organizations. In natural body tissues and organs, cells interact with nanofibrous ECM in 3D. Often, different types of cells are located in distinctive tissue layers. To mimic the specific cell-ECM organizations of human body tissues and organs, cells shall be required to be incorporated in 3D and located into designated positions of scaffold structures. Conventionally, the incorporation of cells within the electrospun tissue engineering scaffolds could be realized by post-electrospinning cell seeding, where the scaffolds were first prepared and the cells were then seeded onto the scaffolds. Both static and dynamic cell seeding methods have been investigated for incorporating cells within electrospun tissue engineering scaffolds.

2.1. *Static cell seeding*

Static cell seeding method is one of the most commonly used methods for preparing electrospun cell-laden scaffolds. In a typical static cell seeding process, cells are manually seeded onto the surface of tissue engineering scaffolds via dripping a cell suspension onto the sterilized scaffolds.[21] After subsequent cell infiltration, cells (either single cell type or multiple cells) are expected to penetrate into the inner structures of the scaffolds to form 3D cell-laden constructs. Since the cell incorporation relies on cell infiltration, the distribution of cells through the thickness of the cell-laden scaffolds built by the static cell seeding method is generally inhomogeneous. The majority of the cells are located near the surface of the scaffolds. Due to the nanofibrous architectures and small sizes of interconnected pores for the electrospun tissue engineering scaffolds, cell infiltration in electrospun scaffolds is particularly low when using the static cell seeding method, resulting in only cell-laden scaffolds with 2D cell-scaffold organization. Although some degrees of successes have been achieved for improving cell infiltration by some strategies to enlarge the pore sizes of electrospun scaffolds such as salt-leaching, sacrificial fiber removal and cryogenic electrospinning, etc.,[22–26] fundamental challenges of constructing thick 3D cell-incorporated structures still remain by means of static cell seeding. Therefore, the electrospun cell-laden scaffolds formed by post-electrospinning static cell seeding can be only potentially used for biomanufacturing or regenerating body tissues with relatively simple structures such as bone, cartilage and skin.[13] The biomanufacturing of cell-laden constructs resembling the structures and anatomies of body tissues and organs with thick and multilayer structures will be a great challenge.[14]

When multiple cells are required to be co-cultured and incorporated within the scaffolds for mimicking the structures and anatomies of complex multicellular tissues and organs, it will be also difficult, if any possible, to be realized by the static cell seeding method. Because different types of cells can be only either simultaneously seeded onto one side or separately seeded onto both sides of the scaffolds by static cell seeding, the limited complexity in cell-scaffold organization for the cell-laden scaffolds formed cannot be comparable to that of native tissues and organs with well-defined multicellular organizations at distinct tissue layers.[27]

For incorporating the cells within the electrospun scaffolds in 3D and precisely controlling the positions of specific cell types in the structures of the scaffolds, a modified manually static cell seeding method has been developed and investigated.[28] Through alternately performing electrospinning and manually cell seeding, multilayer cell-laden constructs with sandwich cell-scaffold structures were fabricated. This method could place cells into specific layers of electrospun scaffolds, which resembled distinct tissue layers of multilayer tissues and organs. However, as the cell seeding procedure and electrospinning process were alternately performed, cell viability might be affected by the evaporation of cytotoxic organic solvents from the polymer solution in the electrospinning process as there are no protection procedures to be implemented for the cells that are to be seeded at the electrospinning intervals. In addition to the alternate manually cell seeding method, the spraying of cell suspension for cell seeding concurrently performed with the electrospinning process has also been developed and investigated for forming nanofibrous electrospun cell-laden constructs with 3D cell-scaffold organizations.[29] Cell suspensions with an addition of a water-soluble polymer were sprayed concurrently with an electrospinning process. After simultaneous depositions of cell-suspended microdroplets and electrospun polymer nanofibers, nanofibrous cell-laden constructs with biomimetic 3D cell-scaffold organizations were finally formed. Despite successful incorporation of cells within structures of scaffolds in 3D and the possibilities of locating different cell types into designated positions, cells handled by this concurrent approach still possess drawbacks as adequate protection to cells for avoiding the influence of residual cytotoxic organic solvents on cell viability was still lacking. Besides, the sprayed cells might also be damaged by the high shear force during the spraying process.

2.2. *Dynamic cell seeding*

Compared to static cell seeding methods, dynamic cell seeding methods can place cells into deeper positions of scaffolds with the assistance of external forces, which have been recently catching increasing attentions for making cell-laden tissue engineering scaffolds with 3D cell-scaffold organization.[30] In a typical dynamic cell seeding process, sterilized porous scaffolds are immersed in a cell suspension under continuous stirring or shaking in a bioreactor for enhancing cell infiltration.[30] Enhanced cell infiltration into the porous structures of scaffolds and high initial cell density could be achieved by using the dynamic cell seeding method.[30] Due to the deep cell infiltration and improved spatial cell distribution, porous scaffolds with incorporated endothelial cells formed by dynamic cell seeding could realize improved vascularization outcomes compared to the conditions of the cell-laden scaffolds built by static cell seeding.[31]

Perfusion strategy is an alternative dynamic cell seeding method, where the cell penetration is stimulated in the resultant cell-laden scaffolds.[32] As the typical procedures of the perfusion strategy, sterilized porous scaffolds are placed in a flow perfusion chamber filled with a cell suspension for cell seeding.[32] By using the perfusion strategy for cell incorporation, mesenchymal stem cells (MSCs) could be deeply seeded into the inner structures of porous silicate-substituted tricalcium phosphate scaffolds in 3D.[32] MSCs in the 3D cell-laden scaffolds seeded by the perfusion strategy exhibited higher initial cell density and enhanced osteogenic differentiation than those in the scaffolds formed by manually cell seeding. The MSC-laden scaffolds formed by the perfusion strategy therefore showed superior performance in assisting bone regeneration.

To further increase the initial cell seeding density and improve 3D homogeneous distribution cells in scaffold structures, one feasible approach is to perform perfusion cell seeding in a shaking or rotating bioreactor chamber.[33] As a more effective alternative, a new dynamic cell seeding method with the assistance with centrifugal forces, termed centrifugal cell immobilization (CCI), have been recently studied.[34,35] As the typical procedures of the CCI method, porous scaffolds were immersed in a cell suspension at a sealed centrifuge tube and then centrifuged to seed cells into scaffolds. Compared to other dynamic cell seeding methods, the CCI methods are particularly favorable to place cells into deep positions of porous scaffolds with relatively small interconnected pores, such as nanofibrous electrospun scaffolds.[36–38] Despite dynamic cell seeding strategies could enhance the cell infiltration and hence realize the deep distribution of cells when used for incorporating cells within electrospun tissue engineering scaffolds, the precise control over the positions of multiple cells in the cell-laden scaffolds for resembling the complex anatomies of multicellular tissues and organs remains challenging. According to the limitations and drawbacks of exiting static and dynamic cell seeding methods for preparing 3D cell-laden scaffolds, new strategies for cell incorporation shall be investigated and developed for better meeting the requirements of biomanufacturing of tissue-mimicking constructs.

3. Cell microencapsulation: Possibilities and challenges of incorporating cells within electrospun scaffolds

3.1. *Forms of cell microencapsulation*

Microencapsulation technologies were effective in producing biocompatible microenvironments for the protection and delivery of bioactive agents, which have been widely investigated in drug delivery, pharmacology, food industry and biomedicine.[39–41] Chang *et al.* first introduced the microencapsulation for bio-encapsulation at 1964.[42] Using a micro-emulsion method, enzyme was successfully encapsulated and protected in semipermeable and structurally stabled microbeads with diameters ranging from 1 to 100 μm, where the encapsulated enzyme showed well-preserved bioactivity both *in vitro* and *in vivo.* Under specific adaptions, the microencapsulation techniques could be extended for cell microencapsulation.[43–45] For instance, through the similar micro-emulsion process to enzyme microencapsulation,[42] islets could also be encapsulated in semipermeable microbeads, which achieved long-term islet survival after transplantation.[46] To date, different cell microencapsulation strategies have been developed and investigated for encapsulating cells into three typical forms (Fig. 1),[16,47,48] including cell embedding within a hydrogel microbead, cell coating directly by a polymer shell, and cell capsule with a liquid-core for cell microencapsulation. Properties of cell-encapsulated structures such as particle size, permeability and degradation behaviors are varied under different cell microencapsulation forms, which could affect the preservation of the viability and phenotype of cells, as well as the perspective of their applications for cell incorporation within tissue engineering scaffolds.

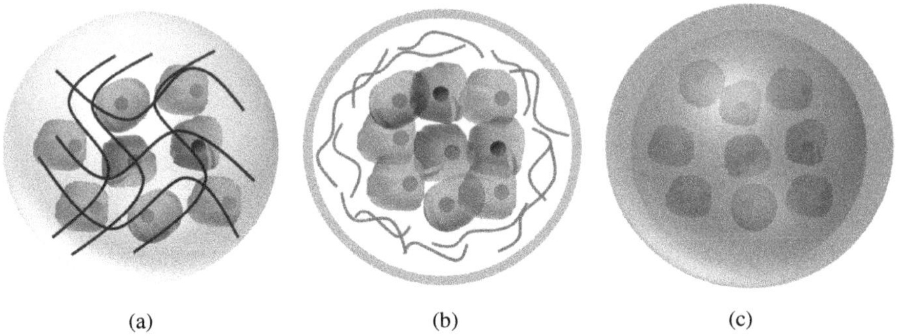

Fig. 1. Schematic illustrations of different forms of cell microencapsulation strategies: (a) Cell embedding, (b) cell coating and (c) cell capsule.

3.1.1. *Cell embedding*

Hydrogel is frequently used in tissue engineering owing to its water-rich contents and tissue-like elastic properties.[49–52] Due to good water swelling and permeability, hydrogel microbeads capable of sufficient nutrients and oxygen exchanges are therefore desirable for cell microencapsulation [Fig. 1(a)].[53] Typical procedures for preparing cell-encapsulated hydrogel microbeads are to mix a cell suspension and a suitable polymer precursor solution firstly, followed by an appropriate gelation process. Different gelation methods applied may result in different properties (e.g., osmolality, mechanical properties and degradation rates) of resultant hydrogel microbeads and hence affect cell encapsulation effects.

Covalent crosslinking is a popular gelation method for forming cell-encapsulated hydrogel microbeads, which is applicable for most of the natural polymers and synthetic polymers. Two major covalent crosslinking approaches have been developed for producing cell-encapsulated hydrogel microbeads, i.e., radical chain polymerization and chemical crosslinking. In the radical chain polymerization process, polymer chains in the precursors are crosslinked to network through the radical groups generated by the stimuli of heat,[54] redox,[55] or light.[56] Radical chain polymerization reaction is often rapid and sensitive so that the whole cell microencapsulation process can be completed in a short time. However, cell viability may be affected by the radical chain polymerization reaction during cell microencapsulation as the chemicals used, radical groups generated and the stimulation methods applied may be harmful to cells. To be specific, for the redox-initiating systems, initiators used for forming active radical groups, such as peroxide oxidizing agents or amine reducing agents, are cytotoxic. As for the heat- and photo-initiating systems, many factors e.g., high temperature, cytotoxic photo initiators and ultraviolet (UV) exposure may influence cell viability.[57] Comparatively, chemical crosslinking, as an alternative gelation method for producing cell-embedded hydrogel microbeads, is relatively cell-friendly since there are no initiators involved. For instance, hyaluronic acids functionalized with thiol-terminal groups could be directly crosslinked to form hydrogel microbeads for encapsulating fibroblasts through disulfide bonding in the presence of air.[58] Besides, through chemical crosslinking reactions among thiolate reactive species in a basic environment, polysaccharides or proteins with thiol-terminal or peptides with cysteine amino acid residues could also be chemically crosslinked to hydrogel microbeads for cell microencapsulation.[59] Chemical crosslinking methods usually have little influence on cell viability. But the relatively slow gelation rate should be a problem. To address this problem, a mix-mode crosslinking (combining radical chain polymerizations with chemical crosslinking) was recently investigated.[60] Whereas the preservation of cell viability and the gelation rate could be balanced by this mix-mode covalent crosslinking method, new challenges in precisely adjusting the structures of the cell-embedded hydrogel microbeads would by brought as the complexity in such gelation process hugely increased.

Cell-embedded hydrogel microbeads could also be formed via ionotropic crosslinking and complex coacervation. Typically, a mixture solution containing polyanionic polymers and cells is dripped into either a salt solution containing divalent cations (termed ionotropic crosslinking) or a polycationic polymer solution (termed complex coacervation) to be crosslinked into cell-embedded hydrogel structures. A natural polymer, alginate, is the most popular polyanionic polymer used for cell encapsulation owing to its good biocompatibility.[61,62] Alginate can be crosslinked by either divalent cations such as calcium and strontium via ionotropic crosslinking,[63,64] or positively charged polymers such as poly(L-lysine) (PLL) or chitosan via complex coacervation.[65,66] It is important to notice that all these alginate-based hydrogel microbeads are effective for cell embedding with high cell viability.

In addition to chemical crosslinking and ionotropic crosslinking/complex coacervation, physical crosslinking methods have also been investigated and developed for the gelation to form cell-embedded hydrogel microbeads when using some polymers of which solubility is sensitive to temperature change. For example, agarose microbeads could be produced from a water-in-oil emulsion upon cooling, which enabled to achieve islet microencapsulation.[67] A thermo-responsive polymer, poly(N-isopropylacrylamide) (PNIPAAm) with reversible gelation-dissolution behaviors at different temperatures, has also been investigated for producing cell-embedded hydrogel microbeads.[68] Controlled cell encapsulation and cell release could be realized by the PNIPAAm-based cell-embedded microbeads owing to their responsive properties.

3.1.2. *Cell coating*

Despite remarkable success of cell embedding methods for cell microencapsulation, the cell-embedded microbeads exhibit an inherent shortage of relatively large bead sizes of hydrogel microbeads (usually hundreds of micrometers). For optimizing the diffusion efficiency of nutrients and oxygen, an alternative strategy of cell microencapsulation, namely cell coating, has been developed, aiming to encapsulate cells within a relatively small microenvironment. In the typical procedures, cells or cell clusters are coated and encapsulated by a thin nanoshell of polymers or bioceramics [Fig. 1(b)], which could be formed using different methods.

The polymer shell for cell coating is generally formed by layer-by-layer (LbL) assembly through the alternant depositions of polycationic polymers and the polyelectrolytes with the reverse electrical charges, resulting in a multilayer polymer shell coated on the cell membrane with negative charges. An early study conducted by Donath *et al.* found that human erythrocytes with glutaraldehyde coating could act as the bio-template for the subsequent adsorption of polyelectrolytes.[69] Using this bio-template, single yeast cell could be coated by a thin polyelectrolyte shell ($\sim$6 nm) assembled by poly (styrenesulfonate sodium salt) (PSS, negative charged) and poly (allylamine hydrochloride) (PAH, positive charged) via an LbL process.[70] When encapsulating cells by cell coating, the preservation of cell viability and phenotype is the major concern. It is therefore important to develop polymers with improved biocompatibility for cell coating. To achieve this goal, poly(vinyl alcohol) (PVA) and phospholipid-conjugated poly(ethylene glycol) (PEG) grafted with maleimide groups were employed for islet encapsulation via LbL assembly.[71] The multilayer ultra-thin shell assembled by PVA and functionalized PEG had good cell affinity and few interventions on cell viability. Besides, poly(L-Lysine) (PLL) and hyaluronic acid have also been studied for the coating of mouse MSCs, which could be coated by a PLL/hyaluronic acid multilayer nanoshell with a thickness of 6–9 nm and exhibited well-preserved viability and pluripotency.[72] To further achieve enhanced immune protection of the encapsulated cells in the cell coating structures, a bioceramic shell was investigated for cell coating.[73] Through bioinspired silicification, multiple types of mammalian cells could be coated by a thin silica shell. There was no significant influence on cell viability by the bioinspired silicification process. The resultant cell-encapsulated structures coated by the silica shell show superior structural stability and enhanced cytoprotective effects.

3.1.3. *Cell capsule*

Although remarkable progresses have been made in cell microencapsulation through either cell embedding using hydrogel microbeads or cell coating by polymer/bioceramic shells, some inherent problems that may influence the perspectives of cell microencapsulation in the applications of cell incorporation within tissue engineering scaffolds are still pending. To be specific, cells are usually immobilized in the structures of the hydrogel microbeads formed by the cell embedding methods, which may limit intercellular communication of organization of cells into multicellular functional structures, while relatively low cell loading amounts shall be a problem for cell-encapsulated structures formed by cell coating. Comparatively, cell capsule where cells are encapsulated in a liquid-core of microcapsule should be more promising as the liquid-core of microcapsule can provide a biocompatible and free microenvironment for cell loading and organization [Fig. 1(c)]. For producing cell capsules, different approaches including interfacial precipitation, sacrificial core method and micro-injection have been studied.

Interfacial precipitation is normally conducted by dripping one phase solution (e.g., an oil-phase polymer solution) into another phased solution (e.g., an aqueous-phase cell suspension) to form liquid-core microcapsules. For example, liquid-core poly(lactic-co-glycolic acid) (PLGA) microcapsules could be formed by interfacial precipitation through dripping a PLGA solution into cell suspension under mechanical stirring and repeated extrusion, which could be used for pancreatic islet encapsulation.[74] But the cell survival rate was not desirable in the resultant PLGA capsules due to direct exposure of cells to cytotoxic organic solvents in the polymer solutions. Besides, through dripping a compound droplet with the outer surfactant-containing alginate aqueous solution and the inner cell suspension into a $CaCl_2$ aqueous solution, the outer alginate phase could be solidified via crosslinking and cell-encapsulated liquid-core microcapsules with alginate-based hydrogel shells were hence produced.[75] Owing to superior biocompatibility of alginate and mild crosslinking conditions, long-term survival and desirable proliferation could be achieved by the cells encapsulated in the alginate microcapsules.

In addition to interfacial precipitation, cell capsules can also be fabricated by using sacrificial core methods.[76] For instance, using cell-embedding alginate-based hydrogel microbeads as templates, core-shell structured microspheres could be formed by subsequently coating a layer of agarose onto the cell-embedding alginate-based hydrogel microbeads. After treating with an alginate lyase to decompose the alginate core, the cell-encapsulated liquid-core microcapsules could therefore be produced.[76] The cell encapsulated in the microcapsules showed desirable viability and well-preserved phenotype.

Alternatively, micro-injection is also a visible method for producing cell capsules where a cell suspension is post-injected into a hollow microcapsule (Fig. 2). The hollow microcapsules for cell micro-injection could also be fabricated by using the sacrificial core method.[77] Specifically, a hollow microcapsule with an alginate-based hydrogel shell could be formed from a core-shell structured microsphere with a carboxymethylcellulose core and an alginate-based hydrogel shell. After the removal of the carboxymethylcellulose core via enzymatic degradation, the hollow alginate-based hydrogel microcapsule was formed, where a cell suspension could be subsequently injected into the hollow core of the microcapsule to result in a cell capsule.[77] Micro-injection method is desirable for the preservation of cell viability in cell microencapsulation although the drawback of low cost-effectiveness is present.

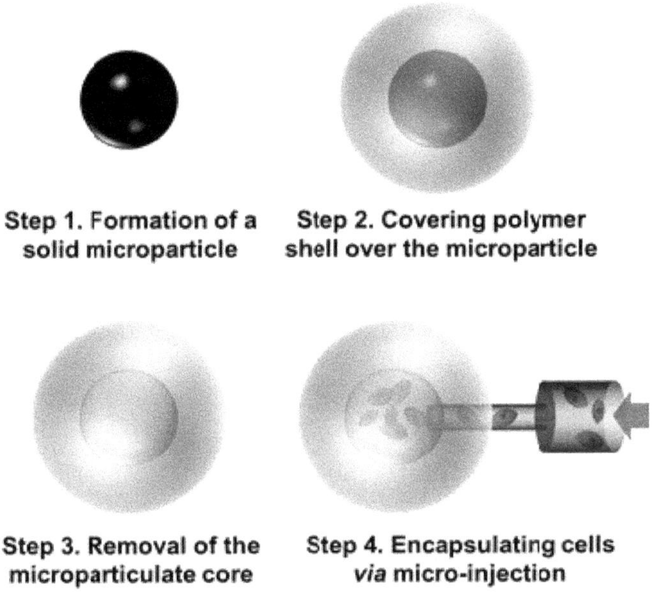

Fig. 2. Schematically illustrating the typical procedures of micro-injection methods for forming cell capsules.

3.2. *Popular technologies for cell microencapsulation*

Cell microencapsulation technologies have shown their various superiorities in protecting cell viability and delivering cells into designated sites for therapeutic purposes.[45] For extending the applications of cell microencapsulation technologies in the fields of cell incorporation within tissue engineering scaffolds and the subsequent biomanufacturing of cell-laden scaffolds with biomimetic cell-scaffold organizations resembling the structures and anatomies of human body tissues and organs, continuous and noncontact approaches for cell microencapsulation shall be preferred. For achieving this goal, different adapted cell microencapsulation techniques, including coaxial aerodynamic-assisted cell microencapsulation and hydrodynamic-assisted cell microencapsulation, have been recently developed and investigated. The possibilities and challenges of applying these adapted cell microencapsulation techniques for cell incorporation within electrospun tissue engineering scaffolds are discussed.

3.2.1. *Aerodynamic-assisted techniques*

Extrusion methods are popular in fabricating spherical hydrogel microbeads for cell embedding.[53] With specific adaptions of the extrusion methods, a new aerodynamic-assisted technique, termed coaxial aerodynamically spraying, has been developed for continuous and noncontact formations of cell-encapsulated structures.[78] In the typical procedures of the coaxial aerodynamically spraying, a pressurized airflow was applied on a cell-suspended polymer solution by using a coaxial device with a concentric nozzle. A cell suspension and a polymer solution (as the carrier solution) passed through the inner capillary and the outer capillary of the concentric nozzle, respectively (Fig. 3). The pressurized airflow was applied outside the concentric nozzle to generate the shear force for forming the cell-encapsulated microspheres.

Since cell suspensions generally possess low viscosity and high surface tension that are hard to be deformed by the shear force generated by the pressurized airflow, a polymer solution with a high

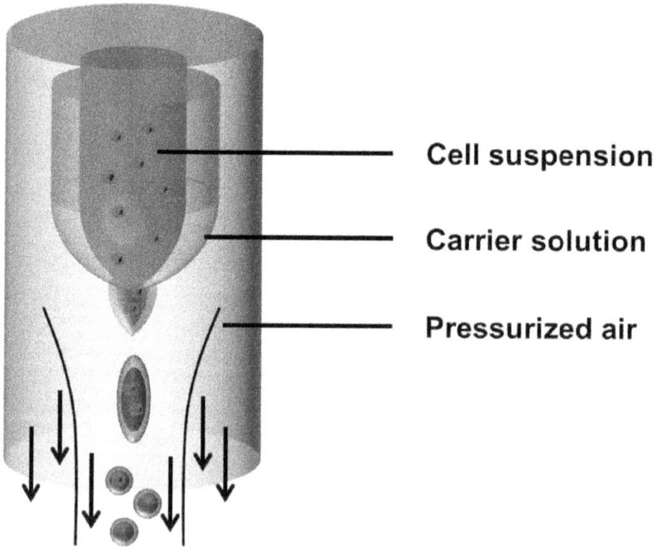

Fig. 3. Schematically illustrating the coaxial device with a concentric nozzle for cell microencapsulation via coaxial aerodynamically spraying.

viscosity is therefore necessary to be used in the aerodynamically spraying process for producing cell-embedded microspheres. It has been found that medical grade poly(dimethyl siloxane) (PDMS) was a suitable candidate for conducting coaxial aerodynamic-assisted cell microencapsulation. Semi-rigid cell-embedded microdroplets could be produced by coaxial aerodynamically spraying using the merged fluids of PDMS and cell suspensions. The flow rates of cell suspension, PDMS polymer solution and pressurized air are crucial for determining the final structure of the as-formed cell-encapsulated structures. By tuning different polymer solution flow rates, either a jetting process forming cell-embedded microbeads or a threading process forming cell-embedded microfibers would occur.[78] Despite cells could be handled and encapsulated in an continuous and noncontact manners by using the aerodynamic-assisted technique, the cell-embedded structures formed are not completely solidified as PDMS would rapidly diffuse in an aqueous environment, which may bring some difficulties when integrating this method with scaffold manufacturing technique such as electrospinning for biomanufacturing biomimetic cell-laden constructs.

3.2.2. *Hydrodynamic-assisted techniques*

Microfluidics provide advanced mini-sized platforms for accurately controlling fluidic flows. With the assistance of microfluidics, complex microstructures with uniform and well-controlled shapes and dimensions can be fabricated.[79] Moreover, microfluidics also offer desirable platforms enabling continuous and noncontact cell microencapsulation via hydrodynamic-assisted approaches.[80] Using different polymer precursor solutions, different cell-encapsulated microstructures can be fabricated on microfluidic platforms via different crosslinking methods (e.g., photo-initiated crosslinking, temperature-induced crosslinking or ion-induced crosslinking).[80] Compared to the light- and temperature-induced crosslinking methods, ion-induced crosslinking using an alginate precursor solution is superior in preserving the viability of the encapsulated cells owing to the mild crosslinking conditions. To form alginate-based cell-encapsulated structures via hydrodynamic-assisted approaches, two typical modes of microfluidic platforms were commonly used (Fig. 4), which include microfluidic platforms of either T-junction mode or flow-focus mode.[80] When employing the T-junction microfluidic platform, the microdroplets of the cell-suspended alginate solution formed outside the junction are solidified after the crosslinking of the alginate by the $CaCl_2$ solution flowing in the main channel, therefore resulting in cell-embedded microbeads [Fig. 4(a)]. Using a flow-focus microfluidic platform, alginate-containing cell suspension and $CaCl_2$ solution respectively flowed through the outer channel and the inner channel of the microfluidic device. Using the flow-focus

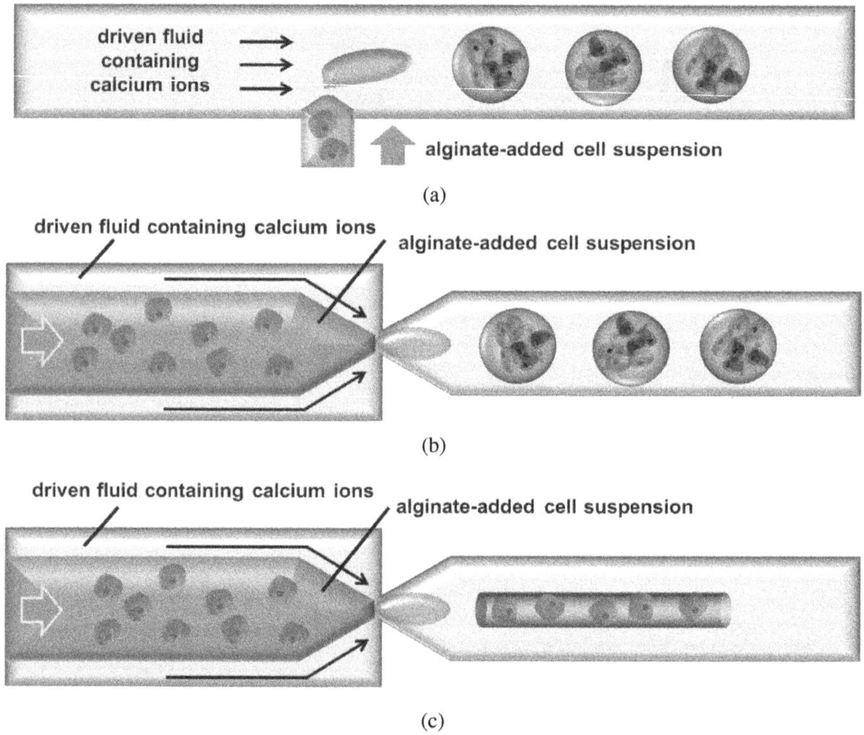

Fig. 4. Schematic illustrations of different modes of hydrodynamic-assisted cell microencapsulation on microfluidic platforms with various device designs: (a) Cell-encapsulated microbeads formed on a microfluidic platform of T-junction mode, (b) cell-encapsulated microbeads formed on a microfluidic platform of flow-focus mode and (c) cell-encapsulated microfibers formed on a microfluidic platform of flow-focus mode.

microfluidic device, the resultant alginate-based cell-encapsulated structures can be well controlled, where either cell-embedded microbeads [Fig. 4(b)] or cell-embedded microfibers [Fig. 4(c)] could be formed by tuning different flowing rates of the inner and outer flows.[81] Recently, a novel 3D flow-focus microfluidic platform was developed for optimizing the cell microencapsulation process, where three concentric microfluidic channels (from the inner channel to the outer channel) were fed by cell suspension, alginate polymer solution and $CaCl_2$ solution, respectively. Using this 3D flow-focus microfluidic platform, cell-encapsulated microcapsule with an alginate-based hydrogel shell and a liquid core could be produced, where cells survived well inside the microcapsules.[82] Cell-encapsulated core-shell structured microfibers with an alginate-based hydrogel shell could also be fabricated using the 3D flow-focus microfluidic platform when a relatively slow fluid flow rate of was employed.[81] Different cells types such as fibroblasts, neutral cells, epithelial cells and endothelial cells could be encapsulated into microfibers with diameters ranging from several micrometers to hundreds of micrometers and well-defined multicellular organizations, which resembled the structures and anatomies of different tube-like tissues such as blood vessels and nerves, holding great promise in tissue engineering and regenerative medicine.

4. Electrospinning and electrospraying with living cells

4.1. *Electrospinning and electrospraying for cell microencapsulation*

In addition to aerodynamic-assisted and hydrodynamic-assisted methods, electrohydrodynamic-assisted methods (i.e., cell electrospinning and cell electrospraying) have also been recently emerging as promising techniques for cell microencapsulation, which will be particularly superior in readily integration with electrospinning for biomanufacturing cell-laden scaffolds with biomimetic cell-scaffold organizations resembling the structures and anatomies of human body tissues and organs.

Electrospinning is effective in producing delivery vehicles and carriers of various types of cargo substances including small molecular drugs, biomacromolecules and nanoparticles.[83,84] Three strategies, i.e., blend electrospinning, emulsion electrospinning and coaxial electrospinning, were commonly used in the encapsulation and delivery of cargo substances (Fig. 5). In blend electrospinning, cargo substances are directly added into a polymer solution to prepare a blend solution [Fig. 5(a)], which is then spun at the high-voltage electrostatic field to form hybrid fibers [Fig. 5(b)]. Through blend electrospinning, polymer nanofibers with incorporated small molecular dexamethasone were formed, which could be used for promoting

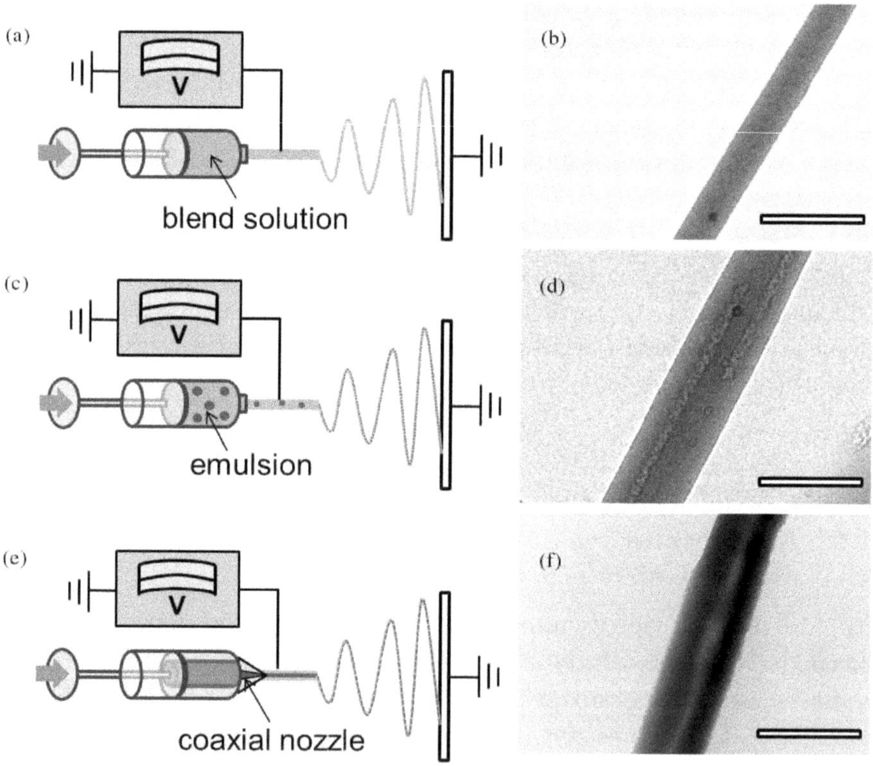

Fig. 5. Schematic illustrations of different electrospinning techniques for producing delivery vehicles or carriers: (a) Blend electrospinning, (b) a representative image of a hybrid fiber formed by blend electrospinning, (c) emulsion electrospinning, (d) a representative image of a core-shell structured fiber formed by emulsion electrospinning, (e) coaxial electrospinning and (f) a representative image of a core-shell structured fiber formed by coaxial electrospinning. Scale bars: 1 μm.

bone regeneration through sustained drug release.[85] Blend electrospinning could also be used for producing hybrid fibers with encapsulated functional nanoparticles such as silver nanoparticles and silica nanoparticles, although the encapsulated nanoparticles could not be released.[86,87] During emulsion electrospinning [Fig. 5(c)], a water/oil emulsion is used where cargo substances are usually suspended in the "water phase". Through emulsion electrospinning, core-shell structured nanofibers with inner water-phase cores could be prepared and the cargo substances are herein encapsulated [Fig. 5(d)], which has widely been investigated for the delivery of biomolecules for diverse tissue engineering applications.[88–90] In addition to emulsion electrospinning, coaxial electrospinning can also result in core-shell structured nanofibers. Unlike a single needle used in blend electrospinning and emulsion electrospinning, a coaxial nozzle with two concentric capillaries is employed in coaxial electrospinning [Fig. 5(e)]. Cargo substances are simply encapsulated in nanofibers through directly adding them into the inner fluid during the coaxial electrospinning process [Fig. 5(f)]. Through coaxial electrospinning, scaffolds with biodegradable core-shell structured nanofibers could be fabricated for the delivery of biomacromolecules such as proteins and enzymes.[91–93]

As for extending the above-mentioned three electrospinning techniques for encapsulating cells, emulsion electrospinning would be inappropriate as cells cannot be exposed to cytotoxic organic solvents usually used in the preparation of emulsions. Blend electrospinning and coaxial electrospinning with specific adaptions have been investigated for cell microencapsulation (Fig. 6). For blend electrospinning, the delivery of cells is also challenging and all the chemicals used in preparing the polymer solution should be noncytotoxic. Using water-soluble polymers such as PVA, microfibers with some concomitant microbeads with diameters approximately 1 μm could be fabricated by blend electrospinning, which could be used for the encapsulation of rod-like bifidobacterial cells (size below 1 μm).[94] To date, the encapsulation of mammalian cells (with diameters beyond 5 μm) via blend electrospinning is difficult due to the diameters of the fibers formed by blend electrospinning are hard

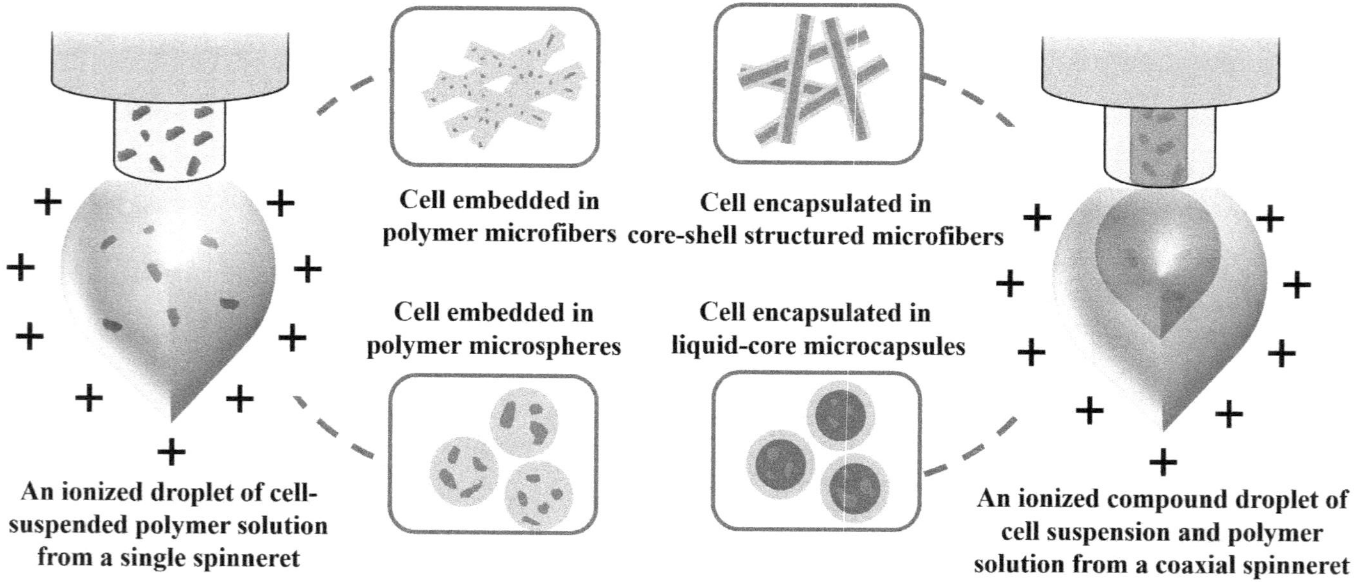

Fig. 6. A schematic illustration of electrospinning and electrospraying for cell microencapsulation: blend electrospinning/electrospray (left) and coaxial electrospinning/electrospray (right) for producing monolithic cell-embedded microfibers/microspheres and core-shell structured cell-encapsulated microfibers/microspheres, respectively.

to reach this value. Besides, the high shear force and the dehydration during the blend electrospinning drying sometimes resulted in massive cell death.[95] Comparatively, coaxial electrospinning is more promising for mammalian cell microencapsulation. During the coaxial electrospinning process, less shear force is applied on the cell suspension fed by the inner capillary, which could be further adjusted through using the outer polymer solutions with appropriate viscosities and polymer concentrations. Owing to its good biocompatibility, low electrical conductivity and high viscosity, medical grade PDMS has been studied and used for mammalian cell microencapsulation via coaxial electrospinning.[96] The merged droplets of PDMS polymer solution and cell suspension formed out of the nozzle of a coaxial spinneret were stretched by the electrostatic force generated from the charged inner liquid (cell suspension) with high conductivity, where the outer PDMS polymer solution could stabilize the electrohydrodynamic atomization process. Semi-rigid PDMS fibers with encapsulated live human astrocytoma cells and dozens of micrometers could be fabricated by coaxial electrospinning, whereas the structure of resultant cell-encapsulated fibers was not solidified and readily to thaw at an aqueous environment.

Electrospraying is another popular electrohydrodynamic technique for the encapsulation and delivery of cargo substances,[97,98] which results in microspherical structures with larger volumes for the loading of cargo substances than those of electrospun fibers and is therefore promising for mammalian cell encapsulation. Two types of electrospraying techniques (i.e., blend electrospraying and coaxial electrospraying) have been investigated and used in producing delivery vehicles or carriers, where microspheres with either monolithic solid structured or core-shell structured are fabricated, respectively.[99] Both the two electrospraying approaches have also been studied for cell microencapsulation, where either cell-embedded microbeads or cell-encapsulated microcapsules were formed accordingly (Fig. 6). For instance, through blend electrospraying, poly (ethylene oxide) (PEO) microbeads with encapsulated rabbit aorta smooth muscle cells could be fabricated when using a submerged system filled with sunflower oil for microbead collection.[100] Cell viability was high in the resultant PEO microbeads as little currents passed through the cell-suspended polymer solution during the blend electrospraying process. Compared to blend electrospraying, coaxial electrospraying can generate core-shell structured microcapsules, of which structures (e.g., diameter and polymer shell thickness) and degradation properties could be well controlled.[99] Through coaxial electrospraying, different types of cell-encapsulated microcapsules could be fabricated. For instance, semi-rigid microspheres with encapsulated primary cardiac cells could be fabricated by coaxial electrospraying using a biopolymer, Matrigel, which was derived from mouse Engelbreth–Holm–Swarm sarcoma.[20] The viability of the encapsulated cells in the final cell-encapsulated microspheres was well preserved, whereas the microspheres were still not solidified yet and would dissolute gradually. For making solidified cell-encapsulated microspheres with stable and durable structures, coaxial electrospraying using an alginate polymer solution as the carrier solution was investigated.[101] Structurally stabled cell-encapsulated alginate-based hydrogel microcapsules could be prepared by coaxial cell electrospraying and a high cell survival rate was finally achieved.

4.2. *Electrospinning and electrospraying for preparing cell-laden scaffolds*

Through electrospinning and electrospraying, the fabrication of nanofibrous tissue engineering scaffolds and continuous live cell microencapsulation can be respectively realized, indicating the potential of developing new cell incorporation strategies for biomanufacturing cell-laden scaffolds with biomimetic cell-scaffold organizations resembling the structures and anatomy of human body tissues and organs. Good preservation of cell activity and cell functions is important perquisites when employing electrospinning and electrospraying for cell incorporation within tissue engineering scaffolds. To avoid contamination, all the materials and reagents used in electrospinning and electrospraying for preparing cell-laden scaffolds must be pre-sterilized by using appropriate methods. One common and effective method is gamma-ray radiation with intensity of 15 kGy for 30 min using a Cobalt 60 source, which could effectively sterilize materials without any alterations on the physicochemical properties. Additionally, *in vitro* investigations should be conducted for evaluating the influence of different factors (e.g., polymer solution properties and processing parameters) of cell electrospinning and cell electrospraying on cell viability and phenotype. Recently, some preliminary *in vivo* trials of applying electrospinning and electrospraying with cells for different therapeutic purposes have also been performed. The results of these *in vitro* and *in vivo* biological investigations into the electrospinning and electrospraying with cells (Table 1) can offer valuable guidelines for extending the technologies in the applications of biomanufacturing.

Since electrospinning process usually involves relatively high shear force which may be harmful to cells to be encapsulated, cell viability is a major concern for the cell electrospinning. As stated previously, live cell microencapsulation in some semi-rigid microstructures made of PDMS or Matrigel could be successfully achieved via blend electrospinning or coaxial electrospinning, where cell viability in these microstructures could be preserved.[19] However, these cell-encapsulated microstructures were both not solidified which bring difficulties for further handling. For making solidified and structurally stable cell-encapsulated microfibers, the blend electrospinning using a mixture solution of cell suspension and polymer solution of water-soluble polymers such as PVA or PEO were conducted,[102,103] which could produce solidified fibers with encapsulated living bacteria. The viability of the encapsulated bacteria in the electrospun fibers could be retained for three months.[103] Through coaxial electrospinning, water-insoluble poly(caprolactone) (PCL) microfibers of with encapsulated *Escherichia coli* could also be formed.[104] Owing to relatively short exposure time of the bacteria to the cytotoxic organic PCL polymer solution during the coaxial electrospinning process, the activity of some encapsulated bacteria could be partially preserved. To reduce the hazards of cytotoxic organic solvent used, a blend electrospinning using a bacteria-suspended aqueous polymer solution containing PEO and Pluronic F127 dimethacrylate (FDMA) was investigated for cell microencapsulation, which resulted in bacteria-

Table 1. Summaries of different electrospinning and electrospraying techniques for preparing cell-laden structures.

Techniques	Carrier materials	Cell types	Cell viability	Limitations	Ref.
Blend electrospinning	PVA	*Escherichia coli, staphylococcus albus*	19–48%	Small diameters, not applicable to mammalian cells, low cell viability	102
	PEO	*Escherichia coli, Micrococcus luteus*	$< 20\%$	Small diameters, not applicable to mammalian cells, low cell viability	103
	PEO and FDMA	*Pseudomonas, Zymomonas, and Escherichia*	$\sim 90\%$	Small diameters, not applicable to mammalian cells	105
	PVA	*Escherichia coli, Micrococcus luteus*	Not mentioned	Small diameters, not applicable to mammalian cells	106
	Matrigel	Mouse lung fibroblasts	$> 90\%$	Nonsolidified structures, quickly diffusing in medium	110
Coaxial electrospinning	PCL	*Escherichia coli*	40%	Small diameters, not applicable to mammalian cells, low cell viability	104
Blend electrospraying	PDMS	Jurkat cells	Not mentioned	Nonsolidified structures, quickly diffusing in medium	19
	PEO	Rabbit aorta smooth muscle cells	70%	Nonsolidified structures, low cell viability	100
Coaxial electrospraying	Matrigel	Neonatal rat cardiac myocytes	$> 90\%$	Nonsolidified structures, quickly diffusing in medium	108
	Matrigel	Mouse embryonic stem cells	$> 90\%$	Nonsolidified structures, quickly diffusing in medium	108
	Matrigel	Mouse hematopoietic stem cells	$> 90\%$	Nonsolidified structures, quickly diffusing in medium	111
	Alginate hydrogel	Human umbilical vein endothelial cells	$> 98\%$	Inhomogeneous cell distribution	101

encapsulated hydrogel microfibers after the following PEO extraction and the subsequent crosslinking of FDMA by a nontoxic regent, glycerol.[105] The fibrous structure formed was stable in an aqueous environment and a cell viability above 40% was attained. The bacteria encapsulated in such hydrogel microfibers created by blend electrospinning could survive for several months and their activities were well maintained. Besides, high cell viability for the bacterial cells in electrospun fibers could be achieved through pre-encapsulating the bacterial cells into crosslinked PVA microbeads prior to the electrospinning process.[106] The bacterial cells to be electrospun and encapsulated could thus be protected, which avoided the direct exposure of cells to the cytotoxic organic solvents and therefore achieved improved cell viability. Although many efforts have been made for live bacteria microencapsulation in solidified electrospun fibers, the electrospinning with mammalian cells to form solidified and structurally stable cell-encapsulated fibers remains challenging as the formation of solidified fibers via electrospinning requires complete dehydration and high electrostatic stretch. Both may significantly damage the viability of encapsulated cells.[95]

Since electrospraying normally employs a precursor solution with a low viscosity and is performed at relatively a low applied voltage, making it more feasible for the microencapsulation of live mammalian cells, some *in vitro* investigations have been conducted for the electrospraying with mammalian cells. For instance, through submerged electrospraying, rabbit aorta smooth muscle cells could be encapsulated in PEO microdroplets with a high cell survival rate (about 70%) at an oil collection bath.[100] Besides, Matrigel microspheres with encapsulated neonatal rat cardiac myocyte could be formed by coaxial electrospraying and collected in a collection bath containing specific cell culture medium.[107] The cell-embedded semi-rigid Matrigel microspheres formed could retain their spherical shapes up to 24 h. The encapsulated cells were then slowly released along with the diffusion of Matrigel in the cell culture medium. It was notable that a very high cell viability (more than 90%) could be attained through such coaxial electrospraying method, demonstrating its high efficiency in live mammalian cell microencapsulation. Moreover, through a similar coaxial electrospraying approach using Matrigel, stem cells including mouse embryonic stem cells and mouse hematopoietic stem cells were also successfully encapsulated.[108] The differentiation and engraftment potentials of the encapsulated stem cells in the electrosprayed structures were investigated, indicating the well-preserved pluripotency of the encapsulated stem cells in the semi-rigid Matrigel microspheres and further verifying the desirable biosafety of this coaxial electrospraying process.

Owing to their superior performances in handling living cells, cell electrospinning and cell electrospraying have recently been emerging as potential alternatives of cell-based therapies for *in vivo* applications. The retention of activities of the cells and potential immunogens problems must be carefully considered for cell electrospun or electrosprayed structures during *in vivo* applications. Allogeneic or homogenous cells shall be used in the cell-laden structures for reducing the risks of immune rejection upon implantation. For instance, in a preliminary trial of stimulating the cutaneous wound healing through cell-based therapies using cell-laden structures formed by cell electrospinning and cell electrospraying, allogeneic mouse primary cells were used to yield cell-laden structures to be transplanted towards mouse skin wound.[109] The neo-formation of skin tissues with normal histological organization of epidermis, dermis and subcutaneous tissues was found to be effectively promoted upon the transplantation of cell-encapsulated structures, which demonstrated that the activities and functions of the cells treated by cell electrospinning and electrospraying could be well preserved. In a trial of treating the hematopoietic dysfunction using hematopoietic stem cells, allogeneic mouse hematopoietic stem cells were encapsulated in the structures made of Matrigel through coaxial electrospraying and then capable of differentiating towards different blood cell lineages once injected into the peripheral vein of a mouse model.[110] The encapsulated hematopoietic stem cells behaved similar pluripotency yet improved duration of activity retention as compared to the cells been directly injected, revealing that there are no obvious side-effects or alterations on the functions of stem cells treated by suitable electrospraying processes. On basis of electrospraying-based stem cell microencapsulation and cell delivery, the possibilities to transport specific active stem cell-encapsulated microstructures into targeting positions of human body tissues and organs as protein factories or genetic materials for various stem cell-based therapies have been demonstrated.[111] Existing *in vivo* investigations into cell electrospraying further confirmed that electrospraying should be a visible and safe approach for cell delivery and cell-based therapies. The formation of advanced cell-laden tissue engineering scaffolds with biomimetic nanofibrous architecture and 3D cell-scaffold organization would be of high possibilities through electrospinning and cell electrospraying.

Recently, coaxial electrospraying using different water-soluble polymers including PVA, gelatin and alginate were investigated for producing solidified cell-encapsulated polymer microspheres.[101] Although solidified microspheres with encapsulated human umbilical vein endothelial cells (HUVECs) with an average diameters of about 5 μm could be successfully made by coaxial electrospraying using a blend polymer solution of alginate and gelatin, the number of cells been encapsulated in microspheres was few and majority of encapsulated cells were dead due to the high electrostatic stretch exerted during the formation of microspheres with small diameters. Given direct electrospraying of cell-suspended polymer solutions for the formation of solidified cell-encapsulated microspheres should be difficult, a new coaxial cell electrospraying method aiming to prepare hydrogel microspheres for live mammalian cell microencapsulation with the assistance of a post-electrospraying crosslinking treatment was then developed and studied.[101] Through this coaxial cell electrospraying process, HUVEC-encapsulated core-shell structured alginate-based hydrogel microspheres with a relatively large average diameter (around 100 μm) were fabricated (Fig. 7). Owing to the little currents (less than 5 nA) passing through the inner cell suspension during the coaxial cell electrospraying process, a very high cell survival rate (over 95%) was finally achieved. After dripping a sodium citrate aqueous solution towards the cell-encapsulated microspheres, the alginate-based hydrogel microspheres would be decomposed and the encapsulated cells could be subsequently triggered and released. Through integrating this coaxial cell

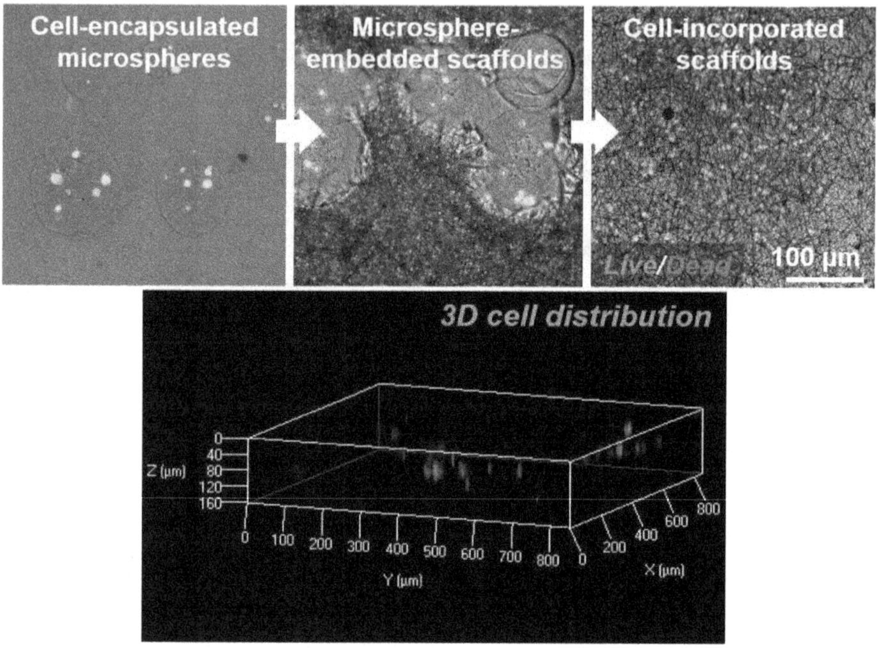

Fig. 7. Formation of nanofibrous cell-laden scaffolds with 3D cell distribution through concurrent emulsion electrospinning and coaxial cell electrospraying. Reprinted from Ref. 22 with permission from Elsevier, copyright 2021.

electrospraying method with emulsion electrospinning, the nanofibrous cell-laden scaffolds with 3D cell distribution could be formed, holding great promise in biomanufacturing of tissue-mimicking constructs for applications in tissue engineering and regenerative medicine.

5. Concluding remarks and outlook

The biomanufacturing of cell-laden scaffolds resembling the structures and anatomies of native tissues and organs has become a new trend in tissue engineering and regenerative medicine, whereas existing scaffold manufacturing techniques and cell incorporation strategies have their respective limitations for realizing this goal. Cell microencapsulation strategies are capable of protecting and delivering cells into designated positions, which have also been verified to be feasible for incorporating cells within tissue engineering scaffolds to form biomimetic 3D cell-laden structures with well-preserved cell viability and phenotype. In particular, with assistances of some advanced cell microencapsulation techniques that could be performed in continuous and noncontact manners, such as coaxial aerodynamic-assisted cell microencapsulation, hydrodynamic-assisted cell microencapsulation and electrohydrodynamic-assisted cell microencapsulation (i.e., cell electrospinning and cell electrospraying), cells could be handled and encapsulated via noncontact ways. It is therefore feasible to combine these advanced cell microencapsulation techniques with scaffold manufacturing techniques such as electrospinning for high-efficiency biomanufacturing of biomimetic 3D cell-laden structures. Among these three advanced cell microencapsulation techniques, electrohydrodynamic-assisted cell microencapsulation (i.e., cell electrospinning and cell electrospraying) show obvious superiorities in the ease of being integrated with scaffold manufacturing techniques for cell microencapsulation and subsequently delivering specific cell types into designated positions of electrospun nanofibrous scaffolds to form the biomimetic 3D cell-laden structures, which can be formed through the concurrent electrospinning of synthetic polymers to form scaffold skeleton and cell electrospinning/electrospraying for incorporating cells within the nanofibrous structures of the scaffolds. The electrospinning and electrospraying with cells for preparing biomimetic 3D cell-laden structures with multiple cell incorporation that can mimic the cell arrangements and anatomies of some thick tissues and solid organs will be a visible target, while the structural, physicochemical and biological properties of the scaffolds should be modulated and optimized for attaining desirable cell viability and interactions between the incorporated cells and the scaffolds that act as the synthetic cell microenvironments.

The recapitulation and reconstruction of the 3D multicellular structures and cell-ECM organizations of some native body tissues and organs shall be the first step in biomanufacturing of cell-scaffold constructs with tissue-mimicking structures for potentially repairing or regenerating such tissues and organs with relatively complex anatomies. It can be further envisioned that there will be a more exciting yet challenging goal of biomanufacturing "living" cell-scaffold constructs having tissue functions that can even be used for replacing native body tissues and organs with disorders or dysfunctions. To achieve this goal, it will require not only the desirable strategies for precisely incorporating multiple cell types within the designated positions of scaffold structures in well-defined and controllable manners, but also well-designed properties (structures, physicochemical properties and bioactivities) of the scaffolds for supporting the ingrowth and arrangements of multiple cells. To meet the specific requirements of tissue regeneration or development at different stages, the scaffolds will even be required to be bio-responsive, which can sense physiological or environmental signals and actuated accordingly at different stages of tissue regeneration processes.[112–114] Besides, recent advances in stem cells and organoids infers that the inclusion of stem cells and organoids, rather than somatic cells, shall be promising for biomanufacturing of cell-scaffold constructs with tissue-mimicking functions.[115] In return, the investigations into stem cells or organoids affected by the biomimetic structural, mechanical and biological cues of the cell-laden scaffolds formed with the assistances of electrospinning and electrospraying with cells may also deepen our understanding of tissue development and regeneration processes.

Acknowledgments

This work was supported by the National Key R&D Program of China (2017YFA0701303), the National Natural Science Foundation of China (51903245), Hong Kong Research Grants Council (HKU 7177/13E, 17201017) and the Natural Science Foundation of Guangdong, China (2114050001067).

References

1. A. Khademhosseini and R. Langer, *Nat. Protocols* **11**, 1775 (2016).
2. S. Badylak and N. Rosenthal, *NPJj Regenerative Med.* **2**, 2 (2017).
3. E. S. Place, J. H. George, C. K. Williams and M. M. Stevens, *Chem. Soc. Rev.* **38**, 1139 (2009).

4. P. Chan and K. W. Leong, *Euro. Spine J.* **17**, 467 (2008).
5. R. O. Hynes, *Science* **326**, 1216 (2009).
6. M. Wang, *Biomaterials* **24**, 2133 (2003).
7. M. P. Lutolf and J. A. Hubbell, *Nat. Biotechnol.* **23**, 47 (2005).
8. S. J. Hollister, *Nat. Mater.* **4**, 518 (2005).
9. K. S. Ogueri and C. T. Laurencin, *ACS Nano* **14**, 9347 (2020).
10. J. Ding, J. Zhang, J. Li, D. Li, C. Xiao, H. Xiao, H. Yang, X. Zhuang and X. Chen, *Prog. Polym. Sci.* **90**, 1 (2019).
11. S. Chen, R. Li, X. Li and J. Xie, *Adv. Drug Deliv. Rev.* **132**, 188 (2018).
12. Q. Zhao, H. Cui, J. Wang, H. Chen, Y. Wang, L. Zhang, X. Du and M. Wang, *ACS Appl. Mater. Interf.* **10**, 23583 (2018).
13. W. Liu, S. Thomopoulos and Y. Xia, *Adv. Health. Mater.* **1**, 10 (2012).
14. S. Khorshidi, A. Solouk, H. Mirzadeh, S. Mazinani, J. M. Lagaron, S. Sharifi and S. Ramakrishna, *J. Tissue Eng. Regen. Med.* **10**, 715 (2016).
15. G. Orive, R. M. Hernandez, A. R. Gascon, R. Calafiore, T. M. S. Chang, P. De Vos, G. Hortelano, D. Hunkeler, I. Lacik, A. M. J. Shapiro and J. L. Pedraz, *Nat. Med.* **9**, 104 (2003).
16. H. Uludag, P. De Vos and P. A. Tresco, *Adv. Drug Deliv. Rev.* **42**, 29 (2000).
17. G. Orive, E. Santos, D. Poncelet, R. M. Hernandez, J. L. Pedraz, L. U. Wahlberg, P. De Vos and D. Emerich, *Trends Pharmacol. Sci.* **36**, 537 (2015).
18. L. A. L. Fliervoet and E. Mastrobattista, *Adv. Drug Deliv. Rev.* **106**, 63 (2016).
19. S. N. Jayasinghe, A. N. Qureshi and P. A. Eagles, *Small* **2**, 216 (2006).
20. S. N. Jayasinghe, J. Auguste and C. J. Scotton, *Adv. Mater.* **27**, 7794 (2015).
21. Q. Zhao, J. Wang, H. Cui, H. Chen, Y. Wang and X. Du, *Adv. Funct. Mater.* **28**, 1801027 (2018).
22. K. Wang, M. Xu, M. Zhu, H. Su, H. Wang, D. Kong and L. Wang, *J. Biomed. Mater. Res. A.* **101**, 3474 (2013).
23. M. C. Phipps, W. C. Clem, J. M. Grunda, G. A. Clines and S. L. Bellis, *Biomaterials* **33**, 524 (2012).
24. J. Rnjak-Kovacina and A. S. Weiss, *Tissue Eng. B. Rev.* **17**, 365 (2011).
25. A. Blakeney, A. Tambralli, J. M. Anderson, A. Andukuri, D. J. Lim, D. R. Dean and H. W. Jun, *Biomaterials* **32**, 1583 (2011).
26. B. M. Baker, A. O. Gee, R. B. Metter, A. S. Nathan, R. A. Marklein, J. A. Burdick and R. L. Mauck, *Biomaterials* **29**, 2348 (2008).
27. S. Place, N. D. Evans and M. M. Stevens, *Nat. Mater.* **8**, 457 (2009).
28. X. C. Yang, J. D. Shah and H. J. Wang, *Tissue Eng. Pt. A.* **15**, 945 (2009).
29. J. J. Stankus, J. Guan, K. Fujimoto and W. R. Wagner, *Biomaterials* **27**, 735 (2006).
30. G. Vunjak-Novakovic, B. Obradovic, I. Martin, P. M. Bursac, R. Langer and L. E. Freed, *Biotechnol. Progr.* **14**, 193 (1998).
31. A. Mathews, S. Colombus, V. K. Krishnan and L. K. Krishnan, *J. Tissue. Eng. Regen. M.* **6**, 451 (2012).
32. M. H. Ng, S. R. Chowdhury, M. Morshed, K. K. Tan, G. H. Tan, M. Y. Phang, B. S. Aminuddin, O. Fauziah and B. H. I. Ruszymah, *J. Biomater. Tiss. Eng.* **4**, 573 (2014).

33. S. Haykal, M. Salna, Y. Z. Zhou, P. Marcus, M. Fatehi, G. FrostMsc, T. Machuca, S. O. P. Hofer and T. K. Waddell, *Tissue Eng. C. Meth.* **20**, 681 (2014).
34. W. T. Godbey, B. S. S. Hindy, M. E. Sherman and A. Atala, *Biomaterials* **25**, 2799 (2004).
35. Z. Z. Zhang, D. Jiang, S. J. Wang, Y. S. Qi, J. Y. Zhang and J. K. Yu, *ACS Appl. Mater. Interf.* **7**, 15294 (2015).
36. X. G. Lv, C. Feng, Q. Fu, H. Xie, Y. Wang, J. W. Huang, M. K. Xie, A. Atala, Y. M. Xu and W. X. Zhao, *J. Biomed. Mater. Res. B* **104**, 1098 (2016).
37. W. J. Li, Y. J. Jiang and R. S. Tuan, *Tissue Eng. Pt. A* **14**, 639 (2008).
38. W. J. Fu, Y. D. Xu, Z. X. Wang, G. Li, J. G. Shi, F. Z. Cui, Y. Y. Zhang and X. Zhang, *J. Biomed. Mater. Res. A* **100a**, 1725 (2012).
39. I. Katouzian and S. M. Jafari, *Trends Food Sci. Tech.* **53**, 34 (2016).
40. M. Pattnaik, P. Pandey, G. J. O. Martin, H. N. Mishra and M. Ashokkumar, *Foods* **10**, 279 (2021).
41. L. M. C. Aguilar, S. M. Silva and S. E. Moulton, *J. Control. Release* **306**, 40 (2019).
42. T. M. S. Chang, *Science* **146**, 524 (1964).
43. J. M. Rabanel, X. Banquy, H. Zouaoui, M. Mokhtar and P. Hildgen, *Biotechnol. Prog.* **25**, 946 (2009).
44. G. Orive, E. Santos, J. L. Pedraz and R. M. Hernandez, *Adv. Drug Deliv. Rev.* **67–68**, 3 (2014).
45. R. M. Olabisi, *J. Biomed. Mater. Res. A.* **103**, 846 (2015).
46. Lim and A. M. Sun, *Science* **210**, 908 (1980).
47. K. Senior, *Drug Discov. Today* **6**, 6 (2001).
48. R. P. Lanza, J. L. Hayes and W. L. Chick, *Nat. Biotechnol.* **14**, 1107 (1996).
49. J. Leijten, J. Seo, K. Yue, G. T. Santiago, A. Tamayol, G. U. Ruiz-Esparza, S. R. Shin, R. Sharifi, I. Noshadi, M. M. Alvarez, Y. S. Zhang and A. Khademhosseini, *Mater. Sci. Eng. R. Rep.* **119**, 1 (2017).
50. S. Ahadian, R. B. Sadeghian, S. Salehi, S. Ostrovidov, H. Bae, M. Ramalingam and A. Khademhosseini, *Bioconjug. Chem.* **26**, 1984 (2015).
51. K. Y. Lee and D. J. Mooney, *Chem. Rev.* **101**, 1869 (2001).
52. X. Du, H. Cui, Q. Zhao, J. Wang, H. Chen and Y. Wang, *Research* **2019**, 6398296 (2019).
53. D. Nicodemus and S. J. Bryant, *Tissue Eng. B. Res.* **14**, 149 (2008).
54. S. Wust, M. E. Godla, R. Muller and S. Hofmann, *Acta Biomater.* **10**, 630 (2014).
55. T. Gold, D. M. Varma, D. Harbottle, M. S. Gupta, S. S. Stalling, P. J. Taub and S. B. Nicoll, *J. Biomed. Mater. Res. A.* **102**, 4536 (2014).
56. M. S. Bae, J. Y. Ohe, J. B. Lee, D. N. Heo, W. Byun, H. Bae, Y. D. Kwon and I. K. Kwon, *Bone* **59**, 189 (2014).
57. C. G. Williams, A. N. Malik, T. K. Kim, P. N. Manson and J. H. Elisseeff, *Biomaterials* **26**, 1211 (2005).
58. X. Z. Shu, Y. C. Liu, Y. Luo, M. C. Roberts and G. D. Prestwich, *Biomacromolecules* **3**, 1304 (2002).

59. X. Z. Shu, S. Ahmad, Y. C. Liu and G. D. Prestwich, *J. Biomed. Mater. Res. A.* **79a**, 902 (2006).
60. C. N. Salinas, B. B. Cole, A. M. Kasko and K. S. Anseth, *Tissue Eng.* **13**, 1025 (2007).
61. Q. Liu, A. Chiu, L. H. Wang, D. An, M. Zhong, A. M. Smink, B. J. de Haan, P. de Vos, K. Keane, A. Vegge, E. Y. Chen, W. Song, W. F. Liu, J. Flanders, C. Rescan, L. G. Grunnet, X. Wang and M. Ma, *Nat. Commun.* **10**, 5262 (2019).
62. H. Hajiali, J. A. Heredia-Guerrero, I. Liakos, A. Athanassiou and E. Mele, *Biomacromolecules* **16**, 936 (2015).
63. A. Garate, J. Ciriza, J. G. Casado, R. Blazquez, J. L. Pedraz, G. Orive and R. M. Hernandez, *Mol. Pharm.* **12**, 3953 (2015).
64. E. P. Herrero, E. M. M. Del Valle and M. A. Galan, *Biotechnol. Prog.* **23**, 940 (2007).
65. T. Maguire, E. Novik, R. Schloss and M. Yarmush, *Biotechnol. Bioeng.* **93**, 581 (2006).
66. M. Chavarri, I. Maranon, R. Ares, F. C. Ibanez, F. Marzo and M. D. Villaran, *Int. J. Food Microbiol.* **142**, 185 (2010).
67. S. Sakai, I. Hashimoto and K. Kawakami, *J. Biomat. Sci.-Polym. E.* **19**, 937 (2008).
68. L. Klouda, K. R. Perkins, B. M. Watson, M. C. Hacker, S. J. Bryant, R. M. Raphael, F. K. Kasper and A. G. Mikos, *Acta Biomater.* **7**, 1460 (2011).
69. E. Donath, S. Moya, B. Neu, G. B. Sukhorukov, R. Georgieva, A. Voigt, H. Baumler, H. Kiesewetter and H. Mohwald, *Chem.-Eur. J.* **8**, 5481 (2002).
70. A. Diaspro, D. Silvano, S. Krol, O. Cavalleri and A. Gliozzi, *Langmuir* **18**, 5047 (2002).
71. Y. Teramura, Y. Kaneda and H. Iwata, *Biomaterials* **28**, 4818 (2007).
72. N. G. Veerabadran, P. L. Goli, S. S. Stewart-Clark, Y. M. Lvov and D. K. Mills, *Macromol. Biosci.* **7**, 877 (2007).
73. Lee, J. Choi, J. H. Park, M. H. Kim, D. Hong, H. Cho, S. H. Yang and I. S. Choi, *Angew. Chem. Int. Edit.* **53**, 8056 (2014).
74. A. Abalovich, C. Jatimliansky, E. Diegex, M. Arias, A. Altamirano, C. Amorena, B. Martinez and M. Nacucchio, *Transplant. Proc.* **33**, 1977 (2001).
75. N. Bremond, E. Santanach-Carreras, L. Y. Chu and J. Bibette, *Soft Matter* **6**, 6207 (2010).
76. S. Sakai, I. Hashimoto and K. Kawakami, *Biotechnol. Bioeng.* **99**, 235 (2008).
77. S. Sakai, S. Ito, Y. Ogushi, I. Hashimoto, N. Hosoda, Y. Sawae and K. Kawakami, *Biomaterials* **30**, 5937 (2009).
78. S. Arumuganathar, S. Irvine, J. R. McEwan and S. N. Jayasinghe, *J. Appl. Polym. Sci.* **107**, 1215 (2008).
79. Q. Zhao, H. Cui, Y. Wang and X. Du, *Small* **16**, 1903798 (2020).
80. A. Rang, J. Park, J. Ju, G. S. Jeong and S. H. Lee, *Biomaterials* **35**, 2651 (2014).
81. H. Onoe, T. Okitsu, A. Itou, M. Kato-Negishi, R. Gojo, D. Kiriya, K. Sato, S. Miura, S. Iwanaga, K. Kuribayashi-Shigetomi, Y. T. Matsunaga, Y. Shimoyama and S. Takeuchi, *Nat. Mater.* **12**, 584 (2013).

82. C. Kim, S. Chung, Y. E. Kim, K. S. Lee, S. H. Lee, K. W. Oh and J. Y. Kang, *Lab Chip* **11**, 246 (2011).
83. T. J. Sill and H. A. von Recum, *Biomaterials* **29**, 1989 (2008).
84. C. Wang and M. Wang, *Front. Mater. Sci.* **8**, 3 (2014).
85. A. Martins, A. R. Duarte, S. Faria, A. P. Marques, R. L. Reis and N. M. Neves, *Biomaterials* **31**, 5875 (2010).
86. S. Liu, J. Zhao, H. Ruan, W. Wang, T. Wu, W. Cui and C. Fan, *Mater. Sci. Eng. C* **33**, 1176 (2013).
87. B. Song, C. Wu and J. Chang, *Acta Biomater.* **8**, 1901 (2012).
88. Y. Zhou, Q. Zhao and M. Wang, *MRS Commun.* **9**, 1098 (2019).
89. Q. Zhao, W. W. Lu and M. Wang, *Mater. Lett.* **193**, 1 (2017).
90. Y. Zhou, Q. Zhao, N. L. Y. Tsai and M. Wang, *MRS Commun.* **9**, 413 (2019).
91. C. Liao and K. W. Leong, *Biomaterials* **32**, 1669 (2011).
92. H. Jiang, Y. Hu, Y. Li, P. Zhao, K. Zhu and W. Chen, *J. Control. Release* **108**, 237 (2005).
93. Q. Zhao and M. Wang, *Mater. Lett.* **162**, 48 (2016).
94. A. Lopez-Rubio, E. Sanchez, Y. Sanz and J. M. Lagaron, *Biomacromolecules* **10**, 2823 (2009).
95. M. F. Canbolat, C. Tang, S. H. Bernacki, B. Pourdeyhimi and S. Khan, *Macromol. Biosci.* **11**, 1346 (2011).
96. A. Townsend-Nicholson and S. N. Jayasinghe, *Biomacromolecules* **7**, 3364 (2006).
97. M. Windbergs, Y. Zhao, J. Heyman and D. A. Weitz, *J. Am. Chem. Soc.* **135**, 7933 (2013).
98. N. Bock, T. R. Dargaville and M. A. Woodruff, *Prog. Polym. Sci.* **37**, 1510 (2012).
99. Q. Zhao and M. Wang, *Polym. Degrad. Stabil.* **162**, 169 (2019).
100. P. Patel, S. Irvine, J. R. McEwan and S. N. Jayasinghe, *Soft Matter* **4**, 1219 (2008).
101. Q. Zhao, Y. Zhou and M. Wang, *Acta Biomater.* **123**, 312 (2021).
102. W. Salalha, J. Kuhn, Y. Dror and E. Zussman, *Nanotechnology* **17**, 4675 (2006).
103. M. Gensheimer, M. Becker, A. Brandis-Heep, J. H. Wendorff, R. K. Thauer and A. Greiner, *Adv. Mater.* **19**, 2480 (2007).
104. S. Klein, J. Kuhn, R. Avrahami, S. Tarre, M. Beliavski, M. Green and E. Zussman, *Biomacromolecules* **10**, 1751 (2009).
105. Y. Liu, M. H. Rafailovich, R. Malal, D. Cohn and D. Chidambaram, *Proc. Natl. Acad. Sci. USA.* **106**, 14201 (2009).
106. M. Gensheimer, A. Brandis-Heep, S. Agarwal, R. K. Thauer and A. Greiner, *Macromol. Biosci.* **11**, 333 (2011).
107. E. Ng, P. Joly, S. N. Jayasinghe, B. Vernay, R. Knight, S. P. Barry, J. McComick, D. Latchman and A. Stephanou, *Biotechnol. J.* **6**, 86 (2011).
108. A. Abeyewickreme, A. Kwok, J. R. McEwan and S. N. Jayasinghe, *Integr. Biol.* **1**, 260 (2009).
109. S. N. Jayasinghe, G. Warnes and C. J. Scotton, *Macromol. Biosci.* **11**, 1364 (2011).

110. K. Bartolovic, N. Mongkoldhumrongkul, S. N. Waddington, S. N. Jayasinghe and S. J. Howe, *Analyst* **135**, 157 (2010).
111. D. Poncelet, P. de Vos, N. Suter and S. N. Jayasinghe, *Adv. Healthc. Mater.* **1**, 27 (2012).
112. Q. Zhao, J. Wang, Y. Wang, H. Cui and X. Du, *Natl. Sci. Rev.* **7**, 629 (2020).
113. Q. Zhao, C. Li, H. C. Shum and X. Du, *Lab Chip* **20**, 4321 (2020).
114. Q. Zhao, Y. Wang, H. Cui and X. Du, *J. Mater. Chem. C* **7**, 6493 (2019).
115. J. A. Brassard, M. Nikolaev, T. Hubscher, M. Hofer and M. P. Lutolf, *Nat. Mater.* **20**, 22 (2021).

https://doi.org/10.1142/9789819809028_0002

Chapter 2

COVID-19 Testing: Frequency Wins over Sensitivity in Control of Disease Transmission*

Francois Berthiaume

Department of Biomedical Engineering
Rutgers, The State University of New Jersey
599 Taylor Road, Piscataway, NJ 08854, USA
fberthia@soe.rutgers.edu

Emerging pathogens have no known therapies or vaccines and therefore can only be controlled via traditional methods of contact tracing, quarantine and isolation that require rapid and widespread testing. The most recent outbreak from an emerging pathogen is due to the highly transmissible SARS-CoV-2 virus causing COVID-19 disease, which is associated with no symptoms or mild symptoms in 80–90% of the infected individuals, while in the remainder of the patients it exhibits severe illness that can be lethal or persist for several weeks to months after infection. The first tests to diagnose infection by SARS-CoV-2 were developed soon after the genome of the virus became known, and use probes to measure viral RNA by reverse transcriptase-polymerase chain reaction (RT-PCR). These tests are highly sensitive and specific but can require several days to return results, which makes contact tracing and more generally efforts to control the spread of the infection very difficult. Furthermore, the sensitivity threshold is orders of magnitude below the viral load necessary for transmission; therefore, individuals recovering from the infection may still be have a positive test and be required to isolate unnecessarily while they are no longer infectious. Antigen tests were subsequently developed that use antibodies mostly targeted to the nucleocapsid protein of the virus. These tests are about 100 times less sensitive than RT-PCR, yes they detect viral loads that are about 1/10 that needed for transmission. Furthermore, such tests are potentially much cheaper than RT-PCR and yield results in 15 min or less.

---

*To cite this article, please refer to its earlier version published in the *Nano LIFE*, Vol. 11, No. 1 (2021) 2030002 (10 pages), DOI: 10.1142/S1793984420300022

Antibody, also known as serological testing, is available and can provide useful information to understand the extent to which a population has been exposed to the virus; however, it is not a good indicator of current infection and not useful for infection control. Viral transmission models that incorporate testing and contact tracing show that infection control is much more readily achieved by increasing testing frequency than by using higher sensitivity testing. For example, compared to no testing at all, testing once every other week has a marginal benefit, while testing weekly can decrease the number of infections to 20–40%, and testing twice weekly or more can bring about a 95%+ reduction in infections. These lessons learned from dealing from the COVID-19 pandemic should guide future planning against potential emerging viruses.

Keywords: COVID-19; SARS-CoV-2; emerging pathogens; zoonoses; testing.

1. Introduction

Animal reservoirs currently harbor a multitude of viruses that have potential to spread to humans.[1] Emerging pathogens have no known therapies or vaccines and therefore can only be controlled via traditional methods of contact tracing, quarantine and isolation that require rapid and widespread testing. Preparedness for potential future pandemics should therefore prioritize the development of reagents and methods that enable rapid testing for those potential pathogens that could be rapidly deployed if and when they emerge into the human population. In this review, we discuss the testing strategies that have been deployed for SARS-CoV-2, a virus believed to have jumped from animals to infect humans in late 2019, leading to a pandemic that disrupted the world through the entire year of 2020.

Approximately, 80–90% of people infected with the SARS-CoV-2 virus are either asymptomatic or exhibit mild symptoms that are similar to that of other common respiratory illnesses.[2] The remainder of the patients, however, experience severe illness that can be lethal or persist for several weeks to months after infection. Therefore, proper mitigation of continued spread of the virus in the general population cannot rely on detection of infection by symptoms, but rather on widespread laboratory testing to identify individuals who are likely to transmit the infection to others. Furthermore, testing of patients who are known to be infected may be useful to monitor the progression of disease and when it is safe to release them from isolation requirements. In this paper, we discuss the different types of tests available, and some recommendations for effective use of testing in the context of controlling SARS-CoV-2 propagation. These recommendations are likely applicable to other emerging viruses that exhibit high transmissibility and nonspecific symptoms.

2. SARS-CoV-2 course of infection

It is widely believed that SARS-CoV-2 is mainly transmitted by microdroplets ejected from the mouth and nose of infected individuals reaching the mucosal membranes (mouth, nose and eyes) of susceptible persons. The viral dose required for infection is estimated to be on the order of $>10^6$ viral particles/mL, based on what is known about other coronaviruses as well as cell culture studies. Possible infection is assumed if one individual is in close proximity (less than 6 ft or 2 m) to an infected individual for 15 min, requiring quarantining and monitoring of symptoms, according to widely accepted guidelines established by public health authorities.

"Super-spreader" events where a large number of individuals were infected seemingly from a single person harboring the virus have been documented. Since it is unlikely that a single person would have been in close contact with some many individuals during that event, it is thought that other modes of transmission, such as via aerosolization and dispersion of virus through ventilation systems, can occasionally take place.[3] Virus deposited on surfaces can also remain infectious for days depending on the surface type; however, it is thought that fomites play a minor role in transmission.

The incubation period of SARS-CoV-2 can be as short as 2 days, and half of the infections declare within 4–5 days, although in some cases it may extend up to 15 days.[4,5] Thus, a 14-day time window is generally used as quarantine period to ensure that an individual has not become infected.

The initial viral replication phase sees rapid exponential growth of the virus to levels ranging from 10^8/mL to 10^9/mL viral particles in a matter of 24–48 h, leading to first symptoms in symptomatic individuals. In a typical infection, virus load then declines monotonically over the next 10 days to 2 weeks [Fig. 1]. As described in a CDC memo "Duration of Isolation and Precautions for Adults with COVID-19" updated September 10, 2020, in severe cases, replication-competent virus cannot be found in 95% of patients 15 days after onset of symptoms, and 100% after 20 days. These times are shorter by about five days in mild cases. It is noteworthy that viral load typically drops below the 10^6/mL threshold for transmission earlier, after approximately one week. In some individuals, symptoms may worsen in the second week after infection; however, this reflects an immune-driven inflammatory phase, which may also be followed by a hypercoagulability phase. Neither are thought to involve further viral replication or cause viral shedding.

3. Surveillance versus clinical COVID-19 testing

Surveillance testing aims to identify individuals who are at risk of transmitting the virus, irrespective of whether or not they have symptoms. It is the cornerstone of public health measures aimed at limiting the spread of highly contagious emerging infections, such as that caused by SARS-CoV-2, for which no vaccine or reliable treatments exist. For it to be effective, the testing must identify, as quickly as possible, individuals in a population who are likely to transmit infection to others. Therefore, this type of testing must be very widely available, and at-risk individuals must be tested as often as possible, which also means that barriers to testing must be minimized. This feat is best accomplished with tests that are very low cost, do not require a prescription, and can be performed at home (akin to pregnancy tests). Although the most sensitive tests may show detectable virus over periods of 2–4 weeks in an infected individual, surveillance testing does not need to be as sensitive because it focuses on the time period when viral transmission is most likely, which corresponds to the ~7 days that the viral load exceeds 10^6 particles/mL [Fig. 1]. Similarly, implementation of quarantine measures should be limited to that period, so as to not unnecessarily prevent non-infectious individuals from engaging in their daily activities.

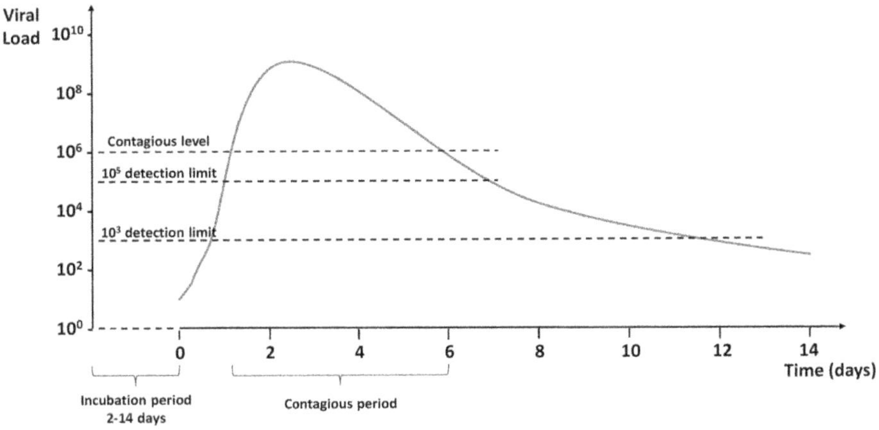

Fig. 1. Dynamics of viral load in typical patient after infection with SARS-CoV-2.

Clinical testing, which may be administered both in out-patient or in-patient settings, aims to determine the cause of disease in an individual who is experiencing COVID-19-like symptoms. High accuracy and sensitivity are both important because test results are used to understand the clinical course of the disease in a particular individual. Although low-cost clinical tests and rapid point-of-care results are obviously preferred to inform treatment approach, they are less critical from a standpoint of public health considerations. Symptomatic patients and other individuals who are quarantining because they were informed of close contact with an infected person, are already isolating at home or in a healthcare facility, and a delay in test results would not lead to further transmission.

One study attempted to model the impact of test sensitivity and frequency of testing, among other variables, on the mitigation of SARS-CoV-2 transmission. Larremore *et al.* compared the impact on individual infectiousness of using two different assays, one with a limit of detection of 10^3 viral particles/mL and 10^5 viral particles/mL, to screen for infected individuals. It was assumed that 35% of infected individuals would be "behaviorally symptomatic", meaning that they were symptomatic and self-isolate within three days. Although the more sensitive tests resulted in lower infectiousness, the difference was quite marginal. In contrast, testing frequency had a dramatic effect.

Testing with either test once every two weeks was about as good as no testing [Fig. 2(a)]. Increasing frequency to weekly testing was already better, and a major decrease in infectiousness was observed if testing was increased to every three days, with even better results with daily testing.

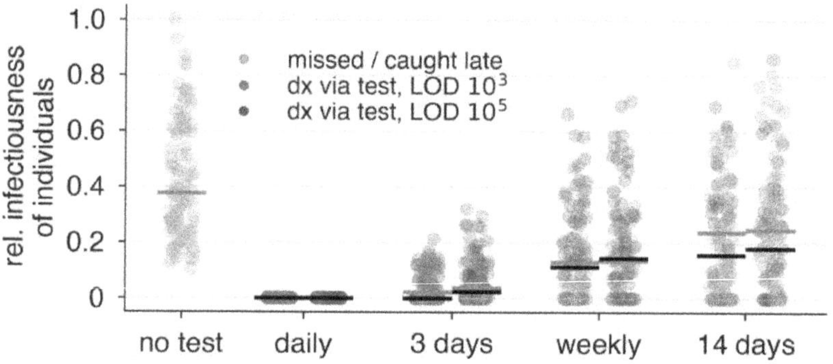

(a)

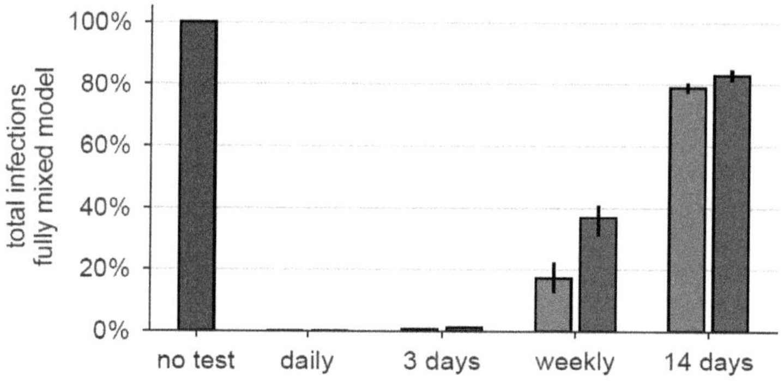

(b)

Fig. 2. (a) Impact of frequency of testing on the infectiousness of 100 individuals, comparing diagnosis (dx) tests with a limit of detection of 10^3 (high sensitivity similar to PCR) versus 10^5 (lower sensitivity similar to antigen tests) viral particles. Red and brown dots denote individuals whose infection was detected by the high sensitivity and low sensitivity tests, respectively. Blue dots denote individuals whose infection was missed. Black lines show medians for detected infections in infectious individuals. (b) Relative number of cases in a population depending on testing frequency for high sensitivity (red) versus lower sensitivity (brown) tests, using 100% as the number of cases if no testing is used. Reproduced, with author's permission, from Figs. 1(d) and 2(c) in Larremore *et al.*,[32] Creative Commons-BY-NC-ND 4.0 International License (color online).

In a simulation where 100 positive individuals were allowed to transmit in a well-mixed population, increasing testing frequency was far more effective than using higher sensitivity tests in decreasing the effective reproductive number Ro (the number of individuals that are infected by a single positive case). In fact, daily testing could achieve a 100% decrease in transmission [Fig. 2(b)]. It was also observed that this finding was unaffected in sensitivity analyses to evaluate the impact of various assumptions in the model (such as effect of viral load on infectiousness, fraction of behaviorally symptomatic individuals, nonwell-mixed population, assay limit of detection). Delays in reporting results of even only 1 and 2 days significantly decreased the effectiveness of the surveillance program. Another majorly important observation was that even accounting for 10% false-negative tests (thus failing to identify 10% infected individuals) and participation of 75% of the population in the testing program, was sufficient to extinguish an epidemic, while 50% participation could significantly decrease the magnitude and duration of an outbreak. Based on these results, the authors have sent an open letter to the New England Journal of Medicine to plead authorities to deploy rapid and inexpensive tests, even if they have worse detection limits than the "gold standard" of nuclcic acid tests.[6]

Another study investigated the impact of testing sensitivity (70–99%) and frequency (every 1, 2, 3 and 7 days), infection reproduction number, and other variables on a simulated college campus with 10 asymptomatic infected individuals in a population of 5000 students.[7] The findings were very consistent with the previous study, in that frequency of testing had a much greater impact on infection control than test sensitivity. It was also noted that symptom-based screening, which is commonly done using noncontact temperature assessment devices and self-reporting of other symptoms (such as cough, sore throat, loss of smell or taste, etc.), is not very effective by itself at containing an outbreak.

Pool sampling is another strategy to test groups of individuals when supplies are limited. For example, if a population of 100 has one positive case (i.e., 1% prevalence), and the population is split into 10 groups of 10, each group getting 1 test, 10 tests will find the group with the infected individual, and an additional 10 tests will find the infected person within that group. Thus, pooling in this fashion uses 20 tests instead of 100 tests that would be needed if all 100 individuals get tested. The number of tests needed would however increase if the prevalence is higher since more groups of 10 would be positive and require follow up. A concern is that multiple samples mixed together may dilute positive cases below detectable levels thus leading to false negatives. However, using high sensitivity tests with a limit of detection of 10^3 viruses/mL, pooled samples from 100 individuals would still detect 10^5 viruses/mL, which is still well below contagious levels. Watkins *et al.* found that if prevalence exceeds 3%, pool samples are preferable; however, at lower prevalence, a pool size of 10–20 would be sufficient.[8]

4. Patient sampling for COVID-19

The vast majority of testing is performed on nasopharyngeal and oropharyngeal swab specimens, which provide samples with high virus titers.[9] The sampling procedure itself is relatively easy and quick when performed by trained medical personnel, and is ideal for individuals who are being tested in a medical care facility. However, it is potentially uncomfortable for the patient, can be difficult to perform on children, and requires extensive use of protective equipment to avoid spreading the virus.

Saliva sampling was developed as an alternative to the nasopharyngeal swab and first rolled out by Rutgers University for testing employees and students returning to campus during a reopening phase beginning in April 2020.[10] Saliva is collected by the patient at home while under the supervision of a nurse during a tele-medicine appointment or in a testing location. A major advantage of this method is that it does not require close interaction of the patient with medical personnel, thus decreasing the risk of viral transmission and the need for personal protective equipment. Furthermore, the minimal supervision required can alleviate one of the major bottlenecks in large-scale sampling of populations. Recent data suggest that this method is as good as the nasopharyngeal swab, and in some cases may be less subject to sampling variability.[2,11]

Sampling of sweat and odor detection by trained dogs has been reported as a means to screen passengers in airports and other public places.[12] The preliminary findings suggest that the dogs can pick individuals with COVID-19 from a mixed group of infected and healthy individuals; however, it is yet unclear whether such tests are specific, in other words whether individuals who have other diseases would be erroneously classified as positive as well.

Serological testing is specifically used for antibody tests, which are not useful for public health management purposes because antibody levels are low during the first week of infection, while the patient is highly contagious.[13] However, such tests may be useful to assess the prevalence of prior infections in a population, and to understand the humoral immune response to the virus. Other markers of infection and disease, such as c-reactive protein levels, white blood cell counts, etc. may be obtained from such samples. The blood sample can be obtained via venipuncture, which is then processed in a laboratory for detection of antibodies using enzyme-linked immunosorbent or chemiluminescence immunoassays. At-home tests have also been developed that use a drop of blood on a testing strip. There is considerable variability in the sensitivity of such tests, which have proliferated due to lack of regulations.

5. Test validation criteria

Validation of new COVID-19 tests is generally done by comparison side-by-side with a well-established and approved reverse transcriptase polymerase chain reaction (RT-PCR) test which uses a chemical lysis step followed by solid phase extraction of nucleic acid (currently viewed as the gold standard). Per current US FDA guidelines (see Templates for EUA submissions of diagnostic tests in Ref. 14), the comparison must be made using a minimum of 30 positive specimens and 30 negative specimens which are randomized and blinded. Furthermore, a minimum of 95% positive and negative agreement is deemed to be acceptable for clinical use. These criteria apply to both nucleic acid tests and antigen tests, although for the former, borderline positive specimens may be added as well. Antigen tests would not be expected to detect virus in borderline positive cases because they are about two orders of magnitude less sensitive than nucleic acid tests.

Other metrics needed to certify a test include the limit of detection, defined as the lowest concentration at which 19/20 replicates are positive, cross-reactivity with a wide range of common human pathogens, including other common coronaviruses (229E, OC43 and NL63), found in the respiratory tract.

The criteria listed above will define the analytical sensitivity and specificity of the test; however, the validation is done under somewhat idealized conditions and does not address the issue of the sampling procedure itself. Inappropriate sampling may lead to false-negative results and evaluation of the test in "real world" conditions is necessary to assess the clinical sensitivity and specificity, and the results so far across various studies show a huge variation, i.e., between 2% and 33% in repeat sample testing.[15] False positives have also been reported, although generally at a lower frequency, i.e., 4% or less,[16] and may be due to contamination with infected material at any step of the sampling or testing procedure.

6. Nucleic Acid Amplification Tests (NAATs)

The current gold standard for the diagnosis of COVID-19 relies on the detection of the SARS-CoV-2 RNA by real-time RT-PCR on samples processed by chemical lysis and solid phase extraction of nucleic acids.[17,18] These tests were developed soon after the genomic sequence for the virus, which became public in early 2020,[19] became known.

RT-PCR is a well-established technique that first involves reverse transcribing the viral RNA into DNA. Then, short synthetic nucleotide sequences called primers that bind specific regions of the viral genome adjacent to regions of interest (ROIs) are used to initiate polymerization of complementary DNA (cDNA) strands thus copying the sequence of those specific ROIs. Primers are preferably designed to target ROIs that are conserved among all strains of SARS-CoV-2 but not with other coronaviruses. Multiple primers targeting multiple regions of the genome may be used simultaneously to increase sensitivity as well as decrease the risk that the test is invalidated due to a mutation or recombination affecting one of the ROIs.[20] Temperature is alternatively raised to melt the cDNA double strand, and cooled to initiate another round of polymerization. Each cycle doubles the number of copies of the targeted nucleotide region. Fluorescent labeling is used to detect the number of copies. The number of cycles to reach the threshold of detection (C_t) is recorded. In general, the reaction is stopped after 40–45 cycles and if no signal is detected at that point the sample is deemed negative.

These tests have a high sensitivity, being able to detect 500 copies of viral RNA per specimen with 95% confidence (in other words the probability of a false-negative result in a sample with this level of RNA would be 5%).[21] They are also highly specific and can discriminate between different strains of SARS-CoV-2. This has enabled the confirmation of a second infection in some individuals that had recovered already once from COVID-19.[22]

RT-PCR tests are currently the most trusted and the ones used to formulate public health polices with regards to requirements for self-isolation, quarantine and travel. However, the testing results require sample processing in specialized laboratory facilities, which can represent a serious bottleneck leading to delays amounting to several days to provide results. In addition, many of the clinical systems operate with an endpoint measurement after 40 or 45 cycles, at which point the sample is declared positive if the fluorescence signal is detected. Therefore, individuals in recovery phase from the disease whose viral load has decreased to 10^3 viral particles/mL, which is not likely sufficient to transmit the virus, will get the same positive test result as someone who is in the active viral replication phase with $>10^6$ viral particles/mL and is highly contagious.

More sophisticated testing locations will record the number of cycles when the sensitivity threshold is reached (C_t). The lower the cycle number needed to reach threshold, the more viral RNA is initially present in the specimen. Thus, knowing this value can differentiate between high positive cases that are more likely infectious from low positive cases. One should keep in mind that these assays do not measure intact infectious viral particles, but rather viral RNA shedding, which can go on for weeks in patients recovering from severe COVID-19 while they are no longer infectious.[23,24]

RT-PCR tests require 3–24 h of laboratory time, and thus results can be made available within a day; however, when testing capacity is strained due to shortage of needed supplies, such as collection swabs, transport media, extraction kits, RT-PCR reagents, etc., as was the cases at certain times during 2020, results can take several days to be made available. Bench-top semiautomated platforms are being developed to bring RT-PCR to the point-of-care; these systems minimize human manipulation by using prepackaged reagents and expandable modular systems, which work as well as "traditional" RT-PCR methods, while shortening time to results to as little as 45 min.[25]

A modification of RT-PCR called reverse transcription loop-mediated isothermal amplification (RT-LAMP) does not require thermal cycling. The DNA products from the DNA polymerase reaction loop backward at their ends, and these loops serve as primers for another round of DNA replication while the temperature remains constant at $\sim 65\,^{\circ}$C. The DNA replication process is self-perpetuating as long as substrates are provided to the reaction. The reaction is allowed to proceed for 30 min to complete, and the readout is a color change from red to yellow that is visible with a naked eye and that can be quantified spectrophotometrically. The assay is less sensitive than

Table 1. Characteristics of COVID-19 major assay methods.

Test category	Sensitivity	Cost ($US per test)
Nucleic acid amplification tests (RT-PCR)	$< 10^3$ viral particles	>$100
Nucleic acid amplification tests (LAMP)	$< 10^4$ viral particles	$25–100
Antigen tests	$< 10^5$ viral particles	$5–50
Antibody tests	Do not detect virus	$15–100

standard RT-PCR, with a detection limit corresponding to $C_t = 30$,[26] although superior to antigen tests, which are described next.

7. Viral antigen tests

Antigen tests measure levels of proteins that make up the SARS-CoV-2 virus and that are present in clinical specimens. The preferred antigen is the nucleocapsid (N) protein because it is the most abundant [Table 2]. This antigen is common to SARS-CoV, thus tests based on that particular target cannot differentiate SARS-CoV from SARS-CoV-2. The test generally involves some type of antibody directed toward the antigen. Creating such assays is not as straightforward as nucleic acid detection because developing the antibodies themselves can take several months. Once the antibodies are available, however, simple assay platforms can be used that give results within minutes. The most common platform used is the lateral flow test, which uses capillarity-induced flow to drive sample content over regions containing different labeling and capture antibodies [Fig. 3]. Positive samples containing the target antigen bind a labeled antibody as they travel further and become trapped on a line containing the capture antibody.[27] Another line further downstream traps unused labeled antibodies and will show as a positive control.

Currently, commercial tests are dispensed by prescription only and not for at-home use; however, it is possible that such tests could be made as routine as pregnancy tests. This would make it possible to perform community-based testing on a massive scale. If the cost can be decreased further (currently $5 being the minimum), daily testing could be used in place of symptom self-evaluation, which is currently one of the parameters in "daily pass" smartphone applications that are used to clear school children and company employees for on-site reporting. Abbott's test BinaxNOW™ COVID-19 Ag CARD can be used in conjunction with the NAVICA™ Mobile APP to display a digital pass when the result is negative, and is one of the first such systems that uses test results in conjunction with a smartphone application.

Table 2. Sample antigen tests for SARS-CoV-2.

Name and manufacturer	Antigen detected	Time to results
COVID-19 Antigen Detection Kit (Beijing Savant Biotechnology) http://www.huaketai.com/en/index.php?c=article&id=315	Nucleocapsid (N) antigen*	15 min
COVID-19 Ag Respi-Strip (Coris BioConcept) https://www.corisbio.com/Products/Human-Field/Covid-19.php#	Not specified	30 min
StrongStep® SARS-CoV-2 Antigen Rapid Test (Nanjing Liming Bio-products) https://www.limingbio.com/sars-cov-2-antigen-kit-product/	Nucleocapsid (N) antigen*	15 min
Biocredit Covid-19 Ag Detection Kit (Rapigen) https://www.biovendor.com/biocredit-covid-19-ag-detection-kit?utm_source=google&utm_medium=organic	Not specified	5–8 min
2019-Novel Coronavirus (2019-nCoV) Antigen Rapid Test Kit (Shenzhen Bioeasy Biotechnology) http://en.bioeasy.com.tr/2019-novel-coronavirus-2019-ncov-ag-test-kit-fluorescence-immunochromatographic-assay/	Not specified	10 min
Sofia SARS Antigen Fluorescent Immunoassay (Quidel) https://www.quidel.com/immunoassays/rapid-sars-tests/sofia-sars-antigen-fia	Nucleocapsid (N) antigen*	15 min
SARS-CoV-2 Ag Test (LumiraDX) https://www.lumiradx.com/us-en/what-we-do/diagnostics/test-technology/antigen-test	Nucleocapsid (N) antigen*	15 min
BinaxNOW™ COVID-19 Ag Card (Abbott) https://www.globalpointofcare.abbott/en/product-details/navica-binaxnow-covid-19-us.html	Nucleocapsid (N) antigen*	15 min

Note: * — cannot differentiate between SARS-CoV-2 and SARS-CoV.

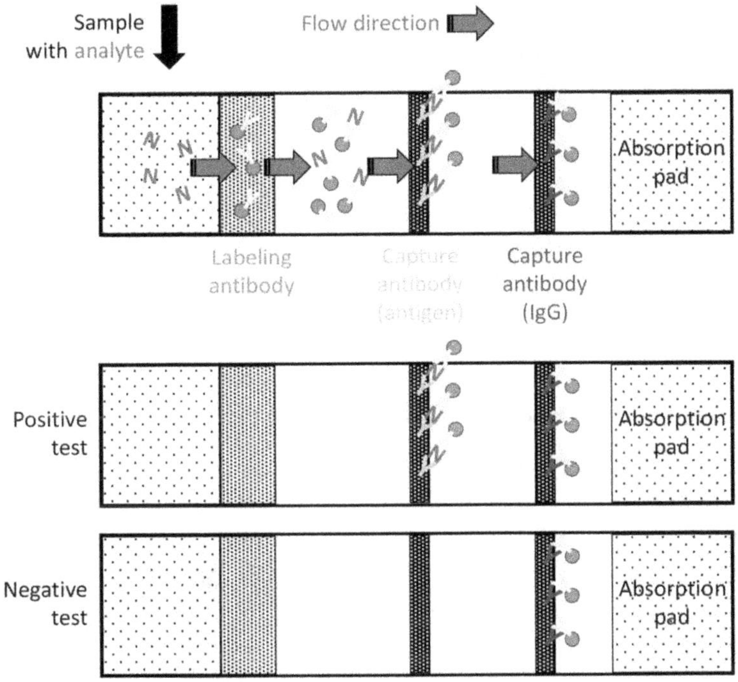

Fig. 3. Principle of the lateral flow assay. Sample is applied on a strip of wicking material which drives flow by capillarity over an area containing free antibodies labeled with gold nanoparticles (or other detectable label). The antibodies bind one antigen on the target analyte, and the complexes, along with unbound antibody, travel to a trap consisting of immobilized antibodies that bind a different antigen on the target analyte. Thus, labeled analytes are captured along a line while excess labeling antibodies continue traveling to another trap, this time consisting of immobilized anti-IgG. The second line traps labeling antibodies even if no antigen is present in the sample, thus providing a positive control for the test (color online).

Antigen tests are gaining in favor and some studies have performed head-to-head comparisons with PCR tests, which typically report a lower sensitivity than PCR.[28] A review of test results that were publicly available by May 25, 2020, reported extremely variable sensitivity among four different antigen tests (ranging from 0% to 94%, with an average of 56%), while specificity was consistently very high, between 95% and 99.9%.[13]

Lower sensitivity for antigen tests versus PCR is no surprise since the same observations have been made with H1N1 influenza and respiratory syncytial virus.[29] In many instances these comparisons are done with leftover clinical samples from multiple patients without considering the dynamics of infection. Time series of clinical samples for individual patients would provide a better basis for comparison. Furthermore, these studies generally interpret the results in the context of diagnostic utility, which is different from population surveillance. This is partly due to the fact that there remains a lack of clarity about acceptable benchmarks for surveillance tests versus diagnostic tests.

8. Antibody tests and serology

Serological tests are tests performed to measure levels of IgG and IgM antibodies in biological fluids, usually blood. Thus, these assays measure the humoral immune response to the virus and can provide evidence of current or past infection. It is likely that antibodies, especially IgG, can remain for weeks post-infection; thus, serological test information is not useful to assess whether an individual is contagious, but large-scale data can be useful to assess the fraction of the population that has been exposed to the virus. Antibodies specific to the viral coat proteins, such as the spike (S) and nucleocapsid (N) proteins, are usually detected in these tests using recombinant S and N proteins as capture antigens. The technologies used include lateral flow tests, which give results in 15–20 min, and enzyme-linked immunosorbent assays, which take a few hours.

The N protein is the most abundant protein in the virus and elicits a strong immune response. Antibodies against the S protein are particularly interesting because they may interfere with the virus binding to the cell surface via the angiotensin-converting enzyme (ACE2), which is thought to be the main mechanism of virus entry into the cell. The role of antibodies in natural immunity to the virus is unclear, especially since convalescent plasma transfusion, which aims to transfer humoral immunity from an individual who has recovered from the virus, to a patient, has not been very effective so far.[30] This does not preclude, however, that vaccines used to engineer immunity could create an effective humoral response against virus infection.

9. Conclusions

Various testing options are now available to identify individuals who have COVID-19 in a population. Diagnostic testing using RT-PCR is well suited for individuals who are strongly suspected to have the disease. However, surveillance testing of large populations is better served with rapid point-of-care inexpensive tests such as antigen tests, even though their sensitivity is inferior. High frequency testing, as much as daily, which may be possible if the costs of such tests can decrease to about $1, and if the tests are made available for at-home use, would bring about the greatest impact on decreasing the spread of COVID-19. Antibody testing is less useful to identify individuals who have an active infection and are contagious, but can provide valuable information on the course of disease in an individual and in assessing the extent to which a population has been exposed to the virus. User-friendly simulation tools which are accessible via the web (such as https://calculator.unitedinresearch.com/) have recently been developed by teams of doctors and scientists that allow schools and businesses develop their own testing strategy optimizing test type, testing frequency and cost.[31] These lessons learned from dealing from the COVID-19 pandemic should guide future planning against other potential emerging viruses.

References

1. M. E. Woolhouse, L. Brierley, C. McCaffery and S. Lycett, *Emerg. Infect. Dis.* **22**, 2037 (2016), doi: 10.3201/eid2212.160123.
2. K. K. To, O. T. Tsang, W. S. Leung, A. R. Tam, T. C. Wu, D. C. Lung, C. C. Yip, J. P. Cai, J. M. Chan, T. S. Chik, D. P. Lau, C. Y. Choi, L. L. Chen, W. M. Chan, K. H. Chan, J. D. Ip, A. C. Ng, R. W. Poon, C. T. Luo, V. C. Cheng, J. F. Chan, I. F. Hung, Z. Chen, H. Chen and K. Y. Yuen, *Lancet Infect. Dis.* **20**, 565 (2020), doi: 10.1016/S1473-3099(20)30196-1.
3. B. Salzberger, F. Buder, B. Lampl, B. Ehrenstein, F. Hitzenbichler, T. Holzmann, B. Schmidt and F. Hanses, *Infection* 1 (2020), doi: 10.1007/s15010-020-01531-3.
4. S. A. Lauer, K. H. Grantz, Q. Bi, F. K. Jones, Q. Zheng, H. R. Meredith, A. S. Azman, N. G. Reich and J. Lessler, *Ann. Intern. Med.* **172**, 577 (2020), doi: 10.7326/M20-0504.
5. X. Nie, L. Fan, G. Mu, Q. Tan, M. Wang, Y. Xie, L. Cao, M. Zhou, Z. Zhang and W. Chen, *J. Infect. Dis.* **222**, 26 (2020), doi: 10.1093/infdis/jiaa211.

6. M. J. Mina, R. Parker and D. B. Larremore, *N. Engl. J. Med.* **383**, e120 (2020), doi: 10.1056/NEJMp2025631.
7. A. D. Paltiel, A. Zheng and R. P. Walensky, *JAMA Netw. Open* **3**, e2016818 (2020), doi: 10.1001/jamanetworkopen.2020.16818.
8. A. E. Watkins, E. P. Fenichel, D. M. Weinberger, C. B. F. Vogels, D. E. Brackney, A. Casanovas-Massana, M. Campbell, J. Fournier, S. Bermejo, R. Datta, C. S. Dela Cruz, S. F. Farhadian, A. Iwasaki, A. I. Ko, N. D. Grubaugh and A. L. Wyllie, preprint, medRxiv (2020), doi:10.1101/2020.09.02.20183830.
9. F. M. Marty, K. Chen and K. A. Verrill, *N. Engl. J. Med.* **382**, e76 (2020), doi: 10.1056/NEJMvcm2010260.
10. K. F. Hung, Y. C. Sun, B. H. Chen, J. F. Lo, C. M. Cheng, C. Y. Chen, C. H. Wu and S. Y. Kao, *J. Chin. Med. Assoc.* **83**, 891 (2020), doi: 10.1097/JCMA.0000000000000396.
11. A. L. Wyllie, J. Fournier, A. Casanovas-Massana, M. Campbell, M. Tokuyama, P. Vijayakumar, J. L. Warren, B. Geng, M. C. Muenker, A. J. Moore, C. B. F. Vogels, M. E. Petrone, I. M. Ott, P. Lu, A. Venkataraman, A. Lu-Culligan, J. Klein, R. Earnest, M. Simonov, R. Datta, R. Handoko, N. Naushad, L. R. Sewanan, J. Valdez, E. B. White, S. Lapidus, C. C. Kalinich, X. Jiang, D. J. Kim, E. Kudo, M. Linehan, T. Mao, M. Moriyama, J. E. Oh, A. Park, J. Silva, E. Song, T. Takahashi, M. Taura, O. E. Weizman, P. Wong, Y. Yang, S. Bermejo, C. D. Odio, S. B. Omer, C. S. Dela Cruz, S. Farhadian, R. A. Martinello, A. Iwasaki, N. D. Grubaugh and A. I. Ko, *N. Engl. J. Med.* **383**, 1283 (2020), doi: 10.1056/NEJMc2016359.
12. D. Grandjean, R. Sarkis, J.-P. Tourtier, C. Julien-Lecocq, A. Benard, V. Roger, E. Levesque, E. Bernes-Luciani, B. Maestracci, P. Morvan, E. Gully, D. Berceau-Falancourt, J.-L. Pesce, B. Lecomte, P. Haufstater, G. Herin, J. Cabrera, Q. Muzzin, C. Gallet, H. Bacqué, J.-M. Broc, L. Thomas, A. Lichaa, G. Moujaes, M. Saliba, A. Kuhn, M. Galey, B. Berthail, L. Lapeyre, O. Méreau, M.-N. Matteï, A. Foata, L. Bey, A.-S. Philippe, P. Abassi, F. Pisani, M. Delarbre, J.-M. Orsini, A. Capelli, S. Renault, K. Bachir, A. Kovinger, E. Comas, A. Stainmesse, E. Etienne, S. Voeltzel, S. Mansouri, M. Berceau-Falancourt, B. Leva, F. Faure, A. Dami, M. A. Costa, J.-J. Tafanelli, J.-B. Luciani, J.-J. Casalot, L. Charlet, E. Ruau, M. Issa, C. Grenet, C. Billy and L. Desquilbet, preprint, bioRxiv (2020), doi:10.1101/2020.06.03.132134.
13. J. J. Deeks, J. Dinnes, Y. Takwoingi, C. Davenport, R. Spijker, S. Taylor-Phillips, A. Adriano, S. Beese, J. Dretzke, L. Ferrante di Ruffano, I. M. Harris, M. J. Price, S. Dittrich, D. Emperador, L. Hooft, M. M. Leeflang and A. Van den Bruel, *Cochrane Database Syst. Rev.* **6**, CD013652 (2020), doi: 10.1002/14651858.CD013652.
14. Administration USFDA, In vitro diagnostics EUAs (2020), https://www.fda.gov/medical-devices/coronavirus-disease-2019-covid-19-emergency-use-authorizations-medical-devices/vitro-diagnostics-euas.
15. I. Arevalo-Rodriguez, D. Buitrago-Garcia, D. Simancas-Racines, P. Zambrano-Achig, R. del Campo, A. Ciapponi, O. Sued, L. Martinez-Garcia, A. Rutjes,

N. Low, P. M. Bossuyt, J. A. Perez-Molina and J. Zamora, preprint, medRxiv (2020), doi:10.1101/2020.04.16.20066787.
16. E. Surkova, V. Nikolayevskyy and F. Drobniewski, *Lancet Respir. Med.* **S2213-600**, 30453 (2020), doi: 10.1016/S2213-2600(20)30453-7.
17. V. M. Corman, O. Landt, M. Kaiser, R. Molenkamp, A. Meijer, D. K. Chu, T. Bleicker, S. Brunink, J. Schneider, M. L. Schmidt, D. G. Mulders, B. L. Haagmans, B. van der Veer, S. van den Brink, L. Wijsman, G. Goderski, J. L. Romette, J. Ellis, M. Zambon, M. Peiris, H. Goossens, C. Reusken, M. P. Koopmans and C. Drosten, *Euro Surveill.* **25**(3), pii=2000045 (2020), doi: 10.2807/1560-7917.ES.2020.25.3.2000045.
18. S. Pfefferle, S. Reucher, D. Norz and M. Lutgehetmann, *Euro Surveill.* **25**(9), pii=2000152 (2020), doi: 10.2807/1560-7917.ES.2020.25.9.2000152.
19. C. Huang, Y. Wang, X. Li, L. Ren, J. Zhao, Y. Hu, L. Zhang, G. Fan, J. Xu, X. Gu, Z. Cheng, T. Yu, J. Xia, Y. Wei, W. Wu, X. Xie, W. Yin, H. Li, M. Liu, Y. Xiao, H. Gao, L. Guo, J. Xie, G. Wang, R. Jiang, Z. Gao, Q. Jin, J. Wang and B. Cao, *Lancet* **395**, 497 (2020), doi: 10.1016/S0140-6736(20)30183-5.
20. C. H. Chau, J. D. Strope and W. D. Figg, *Pharmacotherapy* **40**, 857 (2020), doi: 10.1002/phar.2439.
21. C. B. F. Vogels, A. F. Brito, A. L. Wyllie, J. R. Fauver, I. M. Ott, C. C. Kalinich, M. E. Petrone, A. Casanovas-Massana, M. Catherine Muenker, A. J. Moore, J. Klein, P. Lu, A. Lu-Culligan, X. Jiang, D. J. Kim, E. Kudo, T. Mao, M. Moriyama, J. E. Oh, A. Park, J. Silva, E. Song, T. Takahashi, M. Taura, M. Tokuyama, A. Venkataraman, O. E. Weizman, P. Wong, Y. Yang, N. R. Cheemarla, E. B. White, S. Lapidus, R. Earnest, B. Geng, P. Vijayakumar, C. Odio, J. Fournier, S. Bermejo, S. Farhadian, C. S. Dela Cruz, A. Iwasaki, A. I. Ko, M. L. Landry, E. F. Foxman and N. D. Grubaugh, *Nat. Microbiol.* **5**, 1299 (2020), doi: 10.1038/s41564-020-0761-6.
22. N. M. Duggan, S. M. Ludy, B. C. Shannon, A. T. Reisner and S. R. Wilcox. *Am. J. Emerg. Med.* **S0735-6757**, 30583 (2020), doi: 10.1016/j.ajem.2020.06.079.
23. Y. Liu, L. M. Yan, L. Wan, T. X. Xiang, A. Le, J. M. Liu, M. Peiris, L. L. M. Poon and W. Zhang, *Lancet Infect. Dis.* **20**, 656 (2020), doi: 10.1016/S1473-3099(20)30232-2.
24. R. Wolfel, V. M. Corman, W. Guggemos, M. Seilmaier, S. Zange, M. A. Muller, D. Niemeyer, T. C. Jones, P. Vollmar, C. Rothe, M. Hoelscher, T. Bleicker, S. Brunink, J. Schneider, R. Ehmann, K. Zwirglmaier, C. Drosten and C. Wendtner, *Nature* **581**, 465 (2020), doi: 10.1038/s41586-020-2196-x.
25. M. J. Loeffelholz, D. Alland, S. M. Butler-Wu, U. Pandey, C. F. Perno, A. Nava, K. C. Carroll, H. Mostafa, E. Davies, A. McEwan, J. L. Rakeman, R. C. Fowler, J. M. Pawlotsky, S. Fourati, S. Banik, P. P. Banada, S. Swaminathan, S. Chakravorty, R. W. Kwiatkowski, V. C. Chu, J. Kop, R. Gaur, M. L. Y. Sin, D. Nguyen, S. Singh, N. Zhang, D. H. Persing. *J. Clin. Microbiol.* **58** (2020), doi: 10.1128/JCM.00926-20.
26. V. L. Dao Thi, K. Herbst, K. Boerner, M. Meurer, L. P. Kremer, D. Kirrmaier, A. Freistaedter, D. Papagiannidis, C. Galmozzi, M. L. Stanifer, S. Boulant, S. Klein, P. Chlanda, D. Khalid, I. Barreto Miranda, P. Schnitzler, H. G.

Krausslich, M. Knop and S. Anders, *Sci. Transl. Med.* **12**(556), eabc7075 (2020), doi: 10.1126/scitranslmed.abc7075.
27. K. M. Koczula and A. Gallotta. *Essays Biochem.* **60**, 111 (2016), doi: 10.1042/EBC20150012.
28. T. Weitzel, P. Legarraga, M. Iruretagoyena, G. Pizarro, V. Vollrath, R. Araos, J. M. Munita and L. Porte, preprint, bioRxiv (2020), doi:10.1101/2020.05.27.119255.
29. M. M. Azar and M. L. Landry. *J. Clin. Microbiol.* **56**(7), e00367-18 (2018), doi: 10.1128/JCM.00367-18.
30. K. L. Chai, S. J. Valk, V. Piechotta, C. Kimber, I. Monsef, C. Doree, E. M. Wood, A. A. Lamikanra, D. J. Roberts, Z. McQuilten, C. So-Osman, L. J. Estcourt and N. Skoetz. *Cochrane Database Syst. Rev.* **10**, CD013600 (2020), doi: 10.1002/14651858.CD013600.pub3.
31. G. D. Lyng, N. E. Sheils, C. J. Kennedy, D. Griffin and E. M. Berke, preprint, medRxiv (2020), doi:10.1101/2020.10.11.20211011.
32. D. B. Larremore, B. Wilder, E. Lester, S. Shehata, J. M. Burke, J. A. Hay, M. Tambe, M. J. Mina and R. Parker, *Sci. Adv.* (2020), doi:10.1126/sciadv.abd5393.

https://doi.org/10.1142/9789819809028_0003

Chapter 3

Cancer Cell Surface Negative Charges: A Bio-Physical Manifestation of the Warburg Effect*

Donglu Shi

Department of Mechanical and Materials Engineering
College of Engineering and Applied Science
University of Cincinnati
Cincinnati, OH 45221-0072, USA

The early detection of circulating tumor cells (CTCs) in blood as part of medical diagnosis will give the doctors a head start in the provision and treatment of cancer, and therefore, with the advance in Nano technology, there is an increasing expectation of some form of early detection of circulating tumor cells at a highly sensitive level, without any biomarkers, for both early cancer diagnosis and monitoring disease progression after medical intervention. This technical note reports on the recent development in detection of highly sensitive detection of cancer cells without biomarkers. This novel concept is developed based on a hallmark cancer metabolic pattern: high glycolysis rate. Secretion of high level of lactate acid by cancer cells ultimately results in negative electrical charges on their surfaces, enabling strong binding and capturing by the positively-charged nanoprobes, and subsequent magnetic separation. When nanoprobes are incubated with cancer cells in suspension, binding takes place due to charge differences, and cancer cells are then magnetically separated. The separated cells are enumerated using a flow cytometry and identified by pathological and genome sequencing methods. Preliminary results using the approach have shown exceptionally high cancer cell capture rates, therefore potentially applicable in cancer cell detection in clinical settings.

Keywords: Circulating Tumor Cells (CTCs); Warburg effect; Fe_3O_4 nanoparticles.

---

*To cite this article, please refer to its earlier version published in the *Nano LIFE*, Vol. 7, Nos. 3 & 4 (2017) 1771001 (4 pages), DOI: 10.1142/S1793984417710015

1. Introduction

In cancer diagnosis and therapeutics, extensive effort has been devoted to identifying cancer cells in terms of oncogenic and pathological characteristics. One of the major approaches has been the development of tumor-specific ligands for cell targeting. However, previous studies have shown that two isogenic cancer cell lines differ only by a few proteins.[1] Furthermore, any molecules present on cancer cells are not absolutely absent on normal cells.[2–4] These commonalities between cancer and normal cells at molecular level have been the fundamental problems in any biomarker-based cancer diagnosis and therapeutics. It is, therefore, critical to identify a hallmark characteristic that is shared by all cancers, regardless of the phenotype and molecular differences.

2. Warburg effect and lactate secretion generated cancer cell surface negative charges

As is well-known, cancer cells exhibit the so-called "Warburg Effect" by which they only process glycolysis.[5,6] High levels of glucose uptake and lactate secretion are the two most distinguishable metabolic behaviors not only widely observed in cultured cancer cells but also extensively employed in cancer clinical settings. The levels of glucose uptake and lactate secretion are observed to be thirty times greater than those of normal cells.[7,8] Most of the previous studies on the metabolic patterns of cancer cells have mainly focused on biochemistry and the cross-membrane movement of lactate. Our recent study has shown, from 22 cancer cell lines, a close correlation between the lactate acid secreted and a net of negative electrical charges that appears on cancer cell surfaces. More important, this study has shown a direct relationship between cancer cell surface electrical charges and rate of glycolysis, that is regulated by glucose uptake.

3. Cancer cell binding and capturing by surface charged nanoprobes

To monitor the cancer cell electrical charges, the Fe_3O_4-based nanoprobes are designed and surface-functionalized with the

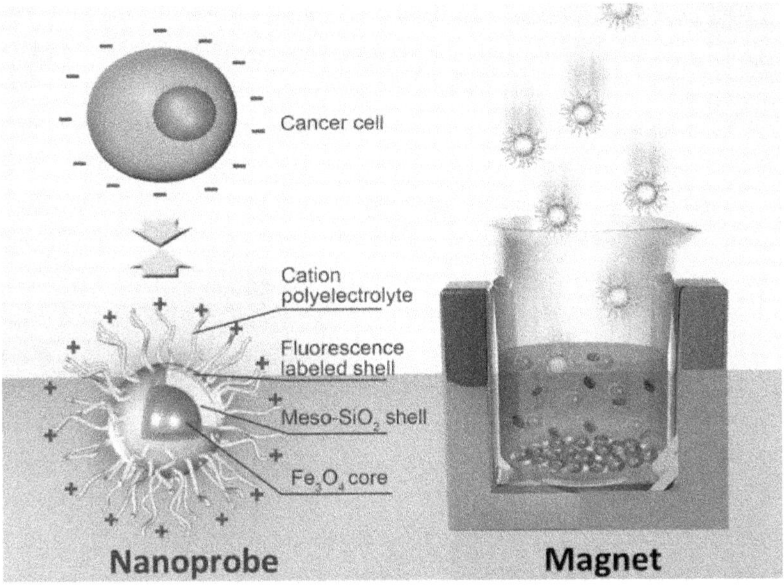

Fig. 1. Schematic diagram showing the nanoprobe design and cancer cell capturing.[9] Mechanism of Cancer Cell Surface Negative Electrical Charges.

polyethylenimine (PEI) molecules, rendering them positively charged for cancer cell electrostatic binding, capturing and magnetic separation, as schematically shown in Fig. 1.[9–12] When mixing the positively-charged nanoprobes with cancer cells of any type, they massively bind onto the cell surfaces due to opposite electrical charges.[9,10] As the Fe_3O_4 nanoprobes are also superparamagnetic, the cancer cells, bound with a high concentration of nanoprobes on their surfaces, are easily magnetically separated. Conversely, if the nanoprobes are negatively charged with the silica functional group, few of them bind on cancer cells, resulting in insignificant cancer cell capture. In this fashion, the nanoprobes can be used to detect the cancer cell surface charges which are associated with lactate secretion, a common metabolic characteristic of all cancer cells. Note that the sizes of cancer cells such as breast cancer cells range 20–30 μm, while the typical dimension of the nanoprobe is on the order of 200–300 nm. The nanoprobe electrostatic binding can therefore take place on cancer surfaces with high concentrations.

Upon strong electrostatic binding, the cancer cells can be sensitively detected, effectively captured, and magnetically removed for both diagnostic and therapeutic purposes.

In a report by Han *et al.*, the Fe_3O_4 nanoparticles were rendered fluorescent and electrically charged either positively (MNCs⊕) or negatively (MNCs ⊖). They carried out systematic *in-vitro* experiments on cell binding of HeLa cells via electrostatic interactions with charged nanoparticles.[10] As shown in Fig. 2, the green fluorescence from the positively-charged nanoparticles (MNCs⊕) is visible around the cancer cells (the blue colored cell nucleus is stained by DAPI) due to strong electrostatic force (middle column in Fig. 2).[10] In sharp contrast, no green fluorescence can be observed on the membrane of cancer cells treated by the negatively-charged nanoparticles (MNCs ⊖). These are strong experimental evidences that show the negatively-charged cancer cell surfaces, consistent with the hypothesis based on the Warburg Effect.

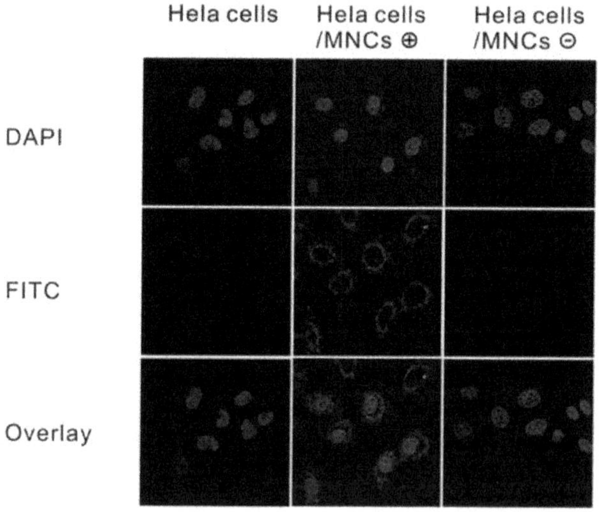

Fig. 2. Confocal fluorescent images showing treated cancer cells (HeLa cells) with positively- (MNCs⊕) and negatively- (MNCs ⊖) charged magnetic nanoparticles. Note the cancer cells are shown in blue fluorescence while the green circles surrounding them are the positively-charged nanoparticles (middle column). No green fluorescent is seen on the right column for the negatively-charged nanoparticles since they do not bind on the cancer cells.[10]

The lactate-secretion-generated cancer cell surface negative changes can be explained by the cross-membrane movement of mobile ions. The charge neutrality of most human cells is maintained by the ion pumps through the plasma membrane. In cancer cells, the cross-membrane movement of lactate is the pathway of glycolysis in hypoxia. The charges of immobile ions can easily encounter massive amount of Na^+ present in the interstitial space and extracellular environment. These immobile ions are fully accessible by Na^+ for charge neutralization. It is the highly elevated level of glycolysis that utilizes sufficient glucose available and secretes a large amount of lactate as a continuous source of mobile anions moving from cell interior to exterior, consequently creating a net of negative charges. Therefore, the perpetuating ion movement is solely responsible for the signature pattern of cancer cell surface negative charges. Our findings mechanistically link one of the most fundamental metabolic pattern, glycolysis, with a hallmark characteristic of cancer cell surface charges. A direct relationship is established between the cancer surface electric charge behavior and the lactate secretion based on a large group of cancer cell lines (22 cell lines). The surface negative charge is found to be a universal property of cancer cells regardless of their molecular and genetic differences. The operating mechanism identified in this study has laid an important foundation for the fundamental understanding of cancer cells. Furthermore, the cancer cell surface charges can be used as an analyte for studying the metabolism of cells since it directly correlates to glycolysis. In conclusion, the cancer cell surface negative change is a bio-physical manifestation of the Warburg effect.

4. Potential in nano detection of tumor cells in clinical blood

The nanoprobes described in Fig. 1 provide a new strategy in highly sensitive detection of cancer cells without any biomarkers. In sharp contrast to the current approaches, cell targeting, binding and capturing can be effectively achieved based on the electrical charge differences between the negative cancer cells and the positively-charged magnetic nanoprobes. This novel concept is developed based on a hallmark cancer metabolic pattern: high glycolysis rate. Secretion of high level of lactate acid by cancel cells ultimately results in negative electrical charges on their surfaces, enabling strong binding and capturing by the positively-charged nanoprobes, and subsequent magnetic separation. As shown in Fig. 1, when nanoprobes are incubated with cancer cells in suspension, binding takes place due to charge differences, and cancer cells are then magnetically separated. The separated cells are enumerated using a flow cytometry and identified by pathological and genome sequencing methods. Our preliminary results using the above approach have shown exceptionally high cancer cell capture rates, therefore potentially applicable in cancer cell detection in clinical settings.

One of the clinical implications, as described in Ref. 9, is the detection of circulating tumor cells (CTCs) in blood. CTCs are defined as those that detach from the primary tumor and enter blood therefore responsible for metastasis as they develop secondary lesions.[13,14] As such, there is an increasing need for early detection of circulating tumor cells at a highly sensitive level for both early cancer diagnosis and monitoring disease progression after medical intervention. The current CTC detection technologies rely on immunomagnetically labeled cells or morphological differences between cancer and normal cells, therefore with limitations due to biomarker non-specificity and morphological non-exclusivity. More important, both methods can only achieve capturing of a few CTCs per 7.5. ml of blood sample. This sensitivity level is still too low, and new detection mechanisms need to be identified for much higher detection sensitivity. The charge-based nanoprobe will serve as a highly promising technology for CTC detection.

References

1. H. Martin *et al.*, *Anal. Chem.* **82**, 2797 (2010).
2. P. L. Bedard *et al.*, *Nature* **501**, 355 (2013).
3. H. Ledford, *Nature* **464**, 972 (2010).
4. J. Bostrom, *Science* **323**, 1610 (2009).
5. M. G. Vander Heiden, L. C. Cantley and C. B. Thompson, *Science* **324**, 1029 (2009).

6. W. H. Koppenol, P. L. Bounds and C. V. Dang, *Nat. Rev. Cancer* **11**, 325 (2011).
7. S. S. Gambhir, *Nat. Rev. Cancer* **2**, 683 (2002).
8. A. Annibaldi and C. Widmann, *Curr. Opin. Clin. Nutr.* **13**, 466 (2010).
9. B. Chen *et al.*, *Theranostics* **6**, 1887 (2016).
10. X. Han *et al.*, *Nanoscale, 2017*, **9**, 1457 (2016).
11. H. S. Cho, Z. Y. Dong, G. M. Pauletti *et al.*, *ACS Nano* **4**, 5398 (2010).
12. D. L. Shi, H. S. Cho, Y. Chen *et al.*, *Adv Mater.* **21**, 2170 (2009).
13. R. A. Ghossein *et al.*, *J. Clin. Oncol.* **13**, 1195 (1995).
14. M. V. Seiden *et al.*, *J. Clin. Oncol.* **12**, 2634 (1994).

https://doi.org/10.1142/9789819809028_0004

Chapter 4

Therapeutic Delivery of Stromal Cell-Derived Factor-1 for Injury Repair*

Agnes Yeboah

Department of Chemical and Biochemical Engineering,
Rutgers University,
98 Brett Road Piscataway, NJ 08854, USA
agnes.yeboah@rutgers.edu

Martin L. Yarmush

Department of Biomedical Engineering,
Rutgers University,
599 Taylor Road Piscataway, NJ 08854, USA

Center for Engineering in Medicine,
Massachusetts General Hospital and Shriners Burns Hospital,
51 Blossom Street, Boston MA, 02114, USA
yarmush@rci.rutgers.edu

Francois Berthiaume†

Department of Biomedical Engineering,
Rutgers University,
599 Taylor Road Piscataway, NJ 08854, USA
fberthia@rci.rutgers.edu

Stromal cell-derived growth factor-1 (SDF1) is a chemokine that is over-expressed at sites of injury and is believed to play an important role in wound repair. At the cellular level, SDF1 regulates the mobilization and trafficking of endothelial progenitors that originate in the bone marrow and functionally contribute to neovascularization and angiogenesis in the

*To cite this article, please refer to its earlier version published in the *Nano LIFE*, Vol. 6, No. 1 (2016) 1530001 (11 pages), DOI: 10.1142/S1793984415300010
†Corresponding author.

wound. Consequently, SDF1 is a potentially interesting therapeutic with the potential to enhance these processes in acute and chronic injuries that otherwise tend to heal poorly, such as spinal cord injury, stroke, myocardial infarction, diabetic skin wounds and acute burns. However, the therapeutic usefulness of SDF1, as many other similar peptide-based growth factors and chemokines, is severely limited due to its short *in vivo* half-life, as it is rapidly degraded by proteases, which are typically very abundant at the wound site. Several studies have reported methodologies to increase SDF1 *in vivo* stability by mutating the protease cleavage sites of the molecule. Another approach has been to incorporate the chemokine into biomaterials that shield it from degradation. Yet another approach would be to develop a system that is inherently stable and could be combined with these aforementioned strategies. For example, self-assembled nanoparticles could shield SDF1 (or one of its forms engineered to be more resistant to proteolysis) from proteolysis and then be incorporated into suitable biomaterials. Nanotechnology-based delivery systems have however been used to a very limited extent for SDF1. This paper aims to provide a summary of the various stabilization and delivery methods available for SDF1, some of which have been already used, as well as others that have been used with other bioactive peptides, but would be potentially applicable to SDF1.

Keywords: Stromal cell-derived factor-1; nanotechnology; proteases; wound healing.

1. Introduction

Stromal cell-derived growth factor-1 (SDF1) is a chemokine encoded by the CXCL12 gene and is so far known to exist in six different isoforms, SDF1α to ϕ, by alternate splicing of the same gene.[1] SDF1α, shown in Fig. 1, is the predominant isoform found in all tissues. It consists of 89 amino acids. The first 21 amino acids make up the signal peptide, while the mature protein spans Lysine 22 to Lysine 89. SDF1α comprised a three β-strands, an α-helix and is bordered by disordered N and C-terminal ends. It is believed that the N-terminus (residues one to nine) is responsible for SDF1's binding to its receptors.[2] Other isoforms of SDF1 share the same N-terminal amino acid sequence, but have different C-termini.

As shown in Table 1, SDF1α has a net positive charge which is attributed to its numerous basic amino acids. It has a molecular weight of about ten kilodaltons.

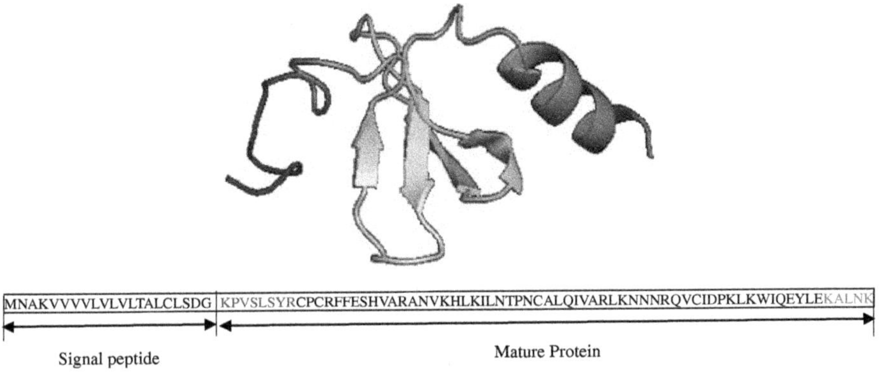

Fig. 1. Image of SDF1α by Ryu *et al.*[3] (RSCB Protein Data Bank ID: 2J7Z). SDF1α monomer was obtained using Pymol. N-terminus is colored in blue and C-terminus colored in red.

Table 1. General properties of SDF1α (obtained using the ExPASy Server[4]).

Molecular Formula	$C_{453}H_{753}N_{129}O_{119}S_6$
Molecular weight/size	~10 kilodaltons
Total number of negatively charged residues (Asp + Glu)	5
Total number of positively charged residues (Arg + Lys)	14
Net charge on protein	Positive (+9)
Theoretical isoelectric point	9.72
Theoretical extinction coefficient	$8730\,M^{-1}\,cm^{-1}$

There are at least two known receptors for SDF1, C-X-C chemokine receptor type four (CXCR4) and type seven (CXCR7).[5] The binding of SDF1 to CXCR4 results in intracellular signaling via guanine nucleotide-binding proteins (G-proteins), which triggers the activation of the MAPK, PI3K and IP3 pathways, as well as intracellular calcium release, resulting in increases in target cell survival, proliferation and chemotaxis.[6] CXCR4 is expressed by several cell types, such as hematopoietic stem cells, endothelial and epithelial cells,[7] as well as cells in the immune and central nervous systems.[8]

SDF1 was originally identified as the factor that promotes the retention of hematopoietic stem cells in the bone marrow.[9] One of the first therapeutic interventions targeting the SDF1 pathway involved blocking SDF1 binding to its receptor to induce the release of bone marrow stem cells, thus increasing their numbers in the circulation. The blood enriched in stem cells could then be used for bone marrow transplantation procedures.[10] SDF1, as other angiogenic factors, is also known to perpetuate cancer tumor growth and progression; therefore, several studies have also evaluated the benefit of blocking this pathway as a potential cancer therapy.[7] Through its binding to CXCR4, SDF1 may also be an endogenous inhibitor of CXCR4-trophic HIV-1 strains.[11]

SDF1 is also known to be implicated in the endogenous response to tissue damage and subsequent tissue repair. For example, SDF1 may be expressed in the local injury area to promote the recruitment of stem cells from the bone marrow to injured tissues/organs.[12] It is believed that SDF1, upon entering the bone marrow environment, induces the release of soluble kit-ligand (sKitL), which induces the release of more SDF1, enhancing mobilization of the CXCR4+ and c-Kit+ cells to the circulation.[13] Once the progenitor cells reach the injury site, it is thought that they participate in the regeneration of damaged blood vessels. Thus, exogenous SDF1 has been explored as a therapeutic molecule to enhance these processes in several acute and chronic injury types that otherwise tend to heal poorly, such as injuries related to the central nervous system, including spinal cord,[14,15] multiple sclerosis,[16] stroke[17] and myocardial infarction.[18–20] It is also being explored for treatment of chronic skin wounds[12,21] and acute burn wounds.[22]

A major limitation in the use of SDF1 as a therapeutic molecule, like many other similar peptides, is its short *in vivo* half-life due to rapid degradation by proteases. Providing a sustained supply of SDF1 in the first two to three weeks of injury healing (proliferative phase) would be clinically beneficial.

Different strategies are being explored to increase the stability of SDF1 *in vivo* in the context of different injury types and disease situations. Some researchers have focused attention on designing derivatives of SDF1 with increased *in vivo* stability.[19,23–27] Other researchers have explored incorporating SDF1 into biomaterials, such as hydrogels and scaffolds in order to prolong its release profile and protect it from degradation. Nanoparticle-based delivery is especially advantageous because the delivery system can be administered in a variety of ways and can be easily incorporated into biomaterials that are already used to enhance tissue repair.

Therefore, here we review the various stabilization and delivery methods available for SDF1, some of which have been already used, as well as others that have been used with other bioactive peptides, but would be potentially applicable to SDF1.

2. Challenges with delivering SDF1

SDF1 has a short half-life *in vivo* as it is readily degraded by multiple proteases, including dipeptidyl peptidase IV, a serine exopeptidase, matrix metalloproteinases,[28,29] cathepsin G[30] and neutrophil elastase,[31] which are activated at the sites of injury and typically attack the chemokine at the N-terminus. Cleavage of the N-terminus of SDF1 results in a loss of binding to its receptor CXCR4 and as such a loss of its chemoattractant activity.

In addition to potential N-terminus cleavage, SDF1α can also be cleaved at the C-terminus by carboxypeptidase N (CPN), which also results in attenuated chemoattractant activity.[32,33] The *in vivo* half-life of SDF1α is known to be about 25.8 min.[34] Due to the presence of additional exons on the C-terminus, the other isoforms of SDF1 are not susceptible to proteolysis by CPN.

Since exogenous recombinant SDF1 is susceptible to the same proteolytic mechanisms as the endogenous one, in the absence of any engineered delivery system, high and repeated doses of the peptide may be needed for therapeutic activity. For example, in studying the effect of SDF1α on model wounds in mice, Sarkar *et al.*[35] demonstrated that a repeated dosing regimen of four daily applications of 1 μg SDF1α was needed to allow for faster reepithelialization of an excisional wound made on wild-type mice.

Repeated application of SDF1 is costly and impractical. Thus, protein engineering technologies and delivery methods that will allow for a stabilization of the growth factor *in vivo* are essential. Below, we first discuss some of the protein engineering approaches being used to alter the structure of the peptide itself and then the delivery systems used to protect the peptide (either native or modified) to allow sustained delivery *in vivo*.

3. Stabilization of SDF1 using protein engineering

3.1. *Fusion proteins and derivatives of SDF1 with longer half-lives*

One way to increase the stability of SDF1 is to construct a fusion protein comprised of the SDF1 gene juxtaposed to another protein or peptide at either the N- or C-terminus (for SDF1α only). As shown in Fig. 2, both the terminal ends of SDF1α are susceptible to degradation. Since the N-terminus is involved in binding to the CXCR4 receptor, fusions are typically made at the C-terminus. "Capping" the C-terminus of SDF1α with a peptide or protein should

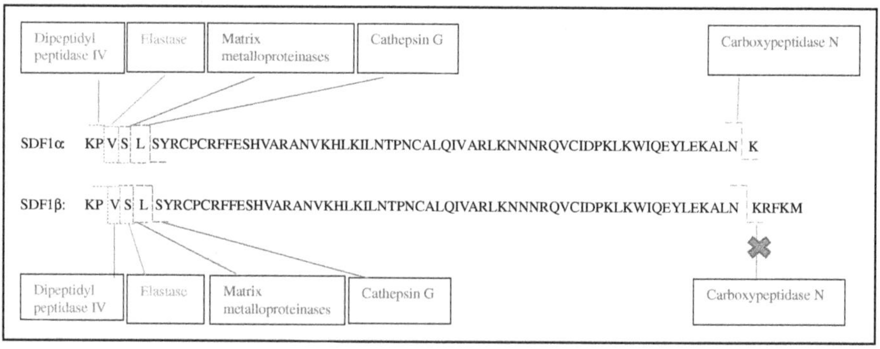

Fig. 2. SDF1α and SDF1β degradation by different proteases. Dipeptidyl peptidase IV cleaves off Lys22 and Pro23 (KP); elastase cleaves off Lys22, Pro23 and Val24 (KPV); matrix metalloproteinases cleave off Lys22, Pro23, Val 24, Serine 25 (KPVS); cathepsin G cleaves off Lys22, Pro23, Val24, Ser25, Leu26 (KPVSL). Carboxypeptidase N cleaves off the lysine at the C-terminus of SDF1α. Due to the presence of an additional exon at the C-terminus, SDF1β is not subjected to degradation by carboxypeptidase N.

help reduce its degradation. For example, SDF1β, which only differs from SDF1α by having a fourth exon at the C-terminus, has a longer half-life *in vivo* and as a result is known to be twice as potent.[1]

Ziegler *et al.*[19] explored this concept with their design of a bispecific SDF1-GPVI fusion protein, consisting of SDF1α and the platelet collagen receptor GPVI. GPVI was fused to the C-terminus of SDF1α (SDF1α-GPVI), as well as the N-terminus of SDF1α (GPVI-SDF1α). This work was done on the assumption that the binding of GPVI to the collagen triple helix in the sub-endothelial matrix would allow for an increased concentration of SDF1 at the site of injury (in this case, injured myocardium), allowing for SDF1α to be persist longer and recruit bone marrow cells to the damaged area, thus resulting in a better healing process. As expected, the activity of GPVI-SDF1α was greatly diminished, while SDF1α-GPVI fusion protein showed a higher binding activity to the CXCR4 receptor, triggered chemotaxis, increased cell survival and enhanced endothelial differentiation. *In vivo*, SDF1α-GPV1, which was injected intravenously, allowed for the recruitment of significantly more bone marrow cells after tissue damage, as compared with recombinant SDF1α.

Other researchers have designed derivatives of SDF1 with "minor" mutations to the N-terminus region in an attempt to change recognizable cleavage sequences for the proteases, while trying to maintain the integrity of the binding region of the chemokine.

Segers *et al.*[23] developed a new version of SDF1α consisting of a modification to the N-terminus region to reduce susceptibility to common proteases (matrix metalloproteinase-2 and dipeptyl peptidase IV). As opposed to SDF1α, whose N-terminus region comprised KPVSLSYR, S-SDF1α(S4V) has a few modifications shown in red: SKPVVLSYR. An additional serine was added in front of the N-terminal lysine, while the serine in the fourth position was changed to valine as shown in Fig. 3.

The team noted that the S-SDF1(S4V) variant of SDF1 was bioactive but resistant to cleavage by DPPIV and MMPs, as compared to native SDF1. S-SDF1(S4V), the protease-resistant variant of SDF1, was then fused at the C-terminus to RAD16-II (RAD), which has the sequence RARADADARARADADA and

N-terminus region of native SDF1α:	KPVSLSYR
S-SDF1:	SKPVSLSYR
S-SDF1 (S4V):	SKPVVLSYR

Fig. 3. Amino acid modifications made to SDF1 by Segars *et al.*[23]

N-terminus region of native SDF1α:	KPVSLSYR
V-(S4V)-SDF1α:	VKPVVLSYR
AAV-(S4V)-SDF1α:	AAVKPVVLSYR

Fig. 4. Amino acid modifications made to SDF1 by Baumann *et al.*[24]

N-terminus region of native SDF1β:	KPVSLSYR
Methionine-SDF1β:	MKPVSLSYR

Fig. 5. Amino acid modifications made to SDF1 by Yang *et al.*[25]

self-assembles into nanofibers. S-SDF-1(S4V) improved cardiac function after myocardial infarction when it was tethered to the self-assembling peptide RAD for controlled delivery.[23]

Similarly, Baumann *et al.*[24] engineered another derivative of SDF1α (AAV-[S4V]-SDF1α) to have a better stability than recombinant SDF1α. As shown in Fig. 4, two alanines and one valine were inserted in front of the N-terminal lysine and the 4th serine was changed to a valine, similar to the approach taken by Segers *et al.* These changes prevented the degradation of the engineered SDF1α derivative by DPPIV and MMP. The engineered protein was delivered using starPEG heparin hydrogels. The hydrogel delivery results are discussed in Sec. 3.2.2.

Likewise, Yang *et al.*[25] demonstrated that inserting a methionine in front of the N-terminal lysine (Lysine 23) of SDF1β as shown in Fig. 5, enhanced its functional activity compared to native SDF1β. While they acknowledged that the modification resulted in a slightly lower affinity of the chemokine to its receptor, they highlighted that the Met-SDF1β induced a significantly higher intracellular calcium flux indicating a much higher bioactivity as compared to native SDF1β. Similar to other researchers, Yang *et al.* explained that placing a methionine in front of

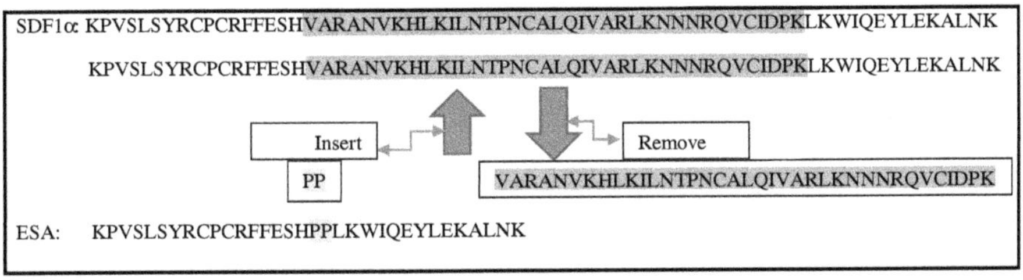

Fig. 6. Amino acid modifications made to SDF1 by Hiesinger *et al.* ESA is a derivative of SDF1 without the large central β sheets of SDF1 but instead two proline residues which connect the N-terminus to the C-terminus.[26,27]

Lysine 23 perturbed the action of DPPIV, allowing the growth factor to be more stable and more bioactive.

In another effort to stabilize SDF1α when used *in vivo*, Hiesinger *et al.*[26,27] engineered an SDF1α polypeptide analog named ESA [Fig. 6], with comparably better activity than recombinant SDF1α. Computational molecular modeling and design was used to cleave off the large central β sheets of SDF1α, replacing them with proline residues, to connect the N-terminus responsible for receptor binding with the C-terminus, so that ESA would have a similar conformation as native SDF1α.

ESA was able to induce EPC migration and improve ventricular performance as compared to the recombinant SDF1α used as a control. The team believes that compared to native SDF1α, the relatively small size of ESA provides enhanced stability and function, allows for easier and cheaper synthesis and perhaps more importantly enhances the diffusion potential and the speed at which the chemotactic signal is deployed.[26]

3.2. *Stabilization of SDF1 using various delivery mechanisms*

3.2.1. *Gene therapy*

Using viral or nonviral constructs encoding for the SDF1 gene can result in an overexpression of SDF1 allowing for a longer protein presence at the injury site.

To this end, Badillo *et al.*[36] made full thickness excisional wounds on diabetic mice and treated them with lentiviral construct containing SDF1 gene fused to green fluorescent protein (GFP) to induce the over-expression of SDF1 in wounds. The viral plasmid with GFP alone was used as a control. The production of SDF1 by transduced cells was confirmed by measuring the total wound mRNA isolated from wounds treated with the SDF1-GFP lentiviral plasmid or the control alone. The research team confirmed that the lentiviral SDF1 treated wound showed an increased production of SDF1 mRNA seven days post injection of the viral plasmid in the wound area. This corresponded to a decrease in wound surface area and an increased granulation tissue seven days post wounding.

Similarly, Sundararaman *et al.*[37] injected different luciferase plasmid DNA (nonviral) encoding human SDF1 into rat heart one month after myocardial infarction. Expression of the gene ranged from five to 32 days. Heart function and immunohistochemistry of the heart tissue was assessed after plasmid injection. Increase in cardiac function was noted four weeks after injection, attributed to increase in blood vessel density. The degree of functional improvement positively correlated with level of vector expression.

3.2.2. *Biomaterials*

Biomaterials have been used for the controlled release, for the prolongation of half-life and enhancement of the therapeutic efficacy of bioactive molecules, including growth factors. Biomaterials have been used to deliver growth factors in a matrix-bound manner as the biomaterial surface allows for the growth factor to be concentrated and delivered locally.[38]

Biomaterials such as alginate scaffolds and hydrogels, degradable poly(lactide ethylene oxide fumarate) (PLEOF) hydrogels, poly(L-lysine) and hyaluronan and starPEG-heparin hydrogels have been used to deliver SDF1.

Rabbany *et al.*[21] and Henderson *et al.*[39] demonstrated the sustained release of SDF1 from alginate hydrogels for wound healing. Rabbany *et al.* loaded alginate hydrogel patches with recombinant human

SDF1 proteins and monitored the *in vitro* and *in vivo* release profile. The hydrogels released about 50% of the protein within the first day and minimally released the rest of the protein over the remaining five days of monitoring period. Wounds treated with SDF1 protein delivered in the hydrogel patch healed faster and showed a significantly faster wound closure as compared to nontreated wounds.

Henderson *et al.* also monitored the release of the SDF1 chemokine from an alginate hydrogel scaffold which was applied directly unto a wound bed made on the dorsum of wild-type mice. The scaffold was designed to allow for a slow release of the growth factor over 18–24 h. The team showed that the SDF1 treated wounds closed rapidly in one to three days after application to the wound bed and much less between three to seven days as compared to the saline control potentially because the SDF1 had been depleted from the scaffold by day three.

In addition to alginate hydrogels, degradable PLEOF hydrogels, poly(L-lysine) and hyaluronan and starPEG-heparin hydrogels have been used to deliver SDF1 in a controlled manner.

He *et al.*[40] developed a macromer made of PLEOF that was cross-linked with different initiators to produce biodegradable hydrogels. Three different hydrogels with different levels of hydrophobicity were evaluated for their SDF1 release profile and its effect on the migration of bone marrow stem cells. The team noted that the hydrogels that were designed to be more hydrophilic had an initial burst release of SDF1 followed by a period of controlled delivery for 21 days. The hydrophobic hydrogels had a less pronounced burst release and displayed a slow but constant release between days one to nine, followed by a fast release from days nine to 18. The migration of bone marrow stem cells closely followed the SDF1 release kinetics out of the hydrogels. That is, the more hydrophilic hydrogels had a higher extent of cell migration initially but finished with the lowest extent of cell migration, while the more hydrophobic hydrogels had a lower extent of initial cell migration but finished off with the highest extent of cell migration.

Dalonneau *et al.*[38] loaded SDF1 into polyelectrolyte multilayer films which was made of poly(L-lysine) and hyaluronan (PLL/HA), to allow for the growth factor to be delivered in a matrix bound manner to myoblast cells. The PLL/HA films exhibited an initial burst release during the first hour, after which the growth factor release was steady. The matrix bound SDF1 enhanced myoblast spreading and considerably promoted cell migration.

Prokoph *et al.*[41] and Baumann *et al.*[24] demonstrated the delivery of SDF1 and its derivative, AAV-[S4V]-SDF-1 (discussed above) using a starPEG-heparin hydrogels. The release profile of native SDF1 from the starPEG hydrogel was highly similar to that of the SDF1 derivative. Both of them were released at a high level (high initial burst) initially, followed by a sustained release. However, the relative migration of endothelial progenitor cells (EPCs) was significantly higher using the engineered derivative of SDF1 delivered via the hydrogel compared with the native SDF1.

4. Overall limitations with existing strategies for therapeutic SDF1 use

While the above strategies and delivery options address some of the challenges in using SDF1 therapeutically, some overall limitations still exist, as highlighted below.

Fusion proteins and derivatives of SDF1 with longer half-lives

- Potential for decrease or loss of activity of growth factor.
- High cost for producing and purifying material.

Gene therapy

- Toxicity and immunogenicity of some of the vectors used were not well understood.
- Concerns about the potential random integration of viral genes into host genome.
- Possibility of sustained transgene expression, which could have detrimental (e.g., cancer-causing) effects.
- Low transfection efficiency of some of the vectors, resulting in low levels of gene expression.

Biomaterials

- High initial burst release from some hydrogels/scaffolds.
- High amount of SDF1 needed for loading into hydrogels due to low loading efficiency of some hydrogels.
- Total fraction of SDF1 released from hydrogels over a period of time relatively low compared to how much was loaded.
- Material of construction for some hydrogels could result in unwanted byproducts when degraded.

5. The ideal delivery system for SDF1

The "perfect" delivery system for therapeutic SDF1 use would therefore be one that encompasses all or a majority of the following characteristics:

- Gradually release SDF1 for about two to three weeks (that is, throughout the proliferative phase of healing after an injury.
- Protect SDF1 from degradation.
- Have minimal to no impact on the bioactivity of the chemokine.
- Can be manufactured less expensively, thus reducing the overall cost of the therapy.
- Allow the right dose of the growth factor to be delivered (typically in the nanogram range).
- Should not be toxic, nonimmunogenic and biocompatible.
- Allow for the growth factor to be readily assessable to its receptor (easy bioavailability).

6. Future perspectives

6.1. *Nanoparticle technologies for SDF1*

A more versatile delivery system would make it easier to translate SDF1-based therapies into reality. Nanoparticles seem to be a viable option to address the shortcomings of the other delivery strategies described above and also encompasses several of the desired characteristics of the ideal delivery system.

The use of nanoparticles to deliver SDF1 offers several advantages. First, formulating SDF1 into nanoparticles will allow the chemokine to be delivered in the same size range as proteins and other macromolecular structures found inside living cells. This is expected to result in improved bioavailability and rapid therapeutic action. Second, it is believed that highly efficient drug delivery system based on nanomaterials could potentially reduce the drug dose needed to achieve therapeutic benefit, which, in turn, would lower the cost and/or reduce the side effects associated with particular drugs. In addition, drugs delivered as nanoparticles have been shown to have prolonged circulation time *in vivo*.[42]

Formulating SDF1 as nanoparticles could allow the growth factor not only to be injected as a suspension but also incorporated as appropriate to topical creams or into existing skin substitutes which have pores in the 10–100 μm range.

Lim *et al.*,[43] Huang *et al.*[44] and Yin *et al.*[45] all incorporated SDF1 into chitosan/chitosan-based nanoparticles. Lim *et al.* noted that their nanoparticle released about 8% of the SDF1 over a period of seven days implying that the delivery system would be suitable for sustained release of the growth factor. The SDF1 enclosed in the nanoparticle delivery system allowed for chemotactic recruitment of adult neuronal progenitor cells (aNPC) by three- to 45-fold relative to hydrogels that lacked SDF1. Similarly, Huang *et al.*[44] highlighted that their chitosan-based nanoparticles protected SDF1 against proteolysis and allowed for a sustained control release up to seven days. Up to 23 ng/ml of SDF1 was released, which retained mitogenic activity, enhanced the migration of mesenchymal stem cells and promoted PI3K expression. Yin *et al.*[45] delivered SDF1 as 700 nm particles in order for the growth factor to reach the alveolus/alveolar duct which is reported to be 25–100 μm in diameter. The incorporated SDF1 in the nanoparticles was slowly released (3% was released over seven days) and was able to cause full chemotactic activity and receptor activation as compared to the native free SDF1. When aerosolized in the lungs, the SDF1 nanoparticles showed a greater retention time than that of free SDF1.

Olekson *et al.*[46] demonstrated the delivery of SDF1 using liposome nanoparticles. Liposome nanoparticles were used to extend the half-life of the growth factor by serving as a local reserve of the chemokine.

The SDF1α lipid nanoparticles were tested for chemotactic activity using HL60 cells (HL60 cells express the CXCR4 receptor). The nanoparticles exhibited similar functional response as free SDF1. When used on an excisional wound created on diabetic mouse, the SDF1 liposomes increased the fractional area of closed tissue by about 15% as compared to free SDF1. This was attributed to the persistence of the SDF1 nanoparticles at the wound area.

6.2. *Nanoparticle technologies for other growth factors*

Thus, despite the potential benefits, few nanotechnology-based delivery approaches have been implemented for SDF1. On the other hand, when considering other growth factors and chemokines, several different nanosystems are potentially available that would exhibit the desirable characteristics for delivering SDF1, some of which are discussed below.

6.2.1. *Release kinetics and protection from degradation*

As shown in Table 2, nanoparticles made of materials, such as silica, elastin and lipids have been successfully designed and used to deliver different types of growth factors. The nanoparticles were only slowly degraded *in vivo*, thus enabling the release of growth factors over an extended period of time. For example, the porous silica nanoparticles designed by Zhang *et al.*[47] allowed for basic fibroblast growth factor (bFGF) to be released for at least three weeks. Similarly, the heparin and ε-poly-L-lysine (PL) nanoparticles designed by LuZhong *et al.*[48] for delivery of nerve growth factor (NGF) and bFGF had a sustained and slow release profile; 43% of bFGF and 60% of NGF were released from the particles within 20 days of use in treatment of peripheral nerve injury.

6.2.2. *Biocompatibility*

All the nanoparticle systems described in Table 2 were designed for eventual use *in vivo*. For example, multiple studies have shown that elastin-like peptide (ELP) used to deliver keratinocyte growth factor

Table 2. Examples of nanoparticles which have been used for other growth factors.

Growth Factor	Disease area/ Application	Type of Nanoparticle Used/Authors	Reasons for Using Nanoparticle Approach
bFGF	Wound healing	Porous silica nanoparticles Zhang *et al.*[47]	Porous silica nanoparticles were used to achieve a prolonged release of bFGF for at least three weeks.
KGF	Wound healing	ELP nanoparticles Koria *et al.*[49]	Designed nanoparticles comprised the fusion of KGF to ELPs which allowed for topical administration of the growth factor to the wound area and also improved the growth factor's bioavailability to the injury site.
NGF and bFGF	Axonal regeneration	Polymeric nanoparticle delivery system composed of heparin and PL	Nanoparticles were prepared for controlled and slow release of NGF and bFGF for the treatment of peripheral nerve injury.
		LuZhong *et al.*[48]	A sustained and no initial burst *in vitro* release profile of growth factors (NGF and bFGF) from the particles was observed.
			For the bFGF, about 43% of the loaded growth factor was released from particles within 20 days. For NGF, about 60% of the loaded growth factor was released from particles within 20 days for the NGF.

Table 2. (*Continued*)

Growth Factor	Disease area/ Application	Type of Nanoparticle Used/Authors	Reasons for Using Nanoparticle Approach
EGF	Wound healing	Lipid nanoparticles Gainza *et al.*[51]	Lipid nanoparticles were used to allow for topical and sustained delivery of recombinant human EGF to chronic wounds.
bFGF	Alzheimer's	Lectins modified PEG-PLGA nanoparticles Zhang *et al.*[56]	The lectin modified PEG-PLGA nanoparticles were used to deliver bFGF to the central nervous system via intranasal administration for treatment of Alzheimer's disease. The growth factor was formulated into nanoparticles to protect it from being degraded within the lumen of the nasal cavity or during passage across the epithelial barrier. The nanoparticle conjugation with lectin allowed for selective binding to N-acetyl glucosamine on the nasal epithelial membrane for its brain delivery.

(KGF)[49] are nonimmunogenic, nonpyrogenic and are biologically compatible.[50] Likewise, the lipid nanoparticles used to deliver epidermal growth factor (EGF) are biodegradable and no adverse reactions were reported by Gainza *et al.*[51] when the nanoparticles were used on mice. Zhang *et al.*[47] demonstrated that the porous silica nanoparticles used to deliver bFGF were not cytoxic. Some studies have described the use of porous silica nanoparticles *in vivo* and reported no adverse events.[52] One concern with the porous silica system, however, is that it is not biodegradable and therefore further *in vitro* and *in vivo* biocompatibility studies may need to be performed if it is to be used in a clinical setting.

6.2.3. *Ease of manufacturing*

Eventual translation of the nanoparticle-based delivery system to the clinic will require large-scale production. For example, the polyethylene glycol-polyactide-polyglycolide (PEG-PLGA) nanoparticles used to deliver bFGF for Alzheimer's treatment are well-established nanocarriers for nanomedicine applications and are relatively simple to manufacture.[53] It is noteworthy that all of the systems described above require the bioactive peptide to be produced on a large scale using traditional methods for expressing and purifying the product. The bioactive peptide-ELP approach has the unique feature that, while the methods to express the fusion protein in bacterial production systems are not fundamentally different from any other peptide, purification can be accomplished through repeated temperature cycles to precipitate the final product by centrifugation, thus avoiding the use of expensive chromatography-based methods.[54] The main challenge in using ELP fusion proteins is that care must be taken to preserve biological activity of the bioactive peptide and as suggested by Hassouneh *et al.*,[55] the specific properties of the bioactive peptide (in this case, the size and charge of SDF1) can be factored into the design of the ELP chain length, and sequence, as well as the type and length of the linker used for the fusion protein, so that aggregation temperature is in a desirable range (usually between 30°C and 40°C).

Acknowledgments

This work was partially supported by the Shriners Hospitals for Children. Agnes Yeboah was supported by a National Institute of Health-funded biotechnology training fellowship and a Schlumberger Faculty for the Future fellowship.

References

1. M. Janowski, *Cell Adh. Migr.* **3**, 243 (2009).
2. P. Loetscher, J. H. Gong, B. Dewald, M. Baggiolini and I. Clark-Lewis, *J. Biol. Chem.* **273**, 22279 (1998).
3. E. K. Ryu, T. G. Kim, T. H. Kwon, I. D. Jung, D. Ryu, Y. M. Park, J. Kim, K. H. Ahn and C. Ban, *Proteins* **67**, 1193 (2007).
4. E. Gasteiger, C. Hoogland, A. Gattiker, S. Duvaud, M. R. Wilkins, R. D. Appel and A. Bairoch, *The Proteomics Protocols Handbook*, ed. J. M. Walker (Humana Press, Totowa, NJ, 2005), pp. 571–607.
5. J. M. Burns, B. C. Summers, Y. Wang, A. Melikian, R. Berahovich, Z. Miao, M. E. T. Penfold, M. J. Sunshine, D. R. Littman, C. J. Kuo, K. Wei, B. E. McMaster, K. Wright, M. C. Howard and T. J. Schall, *J. Exp. Med.* **203**, 2201 (2006).
6. Y. Doring, L. Pawig, C. Weber and H. Noels, *Front. Physiol.* **5**, 212 (2014).
7. B. A. Teicher and S. P. Fricker, *Clin. Cancer Res.* **16**, 2927 (2010).
8. Y. R. Zou, A. H. Kottmann, M. Kuroda, I. Taniuchi and D. R. Littman, *Nature* **393**, 595 (1998).
9. M. Z. Ratajczak, C. H. KIm, A. Abdel-Latif, G. Schneider, M. Kucia, A. J. Schneider, M. J. Laughlin and J. Ratajczak, *Leukemia* **26**, 63 (2012).
10. Y. Kang, B. J. Chen, D. DeOliveira, J. Mito and N. J. Chao, *PLoS ONE* **5**, e11316 (2010).
11. E. A. Berger, *Semin. Immunol.* **10**, 165 (1998).
12. X. Xu, F. Zhu, M. Zhang, D. Zeng, D. Luo, G. Liu, W. Cui, S. Wang, W. Guo, W. Xing, H. Liang, L. Li, X. Fu, J. Jiang and H. Huang, *Cells Tissues Organs* **197**, 103 (2013).
13. I. Petit, D. Jin and S. Rafii, *Trends Immunol.* **28**, 299 (2007).
14. A. Jaerve, F. Bosse and H. W. Muller, *Int. J. Biochem. Cell Biol.* **44**, 452 (2012).
15. H. Takeuchi, A. Natsume, T. Wakabayashi, C. Aoshima, S. Shimato, M. Ito, J. Ishii, Y. Maeda, M. Hara, S. U. Kim and J. Yoshida, *Neurosci. Lett.* **426**, 69 (2007).
16. K. S. Carbajal, C. Schaumburg, R. Strieter and T. E. Lane, *Pub. of Nat. Acad. Sci.* **107**, 11068 (2010).
17. S. Woei-Cherng, L. D. David, L. Shinn-Zong, L. Wen-Wen, S. Ching-Yuan, C. Ying-Chen, W. Hsiao-Jung, W. Hsing-Won, T. Chang-Hai and L. Hung, *J. Clin. Invest.* **118**, 2482 (2008).
18. M. Penn, *Circ. Res.* **104**, 1133 (2009).
19. M. Ziegler, M. Elvers, Y. Baumer, C. Leder, C. Ochmann, T. J. Schonberger, T. Geisler, B. Schlosshauer, O. Lunov, S. Engelhardt, T. Simmet and M. Gawaz, *Circulation* **125**, 685 (2012).
20. S. K. Ghadge, S. Muhlstedt, C. Ozcelik and M. Bader, *Pharmacol. Therapeut.* **129**, 97 (2011).
21. S. Rabbany, J. Pastore, M. Yamamoto, T. Miller, S. Rafii, R. Aras and M. Penn, *Cell Transplant.* **19**, 399 (2010).
22. J. Ding, K. Hori, R. Zhang, Y. Marcoux, D. Honardoust, H. A. Shankowsky and E. E. Tredget, *Wound Repair Regen.* **19**, 568 (2011).

23. V. F. M. Segers, T. Tokunou, L. J. Higgins, C. MacGillivray, J. Gannon and R. T. Lee, *Circulation* **116**, 1683 (2007).
24. L. Baumann, S. Prokoph, C. Gabriel, U. Freudenberg, C. Werner and A. G. Beck-Sickinger, *J. Control. Release* **162**, 68 (2012).
25. O. O. Yang, S. Swanberg, L. Z. Lu, M. Dziejman, J. McCoy, A. D. Luster, B. D. Walker and S. H. Hermann, *J. Virol.* **73**, 4582 (1999).
26. W. Hiesinger, A. Goldstone and J. Woo, *Trends Cardiovasc. Med.* **22**, 139 (2012).
27. W. Hiesinger, J. M. Perez-Aguilar, P. Atluri, N. Marotta, J. Frederick, J. R. Fitzpatrick III, R. C. McCormick, J. R. Muenzer, E. C. Yang, R. D. Levit, L.-J. Yuan, J. W. MacArthur, J. G. Saven and Y. J. Woo, *Circulation* **124**, S18 (2011).
28. C. Durinx, A. M. Lambeir, E. Bosmans, J. B. Falmagne, R. Berghmans, A. Haemers, S. Scharpe and I. De Meester, *Eur. J. Biochem.* **267**, 5608 (2000).
29. G. A. McQuibban, G. Butler, J.-H. Gong, L. Bendall, C. Power, I. Clark-Lewis and C. Overall, *J. Biol. Chem.* **276**, 43503 (2001).
30. M. B. Delgado, I. Clark-Lewis, P. Loetscher, H. Langen, M. Thelen, M. Baggiolini and M. Wolf, *Eur. J. Immunol.* **31**, 699 (2001).
31. A. Valenzuela-Fernández, T. Planchenault, F. Baleux, I. Staropoli, K. Le-Barillec, D. Leduc, T. Delaunay, F. Lazarini, J. Virelizier, M. Chignard, D. Pidard and F. Arenzana-Seisdedos, *J. Biol. Chem.* **277**, 15677 (2002).
32. D. A. Davis, K. E. Singer, M. De La Luz Sierra, M. Narazaki, F. Yang, H. M. Fales, R. Yarchoan and G. Tosato, *Blood* **105**, 4561 (2005).
33. L. Marquez-Curtis, A. Jalili, K. Deiteren, N. Shirvaikar, A.-M. Lambeir and A. Janowska-Wieczorek, *Stem Cells* **26**, 1211 (2008).
34. P. Misra, D. Lebeche, H. Ly, M. Schwarzkopf, G. Diaz, R. Hajjar, A. Schecter and J. Frangioni, *J. Nucl. Med.* **49**, 963 (2008).
35. A. Sarkar, S. Tatildede, S. S. Scherer, D. P. Orgill and F. Berthiaume, *Wound Repair Regen.* **19**, 71 (2011).
36. A. T. Badillo, S. Chung, L. Zhang, P. Zoltick and K. Liechty, *J. Surg. Res.* **143**, 35 (2007).
37. S. Sundararaman, T. Miller, J. Pastore, M. Kiedrowski, R. Aras and M. Penn, *Gene Ther.* **18**, 867 (2011).
38. F. Dalonneau, X. Q. Liu, R. Sadir, J. Almodovar, H. C. Mertani, F. Bruckert, C. Albiges-Rizo, M. Weidenhaupt, H. Lortat-Jacob and C. Picart, *Biomaterials* **35**, 4525 (2014).
39. P. W. Henderson, S. P. Singh, D. D. Krijgh, M. Yamamoto, D. C. Rafii, J. J. Sung, S. Rafii, S. Y. Rabbany and J. A. Spector, *Wound Repair Regen.* **19**, 420 (2011).
40. X. He, J. Ma and E. Jabbari, *Int. J. Pharm.* **390**, 107 (2010).
41. S. Prokoph, E. Chavakis, K. R. Levental, A. Zieris, U. Freudenberg, S. Dimmeler and C. Werner, *Biomaterials* **33**, 4792 (2012).
42. R. Gref, Y. Minamitake, M. T. Peracchia, V. Trubetskoy, V. Torchilin and R. Langer, *Science* **263**, 1600 (1994).
43. T. C. Lim, S. Rokkappanavar, W. S. Toh, L.-S. Wang, M. Kurisawa and M. Spector, *FASEB J.* **27**, 1023 (2013).

44. Y.-C. Huang and T.-J. Liu, *Acta Biomater.* **8**, 1048 (2012).
45. T. Yin, A. R. Bader, T. K. Hou, B. A. Maron, D. D. Kao, R. Qian, D. S. Kohane, D. E. Handy, J. Loscalzo and Y.-Y. Zhang, *Biomacromolecules* **14**, 4009 (2013).
46. M. Olekson, R. Faulknor, A. Bandekar, M. Sempkowski, H. Hsia, S. Sofou, A. Schmidt and F. Berthiaume, *Annual Wound Healing Society Meeting*, Orlando, FL (April 23–27, 2014), *Wound Repair and Regen.* **22**, A54 (2014).
47. J. Zhang, L.-M. Postovit, D. Wang, R. B. Gardiner, R. Harris, M. M. Abdul and A. A. Thomas, *Nanoscale Res. Lett.* **4**, 1297 (2009).
48. Z. LuZhong, Z. YouLang, L. GuiCai, Z. YaHong, G. XiaoSong and Y. YuMin, *Sci. China Life Sci.* **57**, 256 (2014).
49. P. Koria, H. Yagi, Y. Kitagawa, Z. Megeed, Y. Nahmias, R. Sheridan and M. L. Yarmush, *Publ. Natl. Acad. Sci.* **108**, 1034 (2011).
50. D. Urry, T. Parker, M. Reid and D. Gowda, *J. Bioact. Compatible Polym.* **6**, 263 (1991).
51. G. Gainza, M. Pastor, J. J. Aguirre, S. Villullas, J. L. Pedraz, R. M. Hernandez and M. Igartua, *J. Control. Release* **185**, 51 (2014).
52. J. M. Rosenholm and C. Sahlgren, *Nanoscale* **2**, 1870 (2010).
53. E. Locatelli and M. C. Franchini, *J. Nanopart. Res.* **14**, 1 (2012).
54. S. MacEwan, W. Hassouneh and A. Chilkoti, *J. Visual Exp.* **88**, e51583 (2014).
55. W. Hassouneh, T. Christensen and A. Chilkoti, *Curr. Protocols Protein Sci.* (2010).
56. C. Zhang, J. Chen, C. Feng, X. Shao, Q. Liu, Q. Zhang, Z. Pang and X. Jiang, *Int. J. Pharm.* **461**, 192 (2014).

https://doi.org/10.1142/9789819809028_0005

Chapter 5

Novel Brain-Derived Neurotrophic Factor Controlled-Release Formulation Promotes Neuroprotection *In Vitro**

Isabel Perez [†], Elisheva Strauss [‡], Shivani Vyas [†],
Rene S. Schloss [†,§] and Martin L. Yarmush [†]

[†]*Biomedical Engineering, Rutgers,*
The State University of New Jersey,
599 Taylor Rd., Piscataway, NJ 08854, USA
[‡]*Cell Biology and Neuroscience, Rutgers,*
The State University of New Jersey,
604 Allison Rd., Piscataway, NJ 08854, USA
[§]*schloss@soe.rutgers.edu*

Traumatic brain injury (TBI) leads to a cascade of primary and secondary neurodegenerative events, often causing lifelong disabilities. Brain-derived neurotrophic factor (BDNF) is a potential therapeutic for functional recovery of neurons. Unfortunately, BDNF is unstable and expensive, making direct infusion impractical. Therefore, we sought to develop a controlled release formulation to deliver BDNF. Our therapeutic construct encapsulates BDNF in poly(lactic-co-glycolic acid) nanoparticles (PLGA NPs), and further encapsulates these NPs in an alginate hydrogel. Encapsulating BDNF within NPs protects and assists in drug delivery, while further encapsulating the BDNF-NPs in alginate enables localization and sustained release. The BDNF-NPs were synthesized and evaluated for size, stability and BDNF release profile. A MATLAB model was developed to determine the approximate quantity of BDNF-NPs needed to evaluate therapeutic efficacy in neurons injured with hydrogen peroxide. We then compared the therapeutic efficacy and BDNF release profile of these BDNF-NPs to our novel alginate/BDNF-NP formulation. We have successfully designed and fabricated a double encapsulation positionally controllable

*To cite this article, please refer to its earlier version published in the *Nano LIFE*, Vol. 14, No. 1 (2024) 2350016 (18 pages), DOI: 10.1142/S1793984423500162
§Corresponding author.

construct that preserves BDNF bioactivity and extends its release. We also demonstrated that very low dosages of BDNF may be equally effective in promoting neuroprotection, thereby potentially reducing therapeutic costs without compromising efficacy. Our novel formulation offers a promising avenue for treating severe TBI and other neurological disorders which would benefit from a long-lasting and positionally controllable neuroprotective treatment. This approach can easily accommodate additional biologics for localized drug delivery with minimal re-formulation.

Keywords: Sustained release; PLGA nanoparticles; alginate; TBI; neuroprotection; BDNF.

1. Introduction

Traumatic Brain Injury (TBI) is a leading cause of morbidity and mortality worldwide and over 5 million patients live with its subsequent cognitive deficits and motor dysfunctions.[1] TBI progresses from an initial mechanical injury, which leads to secondary physiological responses, such as free radical formation, excitotoxicity, ischemia, hypoxia and neuroinflammation, resulting in tissue and cellular degeneration, which limit or prevent functional recovery. Current therapeutic interventions focus on slowing or stopping the progression of secondary injury to promote neuronal regeneration.[1–3] However, to date, there are no FDA approved pharmacological therapies which adequately promote neuroprotection and/or neuroregeneration and, therefore, in severe TBI cases, functional improvement is minimal at best.[2,4]

Given the complexity of TBI and other chronic neuroregenerative disorders, including spinal cord injury (SCI),[5] Parkinson's disease, Alzheimer's disease, amyotrophic lateral sclerosis (ALS), and Huntington's disease,[6] many studies have evaluated a variety of biological and cellular-based therapeutics. Of these, brain-derived neurotrophic factor (BDNF), a critical member of the neurotrophin family, has been identified as a promising treatment option.[7] It is the most abundant neurotrophic factor in the central nervous system (CNS),[8] plays an important role in neuronal survival and differentiation, axonal growth, and neuronal plasticity,[8–10] has been implicated in the reduction of oxidative stress and apoptosis,[11,12] and BDNF levels are reduced in patients with chronic neuroinflammatory diseases.[13] Thus, many investigators have evaluated BDNF as a therapeutic for complex neuroinflammatory diseases.[14] However, this expensive biologic has failed to reach its clinical endpoints due to its instability and short half-life.[9,15] In addition, high BDNF concentrations introduced via direct bolus injection, can reduce its effectiveness significantly, possibly via downregulation of BDNF receptors, or by inducing neuron over-excitability and/or death.[16]

This has led to the development of methods to protect and extend BDNF delivery including the use of genetically modified cells or drug delivery formulations. Notable limitations of cellular therapies include viability, transfection efficiency, migration to other tissues and potential immunogenic responses.[17] Furthermore, the FDA approval process for cell therapies is significantly more difficult. Thus, a more promising alternative would be to use drug delivery vehicles, which would remove the complexity of a cellular component.

Drug delivery vehicles can help achieve controlled release of encapsulated small molecules and biologics and can protect them from rapid metabolism.[18–21] Important considerations for drug carriers include targeting a region of interest and delivering an appropriate dosage. Ideally, a therapeutic would be delivered for an extended period to minimize dosage administrations, which would ultimately lead to improved patient compliance and cost reduction.[22]

Poly-lactic-co-glycolic acid (PLGA), in particular, has been extensively studied for long-lasting delivery of small molecule pharmaceutics, proteins and other macromolecules.[20,23] In fact, peptide-loaded PLGA particles, such as Lupron Depot® and Zoladex® Depot, are commercially available for cancer treatment.[24]

Hydrogels are another commonly used material for drug delivery applications, consisting of a hydrolysable cross-linked polymer network. By adjusting the hydrogel concentration and changing the degree of cross-linking, properties such as their shape, stiffness and degradation can be fine-tuned for different applications.[25,26] Some of the most used naturally derived hydrogels include collagen, alginate and chitosan.[27] Alginate is commonly used in regenerative medicine applications due to its cost-effectiveness, tunable properties, biocompatibility, biodegradability and it can be found in a variety of

FDA approved products.[28] Others have used alginate for the treatment of CNS diseases and disorders since it is nonimmunogenic.[29] Our group has previously utilized alginate to encapsulate cells and localize them to a region of interest, while simultaneously controlling their differentiation and function.[30] In a pre-clinical SCI model, our construct reduced inflammation, without causing adverse effects.[30,31]

Previous studies in our group have shown that alginate encapsulation of bupivacaine (local anesthetic)-loaded PLGA NPs[32] and liposomes[26,33] can successfully control and extend the release of bupivacaine. However, the chemical complexity of biologics such as BDNF, was not previously tested in our double encapsulation construct. This is an important step in expanding our approach to complex neuroinflammatory injury and diseases where positionally controlled, long-term release of functional, but unstable biologics may further therapeutic development. Thus, the current studies were designed to develop a dual delivery system comprised of PLGA NPs and an alginate hydrogel to enable long-lasting controlled release of BDNF. In addition, we evaluated the diffusion profiles in physiologically relevant conditions which would enable better design parameters for both *in vitro* and *in vivo* studies. The studies described here demonstrate that we can formulate alginate/BDNF-NPs which can be positionally controlled, enabling longer release profiles of bioactive BDNF. Unlike other delivery approaches, our formulation can be easily modified to include not only unmodified complex biologics, but a variety of cellular and molecular therapies in concert, offering another approach to treating complex neuro-inflammatory injuries and diseases.

2. Materials and methods

All cell culture reagents were purchased from Gibco™ unless otherwise stated. All chemicals were purchased from Sigma Aldrich unless otherwise stated.

2.1. *Nanoparticle formulation*

Poly(lactic-co-glycolic acid) (PLGA) nanoparticles loaded with BDNF (BDNF-NPs) were synthesized using a modified double emulsion technique.[18] Briefly, PLGA was dissolved in dichloromethane (DCM) followed by the addition of an aqueous solution containing BDNF (R&D Systems) and bovine serum albumin (BSA) at a ratio 1:50. Prior to emulsification, the concentrations of BDNF, BSA and PLGA were 25 μg/mL (or 100 μg/mL), 5 mg/mL (or 1.25 mg/mL), and 250 mg/mL, respectively. The initial use of 25 μg/mL BDNF was based on the manufacturer's recommendation for reconstitution of lyophilized powder.[34] The 100 μg/mL BDNF was employed to increase the amount of encapsulated BDNF in NPs. The ratios of BSA and PLGA were based on previous studies.[18,19] The solution was placed on ice and emulsified using a digital sonifier for 5 s on and 30 s off for four cycles (SFX150 Sonifier®, Branson Ultrasonics). This emulsion was added dropwise to 1% (w/v) polyvinyl alcohol (PVA) and sonicated again for 5 s on and 30 s off for four cycles. The double-emulsified solution was then added dropwise to a solution of 0.1% (w/v) PVA and placed on a rotary evaporator for 2 h at 45°C and constant rotation of 150 RPM (Rotavapor® R-300, BÜCHI). The synthesized particles were then centrifuged for 10 min at $15,000 \times g$, followed by solution aspiration to leave behind pellet of NPs. Lastly, the particles were resuspended in a 2% (w/v) sucrose solution, lyophilized for 48 h, and subsequently stored at −80°C for future analysis and studies. Control NPs (i.e., empty or BSA only) were synthesized using the same concentrations minus the addition of BDNF. Additionally, NPs containing rhodamine B, a fluorescent dye, were also synthesized for visual confirmation of molecule encapsulation. For NPs containing rhodamine B, an aqueous solution with 0.1 mg/mL rhodamine B was used. For albumin NPs used for preliminary release studies, human albumin was used for a final concentration of 1 mg/mL.

2.2. *Alginate and cross-linking formulation*

Alginate was prepared as previously described by Maguire *et al.*[35] Briefly, a 2.2% (w/v) alginate solution was prepared by slowly mixing 0.132 g of alginic acid sodium salt with 6.0 mL of DMEM (high glucose, no glutamine, no calcium — Life Technologies) at 60°C.

To ensure homogenous mixing, the solution was stirred for approximately 3 h under heat. A calcium crosslinking solution was prepared by combining 5.549 g $CaCl_2$ (Fisher Scientific ACROS Organics), 1.0465 g 3-(*N*-morpholino) propanesulfonic acid (MOPS), 4.2369 g NaCl, and 2.5 g D-(+)-glucose to 500 mL of di-water and adjusted for a final pH of 7.0–7.2. The alginate and cross-linking solutions were then sterilized with 0.22 μm filters.

2.3. *Encapsulation of free albumin and albumin NPs in alginate microbeads*

To prepare the albumin-NPs for encapsulation, they were re-suspended at 200 mg/mL in DMEM. A NP/alginate (1:10) mixture was then run through an electrostatically assisted encapsulation unit at a voltage of 6.4 kV and a flow rate of 20 mL/hr. The alg/albumin-NPs solution was pushed through a 0.35 mm outer diameter needle and the microbeads dropped into the cross-linking solution for stabilization. The microbeads were allowed to cross-link for 10 min, coated with poly-l-lysine (PLL), for enhanced stability, and washed with phosphate buffer solution (PBS). Free albumin was encapsulated in alginate microbeads at a concentration of 1 mg/mL using the method just described.

2.4. *Albumin release study*

Controlled release studies were conducted at room temperature using a 24-well plate transwell system. Bottom wells contained 600 μL of phosphate buffer solution (PBS). A vial of lyophilized albumin-NPs was dispersed in ultrapure di-water at a concentration 3 mg/mL (mg of nanoparticles/mL of di-water). Subsequently, 200 μL of the dispersed albumin-NPs were added to the transwell inserts. The alginate beads containing free albumin or albumin-NPs were formulated immediately before the release studies. Similarly, to the albumin-NPs, 200 μL of alginate beads containing free albumin or albumin-NPs were added to the transwells. The transwells for all groups (albumin-NPs, alg/albumin-NPs and alg/albumin) were then inserted into the wells. At each selected time-point, the PBS solution from all conditions was collected and the samples were then frozen at −80°C for future quantification via an albumin Enzyme Linked Immunosorbent Assay, (ELISA, R&D Systems). The ELISA was performed according to the manufacturer's instructions.

2.5. *Nanoparticle characterization*

Studies were designed to characterize BDNF-NP qualitatively via imaging and quantitatively via dynamic light scattering (DLS) (Malvern Zetasizer Nano ZS, UK). DLS provides quantitative data by measuring Brownian motion of molecules in solution and correlating it to particle size and charge. Brownian motion is dependent on molecule size, temperature, and solvent viscosity.[36] Using a 3 mL syringe, a disposable capillary cell was initially flushed with ethanol to facilitate wetting. This was followed by flushing the cell with distilled water at least four times. Lyophilized BDNF-NPs were then re-suspended in ultrapure deionized (di)-water at a concentration of 5 mg/mL. Approximately 1 mL of sample was then placed in the capillary, the experiment was run at room temperature and the refractive index parameter was set to 1.47.

Further studies aimed to characterize the degradation properties of the BDNF-NPs at both room and body temperatures. Lyophilized BDNF-NPs were re-suspended in di-water at a concentration of 5 mg/mL. BDNF-NPs were then incubated at 25°C and 37°C and changes in mass and size were evaluated over the course of 25 days and 16 days, respectively. Change in BDNF-NP mass was determined by weighing the tubes containing BDNF-NPs at each time point and sample volume was also considered in the calculation. The calculation and corresponding variables are summarized below:

- t = time point (day),
- NP_0 = BDNF-NPs (mg), $t = 0$,
- NP_t = BDNF-NPs (mg),
- S_t = sample volume (μL),
- % NP_t decrease $= 1-[(NP_t - S_t)/NP_0]$,

NP size was measured by taking an 80 μL sample which was diluted to 10× for DLS analysis.

2.6. *Release study of BDNF-NPs and alginate/BDNF-NPs*

Release studies were conducted at room temperature using 24-well plate transwell system. Each well contained 600 μL of phosphate buffer solution (PBS) with 1% (w/v) BSA, as a protein stabilizer. A vial of lyophilized BDNF-NPs was dispersed in ultrapure di-water at concentrations of 3 mg/mL or 6 mg/mL (mg of nanoparticles/mL of di-water). Subsequently, 200 μL of the dispersed particles were added to the transwell inserts. For the alginate/BDNF-NP (alg/BDNF-NP) group, dispersed BDNF-NPs were mixed with 2.2% alginate in a one-to-one ratio. Then, 400 μL of alg/BDNF-NPs (to have the same quantity of NPs as the BDNF-NPs group) was added to transwells. The inserts were then submerged in the calcium cross-linking solution for 10 min. Next, the cross-linked alg/BDNF-NPs were washed in PBS for 10 min. The transwells for all groups (BDNF-NPs and alg/BDNF-NPs) were then inserted into the wells. At each selected time-point, the 1% BSA in PBS solution was collected and replenished for collection at a later timepoint. The collected samples were then frozen at −80°C for future quantification via a BDNF ELISA Enzyme Linked Immunosorbent Assay, (ELISA, R&D Systems). The ELISA was performed according to the manufacturer's instructions.

2.7. *Characterization of nanoparticle stability in alginate hydrogel*

Additional studies were executed to evaluate if the addition of alginate barrier protects NPs from rapid degradation. These studies were conducted in a 24-well plate transwell system, similar to the release described above. However, for visual confirmation, rhodamine B NPs were encapsulated in alginate and the lyophilized NPs were re-suspended at a concentration of 2 mg/mL or 3 mg/mL. Fluorescent Z-stack images were taken using a confocal microscope at Day 0, Day 2, and Day 3. The z-stack images were processed using Image-J software to quantify the number of particles encapsulated in alginate.

2.8. *MATLAB model of BDNF release profile*

As a guide for future experiments, we developed a computational model in MATLAB to predict the amount of BDNF released daily from the 100 μg/mL BDNF-NPs based on the number of NPs used. The built in MATLAB 'polyfit' function was used to generate a least squares fit polynomial using empirical data generated from the release studies described above. Using the first 7 days of data, the curve was broken down into two-piecewise polynomial functions (days 0–2 and days 2–7). Once the polynomial variables were generated, the 'polyval' function was used to produce theoretical BDNF release data. A 'for loop' was then implemented to predict the amount of BDNF released when different amounts of NPs are used.

2.9. *E18 rat cortical neuron culture*

For neuronal cultures, cortical tissue from Sprague Dawley rat embryos was purchased from BrainBits, LLC (Springfield, IL). Prior to neuron isolation, 24-well plates were coated with 200 μL of 0.1 mg/mL poly-d-lysine (PDL) for at least 4 h at room temperature and then washed three times with di-water. Once received, the tissue was immediately dissociated for E18 cortical neuron isolation. Briefly, the media in which the tissue was preserved was removed and stored for a later step. The tissue was then incubated in 2 mL of cell dissociation media comprised of hibernate-E without calcium (BrainBits) media containing 2 mg/mL of papain (BrainBits) for 10 min at 37°C. The cell dissociation media was removed, and the preservation media was re-added to the tissue. The tissue was then mechanically dissociated for 1 min with a fire-polished Pasteur pipette. The cell suspension was collected, spun down (200 RCF for 1 min) and the supernatant was aspirated. The cells were then re-suspended in 3 mL of "complete neurobasal media" composed of Neurobasal Medium, 2% B-27™ Supplement (50×), 1% penicillin–streptomycin (10,000 U/mL) and 1% GlutaMAX™Supplement. The isolated neurons were then plated on PDL coated 24-well plates at a density of 25,000 cells per well with 500 μL of "complete neurobasal media". Half the media was changed every 4–5 days. On days *in vitro* (DIV) 14–15, neurons were used for the following experiments.

2.10. *Hydrogen peroxide dose response*

On DIV 14, neurons were placed under oxidative stress with H_2O_2. Right before the injury, a stock solution of 1000 μM H_2O_2 was prepared in "complete neurobasal media". This H_2O_2 dilution is effective for only 30 min, after which the H_2O_2 will destabilize and not induce injury to the cells. To determine an adequate level of toxicity, neurons were exposed to various concentrations of H_2O_2 ranging from 0 μM to 200 μM. To ensure each group was subjected to injury for the same amount of time, first, fresh neurobasal media was added to each group. Then a specified amount of 1000 μM H_2O_2 would be added to achieve the desired final concentration of H_2O_2. Neurons were incubated with H_2O_2 media at 37°C for 30 min. The injury media was then aspirated, and the cells were washed three times with complete neurobasal media.

2.11. *Live/dead assay*

Cell viability was measured immediately and 24 h after injury according to the manufacturer's instructions. Briefly, neurons were incubated with 1.5 μg/mL calcein-AM, 1.3 μg/mL ethidium-homodimer-1, and 2 μg/mL Hoechst-33342 (Invitrogen) for 10–15 min, followed by three washes with "complete neurobasal media". The cells were then imaged using fluorescent microscopy and viability was quantified using ImageJ software. The neurons were subsequently fixed with 200 μL of 4% paraformaldehyde (PFA) per well. After 15 min of PFA incubation, 600 μL of phosphate-buffered saline (PBS) was added to each well to dilute the PFA to 1%. After fixation, the plate was stored at 4°C for any future analysis.

2.12. *BDNF dosage and temporal response*

For the BDNF dosage study, DIV14 neurons were injured with 200 μM H_2O_2 as described above. Following H_2O_2 injury, neurons were immediately treated with BDNF at concentrations ranging from 0 ng/mL to 100 ng/mL. This range was chosen based on the literature review of *in vitro* studies that add bolus BDNF as a treatment.[37–40] For the temporal study, neurons were also injured with 200 μM H_2O_2

and subsequently treated with 25 ng/mL BDNF at different times post-injury (i.e., 0, 1, 2, 3, 4, 6, and 7 h). The concentration of BDNF used for this study was determined based on the results from the BDNF dose response. For both studies, viability was evaluated 24 h post-injury as described above.

2.13. *BDNF depletion studies*

Additional studies were designed to determine the rate at which BDNF is depleted with and without cells. For the studies with cells, neurons were plated on DIV0 at densities ranging from 0 to 25,000 cells/well. Cells were then injured with 200 μM H_2O_2 and incubated with 25 ng/mL BDNF for 24 h. As a control, healthy cells also received 25 ng/mL BDNF. For the studies without cells, 25 ng/mL BDNF in cell culture media was added to 24-well plates and incubated at room and body temperature. After 24 h, supernatants were collected and evaluated via BDNF ELISA. For experiments without cells, supernatants were also collected at 2 h and 4 h.

2.14. *BDNF nanoparticle in vitro study*

Prior to testing for bioactivity of the BDNF-NPs, empty NPs were evaluated to ensure they were not cytotoxic. For cytotoxic studies, different concentrations of empty NPs (2, 5, 10 mg/mL) were incubated with neurons for 24 h followed by evaluation of neuronal viability. Following these studies, BDNF-NPs were tested on neurons injured with 200 μM H_2O_2 as described above. For studies using BDNF-NPs, the amount of BDNF-NPs needed was determined by taking into consideration results from BDNF *in vitro* and diffusion studies previously described. The MATAB model described above was instrumental in designing these studies. The calculations considered the percentage of BDNF depleted after 24 h in the presence of cells and the smallest BDNF dosage needed for therapeutic effect, based on our studies, the calculations will be discussed in greater detail later. Following injury, 100 μL of 10 mg/mL of BDNF-NPs (i.e., 1 mg NPs) were added to transwells and viability was evaluated after 24 h.

2.15. *Alg/BDNF-NPs in vitro study*

To evaluate the efficacy of alg/BDNF-NPs neurons were injured with 200 μM H_2O_2 and then treated with alg/BDNF-NPs (1 mg NPs), BDNF-NPs (1 mg NPs) or bolus BDNF (25 ng/mL). Alg/BDNF-NPs formulation was prepared as described above. Groups that received BDNF or alg/BDNF-NPs also had the same quantity of NPs. After 24 h of treatment, cell viability was evaluated, and supernatants were tested for BDNF levels via an ELISA. Additionally, glutamate release levels were analyzed using a colorimetric assay (Abcam).

2.16. *Microtubule-associated protein 2 immunocytochemistry*

Blocking solution containing 5% (v/v) donkey serum, 0.2% (w/v) sodium azide, and 0.1% (v/v) triton-x 100 in 1× PBS was prepared and stored in 4°C. For a 24 well plate, each well was filled with 0.3 mL blocking solution and incubated on a rocker for 2 h at room temperature. Afterward, the blocking solution was aspirated and 0.2 mL primary antibody solution was deposited in each well, samples were incubated on the rocker for 1 h at room temperature. The anti-MAP2 mouse monoclonal primary antibody (Invitrogen) was diluted to 10 μg/mL in blocking solution. The wells were rinsed three times with 0.3 mL 1× PBS with a 5-min incubation on the rocker between each rinse, aspirating after every rinse. PBS was aspirated after the final wash, and 0.2 mL of secondary antibody solution was deposited in each well and incubated on a rocker for 1 h at room temperature. Alexa Fluor 488 donkey anti-mouse secondary antibody (Invitrogen) was diluted to 2 μg/mL with blocking solution. Cells incubated with secondary antibody alone served as a negative control for nonspecific binding. The wells were rinsed three times with 0.3 mL 1× PBS with a 5-min incubation on the rocker between each rinse. Nuclei staining was also performed as described above with 2 μg/mL Hoechst-33342. Images were then acquired using a fluorescent microscope.

2.17. *Statistical analysis*

Statistical differences among data sets were determined via analysis of variance (ANOVA) followed by Fisher's least significant difference

(LSD) post hoc test, unless otherwise stated. Significance level was $\alpha = 0.05$ in Prism 9 (GraphPad Software, San Diego, CA, USA). For NP characterization, the minimum number of replicates was $n = 3$ and for cell culture studies the minimum number of replicates was $n = 6$; each figure indicates the number of replicates utilized. Data points represent the mean $\pm$ the standard error of the mean (SEM) for the indicated number of independent observations (n) unless otherwise stated.

3. Results

3.1. *Development and characterization of BDNF-loaded PLGA nanoparticles*

With the goal of improving long-term stable and cost-effective BDNF delivery, our initial studies focused on encapsulating protein in PLGA nanoparticles and characterizing the effect of encapsulation on overall nanoparticle stability and protein release.

3.1.1. *Characterization of protein-loaded PLGA NPs*

As an initial proof-of-concept, PLGA NPs were synthesized [Fig. 1(a)] and molecular encapsulation was qualitatively confirmed with rhodamine B, a fluorescent dye [Fig. 1(b)]. For proof of concept, release profiles of albumin, a model protein, in different formulations were evaluated (i.e., PLGA NPs, alginate, alginate/PLGA NPs). As shown in Fig. 1(c), when albumin was encapsulated in PLGA NPs, there was rapid release within the first 24 h. When albumin was encapsulated in cross-linked alginate, the release was slowed for at least 7 days. However, when PLGA-NPs loaded with albumin were encapsulated in alginate, the release was slower than with either component alone, and this was observed for 14 days. Thus, these studies confirm that dual encapsulation of a protein allows it to be released consistently over a prolonged period.

Following the albumin release studies, the formulation was optimized for encapsulating BDNF, which included adding BSA as a stabilizer. NPs were fabricated using two pre-emulsification concentrations of BDNF (i.e., 25 μg/mL and 100 μg/mL). NPs were

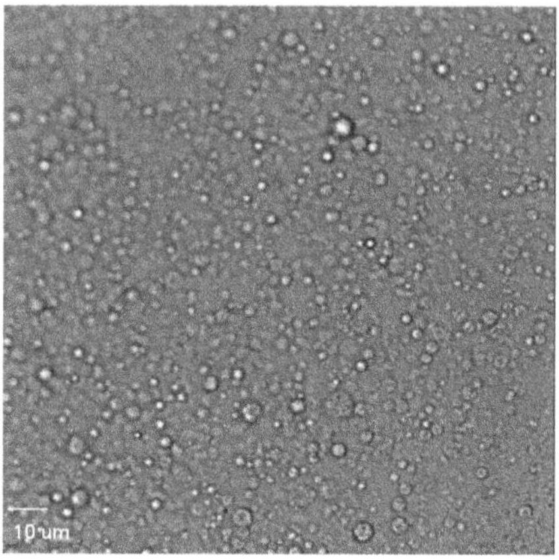

(a)

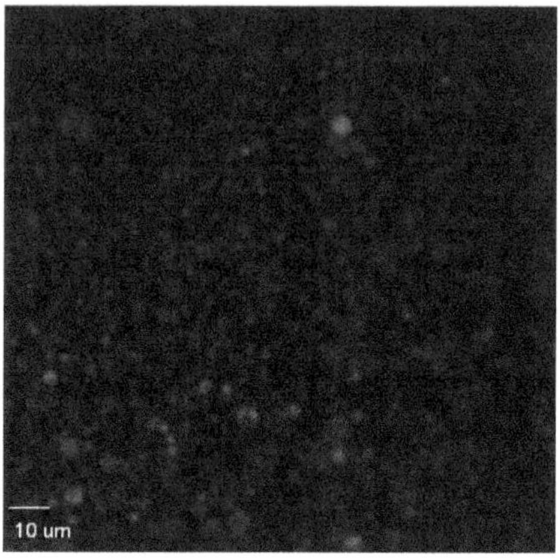

(b)

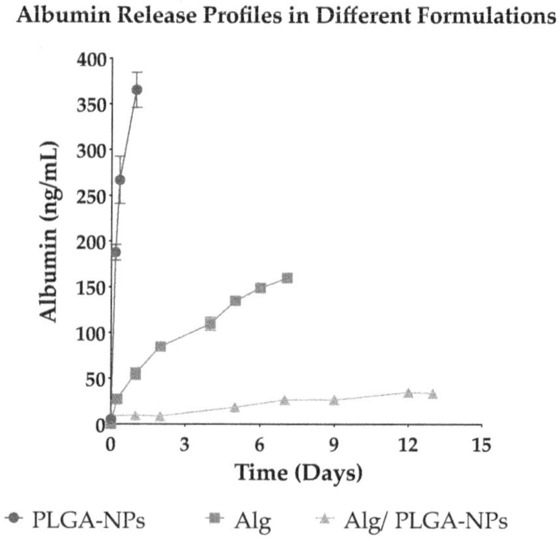

(c)

Fig. 1. NP formulation and release of albumin from different formulations. PLGA NPs were formulated using a double emulsion technique.[18,20] (a) Differential interference contrast (DIC) images of rhodamine-B NPs; (b) fluorescent images of rhodamine-B NPs were taken with an Olympus spinning disk confocal microscope; (c) concentration of albumin released from different formulations (i.e., PLGA NPs, alginate and alginate/PLGA NPs) measured by ELISA. The data is represented as mean $\pm$ standard deviation of $n = 3$ independent observations.

Table 1. NPs remain stable regardless of encapsulated molecule and molecule concentration. The data is represented as the mean ± standard error mean ($n = 3$–6). $^{**}p < 0.05$, $^{***}p < 0.001$.

	Empty NPs	BSA NPs	25 μg/mL BDNF-NPs	100 μg/mL BDNF-NPs
Particle size (nm)	469.5 ± 18.05	498.3 ± 39.87	530.0 ± 88.62	$304.0 \pm 34.83^{**}$
Zeta potential (mV)	-22.48 ± 0.6270	-22.33 ± 0.2030	$-29.43 \pm 1.397^{***}$	-19.37 ± 1.017

then characterized via dynamic light scattering (DLS) for size and zeta potential. Our results indicate that encapsulation of BDNF at a higher concentration resulted in significantly smaller particles (Table 1). However, as indicated by the zeta potential results, NPs remained stable regardless of the amount of protein encapsulated. Furthermore, the size of the NPs remained uniformly distributed.

Additional studies were executed to better understand the degradation and release properties of BDNF-NPs. As demonstrated in Fig. 2(a), the overall mass of BDNF-NPs decreased ~80% by day 25 and temperature did not appear to impact the change in mass. Next, the change of BDNF-NP size was evaluated, and the results indicate that while BNDF-NP size decreased slightly within the NP population over time, the change is not as prominent when comparing size changes to the change in mass [Fig. 2(b)].

3.1.2. *BDNF release from PLGA NPs*

We then characterized the release profile of BDNF encapsulated at two different concentrations (100 μg/mL and 25 g/mL). As shown in Fig. 3(a), regardless of the amount of BDNF encapsulated, the release profiles are very similar. There is a small "dose-dump" within the first 48 h, followed by a steady daily release of BDNF for the following 5 days (Table 2). In addition, the amount of BDNF released by the 100 μg/mL BDNF-NPs was ~3.5 times the amount of BDNF released by the 25 μg/mL BDNF-NPs. We also evaluated the release profile

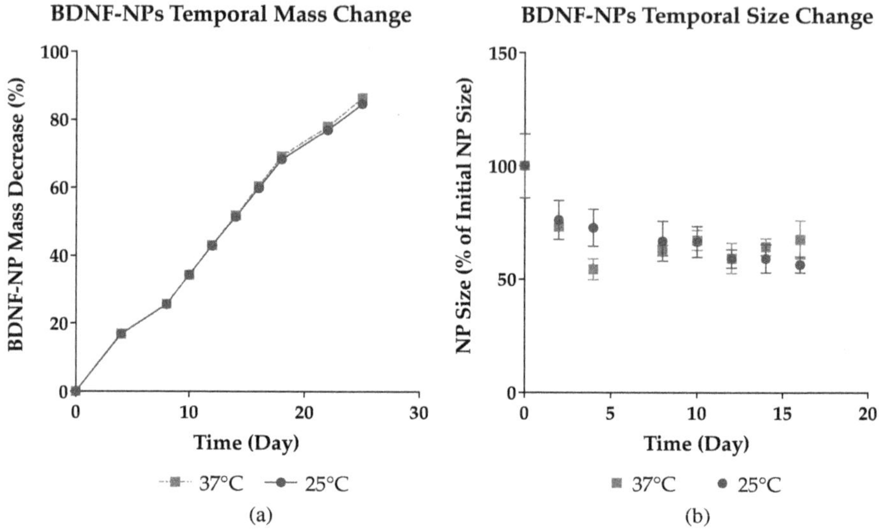

Fig. 2. BDNF-NP degradation at room temperature and body temperature is not significantly different. (a) The percent decrease in BDNF-NP mass over time at room temperature and body temperature. (b) Change in BDNF-NP size over time at room temperature and body temperature. The data is represented as mean $\pm$ standard deviation of $n = 3$ independent observations.

of the 100 μg/mL BDNF-NPs for an additional 4 weeks [(Fig. 3(b)]. Following the first week, the daily release of BDNF is slowly reduced until the 4-week time point. During the fourth week, the amount of BDNF released declined at a much faster rate (Table 3). Therefore, the BDNF-NPs have a steady release profile for $\sim$ one month using these starting conditions. This data was then utilized in a MATLAB model to generate theoretical release profiles when using different starting concentrations of BDNF-NPs. The MATLAB model generated a curve that accurately fit the release profile of the 100 μg/mL BDNF-NPs [(Fig. 3(c)].

3.2. *Evaluation of BDNF-NP functional properties*

Having successfully encapsulated BDNF into PLGA NPs, experiments were designed to evaluate its functional stability and efficacy using an *in vitro* neuronal injury model.

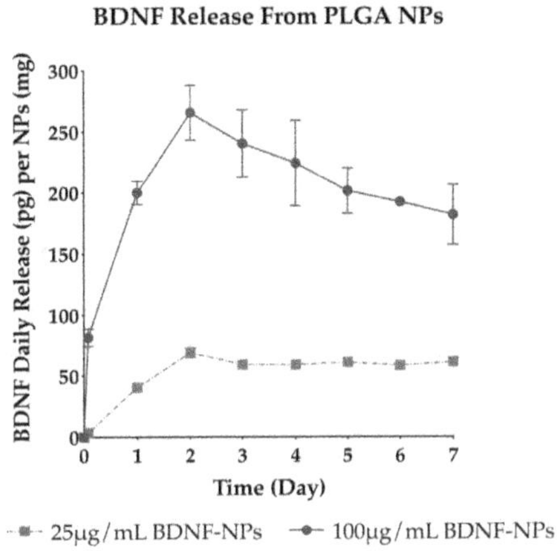

(a)

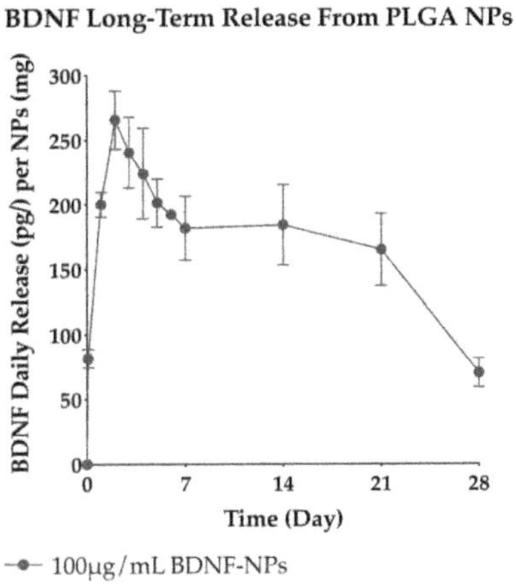

(b)

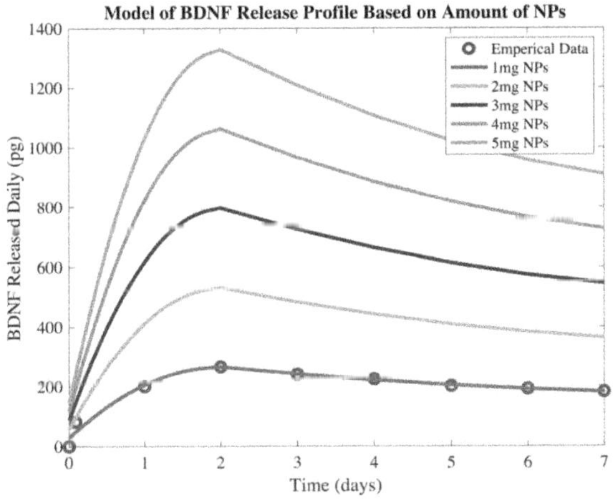

(c)

Fig. 3. Encapsulated BDNF is slowly released from PLGA NPs. Each data point represents the daily amount of BDNF (pg) released at that point in time as measured by an ELISA. (a) Release profile of BDNF synthesized using two distinct concentrations (i.e., 25 μg/mL and 100 μg/mL). These concentrations are pre-emulsification; (b) Long term release of BDNF-NPs synthesized with a starting concentration of 100 μg/mL; (c) MATLAB model prediction of BDNF daily release based on the quantity of NPs used. The data is represented as the mean $\pm$ SEM of $n = 6$–9 independent observations.

Table 2. BDNF is steadily released from NPs for three weeks. The data is represented as the mean ± standard error mean ($n = 5$).

BDNF-NP formulation	Average BDNF daily release (pg) Normalized by the quantity of NPs (mg) (mean ± SEM)
25 μg/mL BDNF-NPs	59.79 ± 1.24
100 μg/mL BDNF-NPs	208.18 ± 23.94

Table 3. BDNF release rate decreases after 3 weeks.

Time period (days)	Slope (BDNF (pg)/ NPs (mg)/day)
0–7	0.36
7–14	−2.73
14–28	−13.55

3.2.1. *BDNF promotes neuroprotection from hydrogen peroxide-induced cytotoxicity*

To ultimately evaluate therapeutic efficacy of BDNF-NPs, a baseline neuronal injury culture was established using H_2O_2. Cells were first dosed with varying levels of H_2O_2 for 24 h. As shown in Fig. 4(a), dosing cells with 100 μM and 200 μM H_2O_2 led to an initial significant reduction in viability. However, after 24 h neuronal viability decreased at least 2-fold for any group that received H_2O_2. Furthermore, both the 100 μM and 200 μM H_2O_2 groups had the most drastic drop in viability after 24 h. Thus, for future studies 200 μM H_2O_2 was used as it has a more detrimental effect on neuronal viability.

We then evaluated different doses of bolus BDNF on chemically injured neurons to determine a therapeutic *in vitro* threshold. Following 24 h of treatment with BDNF the results indicate that all the tested doses of BDNF were neuroprotective [(Fig. 4(b)]. However,

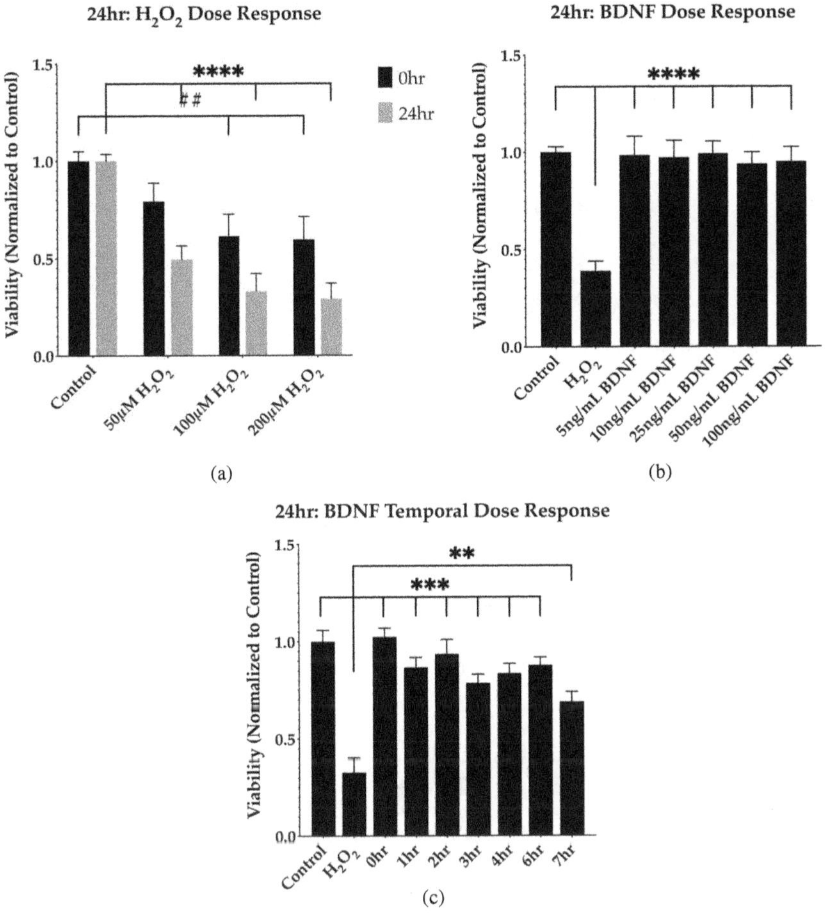

Fig. 4. Bolus dose of BDNF is neuroprotective for at least 24 h. Each bar represents neuronal viability determined via calcein-AM and ethidium-homodimer-staining. (a) Viability of neurons dosed with varying concentration of H_2O_2; (b) Viability of neurons dosed with 200 μM H_2O_2 followed by treatment with varying concentrations of BDNF; (c) Viability of neurons injured with 200 μM H_2O_2 and treated with 25 ng/mL BDNF at various times post-injury. The data is represented as the mean $\pm$ SEM of $n = 9$ independent observations. $^{**}p < 0.01$, $^{***}p < 0.001$, $^{****}p < 0.0001$, $^{\#\#}p < 0.01$.

for subsequent studies, 25 ng/mL BDNF was chosen as an intermediate concentration. Additionally, since the release profiles show the BDNF-NPs release a small amount of BDNF initially, and that therapeutic doses may not be achieved as quickly as bolus applications, additional studies were executed to ensure that BDNF could provide neuroprotection after delayed addition. As shown in Fig. 4(c), after 24 h, the addition of BDNF at 0–7 h post-injury led to significantly higher viability relative to the group that only received H_2O_2. Thus, our studies indicate that BDNF could be delivered for at least 7 h post chemical injury.

3.2.2. *BDNF in vitro depletion rate*

Since neuroprotective function is dependent upon BDNF bioavailability, experiments were designed to determine the depletion rate of BDNF levels in the presence and absence of cells. As shown in Fig. 5(a), after 24 h cells plated at 25,000 cells/well utilized approximately 70% of the bolus BDNF. As expected, at lower densities, the amount of BDNF used was significantly lower. However, it plateaued at around 40% regardless of cell density. Furthermore, BDNF's apparent consumption rate by cells was not affected by

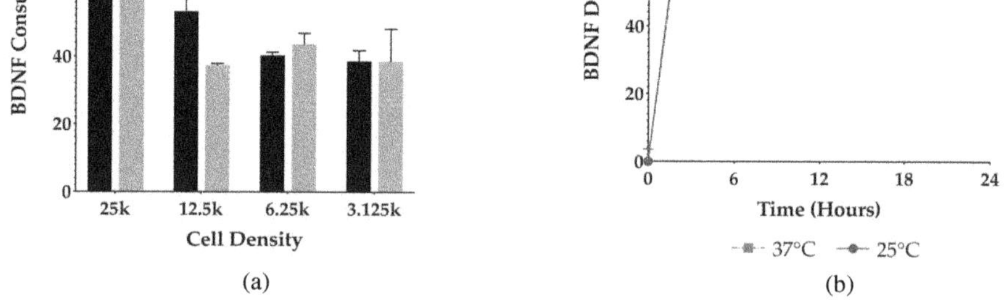

Fig. 5. BDNF depletion rate is slower in the presence of cells. Each data point represents the percentage of BDNF used as determined via an ELISA. (a) BDNF levels in the presence of stimulated and non-stimulated cells; (b) BDNF levels in the absence of cells and different temperatures (room and body temperature). The data is represented as the mean ± SEM of $n = 6$–12 independent observations. $^{*}p < 0.05$, $^{\#\#}p < 0.01$.

exposure to H_2O_2. In the studies without cells, the results indicate that temperature does not impact the degradation rate of BDNF. In both cases approximately 80% of BDNF had degraded within 5 h as shown in Fig. 5(b) and was completely depleted by 24 h, further substantiating the need for a protective drug delivery approach.

3.2.3. *Encapsulated BDNF remains bioactive in vitro*

Having evaluated the effectiveness of bolus BDNF concentrations and its stability in our *in vitro* model, we quantified the bioactivity of BDNF-NPs relative to bolus BDNF. Neurons were initially dosed with empty PLGA NPs at multiple concentrations and no detrimental effect on viability was seen [Fig. 6(a)]. Next, efficacy of BDNF-NPs *in vitro* was evaluated, and the amount of NPs used was

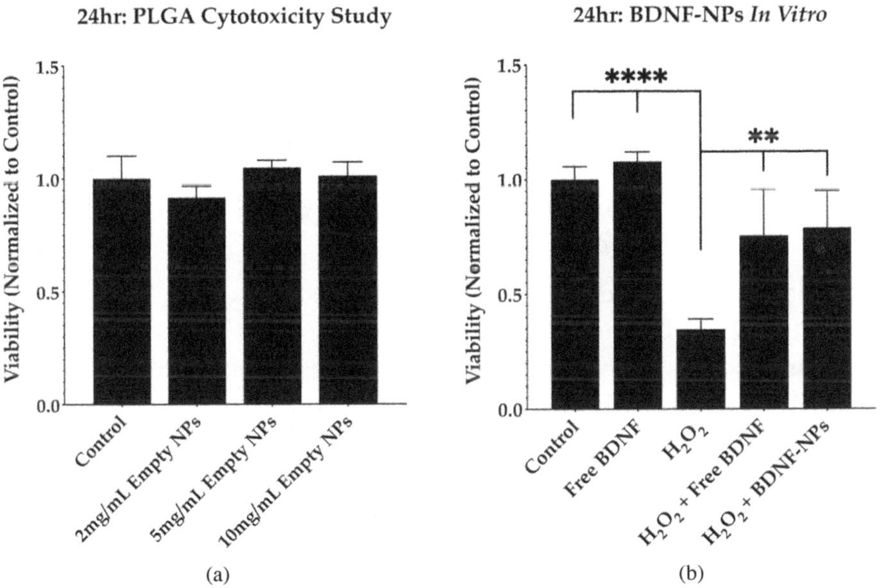

Fig. 6. BDNF-NPs are neuroprotective *in vitro*. Each bar represents neuronal viability determined via calcein-AM and ethidium-homodimer-staining. (a) Viability of neurons exposed to empty PLGA NPs and (b) Viability of neurons injured with H_2O_2 followed by treatments with bolus BDNF and BDNF-NPs. The data is represented as the mean $\pm$ SEM of $n = 6$–9 independent observations. $^{**}p < 0.01$, $^{****}p < 0.0001$.

determined based upon the results from studies described above. Briefly, after a bolus treatment with 5 ng/mL of BDNF, there is about 1.5 ng/mL or 0.9 ng of BDNF after 24 h (~70% depletion), thus we designed our experiments to target this range of BDNF. Using the release profile of 100 μg/mL BDNF-NPs, as well as the MATLAB model, we estimated that the NPs released around 0.2 ng of BDNF per mg of NPs after 24 h. Therefore, around 4.5 mg of NPs would be needed to achieve this level [Fig. 3(c)]. However, in fact, we decided to further reduce the NP amount to conserve supply and to assess if even less would be effective. Therefore, only 1 mg of NPs was used in these experiments. The results indicate BDNF-NPs were equally protective as bolus BDNF within the first 24 h [(Fig. 6(b)].

3.3. *Characterization of alg/BDNF NPs formulation*

Once BDNF-NPs were shown to be efficacious *in vitro*, they were encapsulated in alginate to determine if that would enable a longer controlled release profile and to evaluate its neuroprotective properties.

3.3.1. *BDNF release further delayed by the addition of an alginate hydrogel barrier*

For these studies, the same quantity of NPs was used. As shown in Fig. 7(a), BDNF-NPs release BDNF at a much faster rate when compared to alg/BDNF-NPs, with 5% being released within the first 24 h. After 5 days, BDNF-NPs released ~3 times the amount of BDNF released by alg/BDNF-NPs. Thus, our results indicate that BDNF release is slowed down and potentially released for a longer time with the addition of an alginate hydrogel barrier.

In addition, we also looked at the release profiles at physiologically relevant conditions. We evaluated the effect of cell culture media vs PBS 25°C vs 37°C. The results suggest that BDNF diffusion is slowed in both PBS and cell culture media at 37°C [(Fig. 7(b)]. Additional studies demonstrated that the number of NPs encapsulated in alginate remains consistent, indicating that alginate does slow the

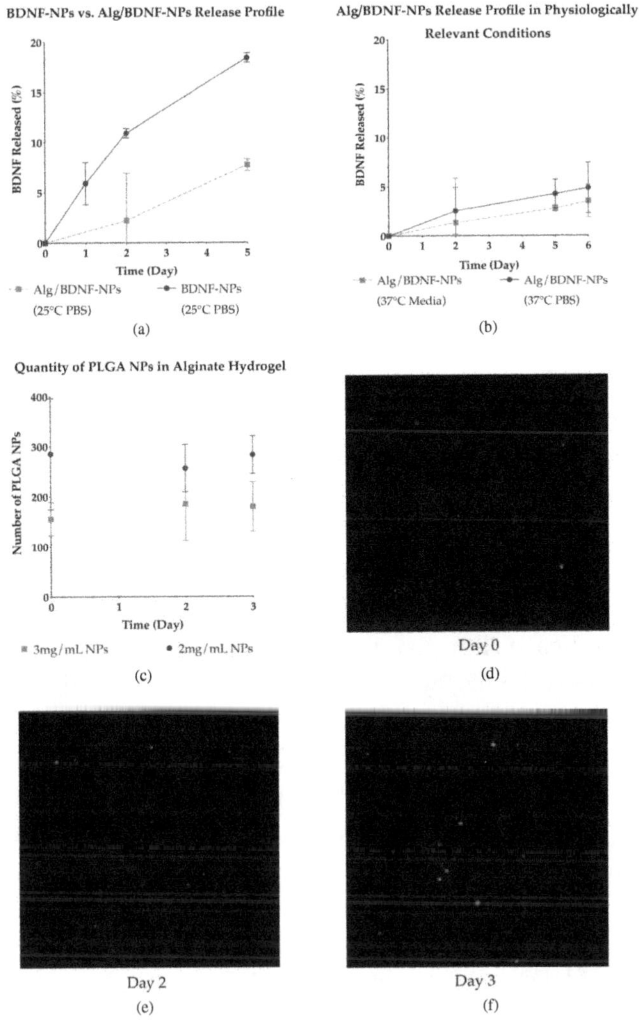

Fig. 7. Alginate/BDNF-NP yields uniform particles and slow release of BDNF. (a) Comparison of percentage of BDNF release from BDNF-NPs and alg/BDNF NPs, where BDNF-NPs resulted in faster BDNF release; (b) Alg/BDNF-NP release profile under physiological relevant conditions. Each data point represents the percent of BDNF released at that time point; (c) PLGA NPs encapsulated in alginate at two different concentrations were quantified over a 3-day period; (d–f) Representative fluorescent images of 2 mg/mL NPs suspended in alginate. (d) Day 0 of NPs encapsulated in alginate; (e) 2 days following NP encapsulation in alginate; (f) 3 days following NP encapsulation in alginate. Quantified data in represented as the mean ± SEM.

release of BDNF [(Fig. 7(c)]. This was also qualitatively confirmed via fluorescent imaging of the encapsulated NPs over a period of 3 days [Figs. 7(d)–7(f)].

3.3.2. *Alg/BDNF-NPs are neuroprotective in vitro*

Next, the alg/BDNF-NPs were evaluated for therapeutic efficacy, especially given the low release profile of alg/BDNF-NPs. Figure 8(a) demonstrates that alg/BDNF-NPs are just as neuroprotective as BDNF-NPs and bolus BDNF-NPs. Furthermore, we also quantified levels of BDNF released from both vehicles after 24 h [Fig. 8(b)]. The results were consistent with previous diffusion studies and showed that alg/BDNF-NPs release significantly lower levels. However, even with a 2-fold reduction in BDNF concentration, the alginate/BDNF NP vehicle was still protective.

Glutamate levels were also measured 24 h after injury with H_2O_2 and treatment with BDNF, BDNF-NPs, or alg/BDNF-NPs [Fig. 8(c)]. The results indicate that groups that received H_2O_2 had significantly higher glutamate levels, while only treatment with alg/BDNF-NPs led to a significant reduction in glutamate levels relative to other groups that received H_2O_2. As an additional characterization metric, cells were stained with anti-MAP2, a marker for dendritic branching, and images were acquired. As seen in Fig. 8(d), neurons which were neither injured nor treated are characterized with a high degree of branching, while neurons treated with H_2O_2 have reduced dendritic branching [Fig. 8(e)]. However, when treated with any form of BDNF (bolus, BDNF-NPs, alg/BDNF-NPs) the dendritic branching is more prominent when compared to the H_2O_2 injured group [Figs. 8(f)–8(h)].

Collectively our studies indicate that we can fabricate stable PLGA NPs which effectively release BDNF for at least 30 days. In addition, by including an alginate barrier the release profiles can be further controlled. Our NPs can reduce neuronal damage and can be designed for quantitative controlled release of BDNF for therapeutic efficacy.

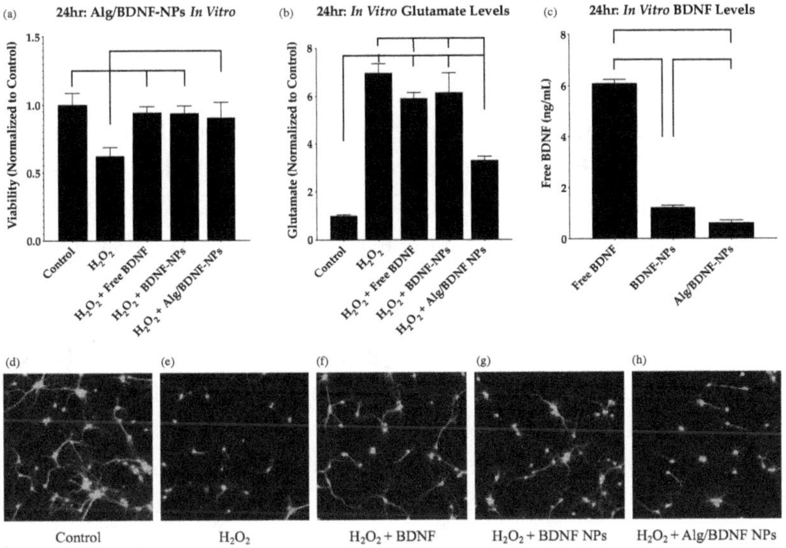

Fig. 8. Alg/BDNF-NPs formulation is neuroprotective *in vitro*. (a) Viability of neurons treated with alg/BDNF-NPs, BDNF-NPs, or bolus BDNF following injury. Each bar represents neuronal viability determined via calcein-AM and ethidiumhomodimer-staining; (b) BDNF concentration present *in vitro* after 24 hr incubation with bolus BDNF, BDNF-NPs, and alg/BDNF-NPs; (c) Concentration of glutamate present *in vitro* after treatment with alg/BDNF-NPs, BDNF-NPs, or bolus BDNF following injury. Glutamate levels were measured via a glutamate colorimetric assay. (d–h) Representative images following Anti-MAP2 staining. (d) Anti-MAP2 staining of control neurons (i.e., no injury and/or treatment). (e) Anti-MAP2 staining of neurons injured with 200 μM H_2O_2; (f) Anti-MAP2 staining of neurons injured with 200 μM H_2O_2 and treated with bolus BDNF; (g) Anti-MAP2 staining of neurons injured with 200 μM H_2O_2 and treated with BDNF-NPs; (h) Anti-MAP2 staining of neurons injured with 200 μM H_2O_2 and treated with alg/BDNF-NPs. Green represents MAP2 and blue represents nuclei. Quantitative data is represented as the mean $\pm$ SEM of $n = 9$–12 independent observations. $^{*}p < 0.05$, $^{**}p < 0.01$, $^{****}p < 0.0001$.

4. Discussion

BDNF has been extensively investigated as a treatment for TBI and other neurological disorders due to its neuroprotective and neuroregenerative properties. However, the main concern with bolus dosage of BDNF is its relatively short half-life which resulted in its failure in clinical trials for ALS.[41] This has led to the development of polymer-based formulations for long-term delivery of BDNF.[20] These formulations are typically composed of chitosan, alginate, poly-lactic acids, or polyethylene glycols.

These vehicles have been explored to extend BDNF release and provide appropriate pharmacodynamics needed for therapeutic efficacy.[9,18,19] BDNF has been successfully encapsulated into polymer-based and hydrogel vehicles. In prior studies, BDNF release was only seen for 7–14 days, while BDNF encapsulated in hydrogels was released for 3–4 weeks.[20] In these studies, PEG was used as a delivery vehicle for PLGA-BDNF. Some of these formulations have been evaluated *in vivo* rodent models and demonstrated promising effects.[19,42,43] However, free delivery vehicles that are not positionally targeted, may introduce unwanted off-target effects, and will require increased initial drug loading to compensate for systemic dilution.[44] Thus, higher quantities of NPs would be necessary for clinical applications, thereby making it an expensive therapy. Therefore, other hybrid material systems that can deliver controlled BDNF levels to a localized region, must still be developed.[45–47]

Although others have been able to synthesize vehicles containing BDNF, they are delivered systemically or are directly injected into the injury site.[18,19,43,48–50] Systemic delivery of the vehicles will reduce the amount of BDNF available and direct injection may further exacerbate the injury which could lead to faster degradation of BDNF and longer recovery time.

These approaches can be enhanced by adding an additional layer to enable positional control for BDNF delivery. Thus, we have developed a controlled release formulation comprised of BDNF-NPs encapsulated in an alginate hydrogel. The hydrogel is a secondary barrier that enables BDNF to be localized near a site of injury in addition to prolonging the delivery of BDNF. With this in mind, these studies were designed to ensure our novel BDNF delivery formulation provides stable and bioactive BDNF for continuous delivery over an extended period.

The present studies indicate that our BDNF-NPs can release BDNF for at least one month and the added hydrogel layer reduces the release rate. We also evaluated the degradation properties of the BDNF-NPs and found that NP size decreases by about 30% over the course of the first two days and remains approximately the same size for an additional 2 weeks, regardless of the incubation temperature. This initial reduction in size correlates with the initial burst release seen in the BDNF release studies. This biphasic release pattern is commonly seen in small PLGA NPs.[51] Also, while the release of BDNF was relatively consistent during the initial 2 weeks, it began to slow down after the third week. This can be due to the reduction in BDNF-NP mass that was quantified. While NP size remains constant, NP mass decreases linearly for 25 days and this reduction in mass can be due to NP swelling which may cause them to either burst or degrade via hydrolysis.[51] Overall, our data suggest that BDNF is released via diffusion from the NP, as well as PLGA particle degradation/hydrolysis over time. In contrast, our results demonstrate that release from alginate encapsulated NP is likely protected from environmental hydrolysis and therefore, BDNF release profiles are relatively linear for at least 5 days [Fig. 7(a)].

Prior to the therapeutic evaluation of different BDNF delivery modalities, an injury model consisting of H_2O_2 was optimized. H_2O_2 was chosen given that secondary injury in TBI is exacerbated by the release of reactive oxygen species (ROS) and nitric oxide (NO).[52] Additionally, H_2O_2 is commonly used *in vitro* to induce oxidative stress in other models of neurological disorders, such as ischemia, Alzheimer's disease and Parkinson's disease.[53–55] While stretch and strain injury may characterize initial TBI events more accurately,[56] and ultimately *in vivo* studies are needed to evaluate therapeutic efficacy, our initial model focused on chronic injury-related events. Using this injury model, our studies demonstrated that very small doses of BDNF released from the alginate/NP formulation are neuroprotective in our *in vitro* system. This was demonstrated by evaluating viability, glutamate levels, and MAP2 expression. Interestingly, while glutamate release following injury is expected, only treatment with alg/BDNF NPs resulted in reduced levels of neurotoxic glutamate. Qualitative analysis of MAP2 expression demonstrated decreased expression in H_2O_2 injured groups relative to controls. However, treatment with any form of BDNF minimized reduction in dendritic branching. Therefore, while BDNF certainly provides viability neuroprotection, our studies indicate that treatment may also improve structural/functional characteristics.

Our initial studies only evaluated the efficacy of bolus BDNF at a limited range of concentrations (5–100 ng/mL). These concentrations were chosen based on previous studies evaluating bolus BDNF efficacy *in vitro*. However, for studies evaluating the efficacy of the BDNF-NPs and alg/BDNF-NPs, we used MATLAB to extrapolate our data and predict the amount of BDNF released depending on the amount of BDNF-NPs used. As described above, we aimed to target for a range that would mimic the neuroprotective effects seen when 5 ng/mL BDNF bolus dose was utilized immediately after injury. However, our results indicated that after 24 h the BDNF-NPs and alg/BDNF-NPs released a dosage of 1 ng/mL (0.6 ng) and 0.3 ng/mL (0.09 ng), respectively. This suggests that even lower dosages of BDNF that we evaluated can provide therapeutic effects if it is continuously delivered. Given the flexibility of our construct design, concentrations can be easily varied by either adjusting the starting concentration per NP or increasing the number of NP within the alginate.

Together, these findings have very important implications for clinical translation considering that, for example, in ALS clinical trials patients were continuously infused with 25 or 100 μg/kg BDNF daily for 9 months.[11] This indicates that a person of average weight would need about 1.7–6.8 mg of BDNF daily, which can be very expensive and inconvenient. It is also important to note that we determined that the delayed addition of BDNF can be neuroprotective. This makes it more feasible to treat patients with traumatic injuries since they may not be able to receive treatment immediately. Therefore, our formulation can be a more cost-effective long-term treatment option and our findings suggest a lower dosage may be effective.

In addition, our formulation can be customized depending on the patient and application. For these studies, our construct's shape was designed to enable optimum gas exchange *in vitro*, which was decided based on the manufacturer's recommendation for the maximum working volume allowed in a transwell. However, the construct's shape, size and degree of cross-linking can be adjusted. For example, previous studies in our group have used alginate microspheres as opposed to an alginate sheet as a mode of therapeutic delivery for spinal cord injury applications.[30] Freudenberg *et al.* developed a star-shaped PEG gel to address the importance of using mechanical and biochemical cues in neurological applications.[57] Therefore, molds can be fabricated and utilized to personalize treatment for patients based on the location and severity of their injury. For example, nanoparticle delivery systems can be optimized for intra-ocular or cochlear implantation.[16] Furthermore, by adjusting the method and degree of cross-linking, the pore size and rigidity of the formulation can be modified to allow for slower or faster release times. Currently, our formulation is intended for severe TBI which can require invasive intervention to reduce intracranial pressure, which would provide an opportunity to administer the formulation. However, future work could focus on modifying the hydrogel to a self-assembly formulation to administer as an injection for a minimally invasive procedure.[29]

Our additional experiments also demonstrated that bolus BDNF is almost completely depleted after 24 h both with and without cells. Our results also indicate that in the presence of cells, BDNF depletion rate is actually slower. This phenomenon may be due to neurons naturally releasing some molecules that protect BDNF, considering the rate of depletion was the same in healthy and injured neurons. However, even though the degradation rate is different when there are cells present, this does not impact our alginate/BDNF-NPs formulation's ability to continuously deliver BDNF. This supports our hypothesis that an alginate barrier will protect the BDNF-NPs and it will enable positional control for BDNF delivery.

We were able to synthesize an alginate-NP formulation for controlled release of the relatively unstable neurotrophic factor, BDNF, and we demonstrated its stable neuroprotective efficacy *in vitro*, even after double encapsulation. We recognize that these initial characterization studies were limited to a short-time frame. Thus, future work must include evaluation of our system in an *in vivo* model of TBI.

It is important to recognize that since complex neuroinflammatory diseases result from multi-pathway dysregulation, targeting only one pathway is likely to be ineffective. Therefore, the development of multi-drug formulations is warranted.[58] Our formulation is perfectly suited for this approach since it may be optimized to encapsulate other molecules which are essential in treating TBI and other neurological diseases and disorders. For example, the small molecule BDNF mimetic available, 7,8,-dihydroxyflavone, may significantly reduce the cost of treatment while providing the same benefits as BDNF. Vascular endothelial growth factor (VEGF), fibroblast growth factor (FGF) and epidermal growth factor (EGF) have also been shown to be potential therapeutics for neurological disorders[59] and they, as well as anti-oxidants, could be encapsulated using our formulation as well, without complex design changes. Furthermore, we have already demonstrated that our alginate formulation can encapsulate MSC for SCI treatment and co-encapsulation of MSC with PLGA-NP did not compromise MSC function (unpublished observations). Our localized delivery approach also reduces the potential for off-target side effects. Thus, the work presented here can be easily translated to address multiple pathways that are affected when suffering from neurological disorders.

5. Conclusions

Severe TBI can result in life-lasting complications and there are currently no commercially available products that provide long-term benefits. While biologics provide a promising outlook for TBI therapeutics, two main concerns need to be addressed, (1) stability of the therapeutic and, (2) long-lasting, localized therapeutic delivery. With this in mind, we developed a novel formulation to enhance BDNF bioavailability by protecting it from the environment and enabling controlled release, thus making BDNF a more effective treatment option for TBI and other neurological disorders. Our neuronal *in vitro* studies demonstrate our formulation's ability to deliver bioactive BDNF. Moreover, this formulation can be easily modified to deliver not only BDNF but other relevant drugs, thereby minimizing the overall cost of drug development. Thus, our novel formulation is applicable to a wider range of therapeutics for TBI and other diseases and disorders.

Acknowledgments

Research reported in this manuscript was supported by the National Institute of General Medical Sciences of the National Institute of Health (T32 GM135141) and The New Jersey Commission on Spinal Cord Research (CSCR18IRG007).

Conflict of interest

Martin Yarmush declares that, as co-Editor-in-Chief of Nano LIFE, there is a conflict of interest regarding this manuscript. However, he confirms that he was not involved in the peer review process of the manuscript, and therefore he has not had any influence on the editorial decision-making process. The conflict of interest was disclosed to the editorial team, and appropriate steps were taken to ensure that the peer review and decision-making process for this manuscript were handled impartially and transparently.

Author contributions

The contributions for each author were substantial and are as follows:

Isabel Perez: Conceptualized all studies, performed experiments, analyzed data, drafted and revised the manuscript.

Elisheva Strauss: Performed experiments, analyzed data.

Shivani Vyas: Performed experiments, analyzed data.

Martin L. Yarmush: Conceptualized and supervised all studies, provided funding.

Rene S. Schloss: Conceptualized and supervised all studies, analyzed data, revised the manuscript.

Each author also reviewed and approved the manuscript content.

Authors' note

Each of the authors was included within the online submission portal and form. During the conversion from the online form to the PDF, only two authors were subsequently transferred from the portal. At the final stage in the publication process the authors have requested that the error be corrected with the author's names and affiliations included as originally listed.

ORCID

Isabel Perez https://orcid.org/0000-0002-4149-8613
Elisheva Strauss https://orcid.org/0009-0000-0699-9060
Shivani Vyas https://orcid.org/0000-0003-4452-8627
Rene S. Schloss https://orcid.org/0000-0002-1210-4099
Martin L. Yarmush https://orcid.org/0000-0003-4986-8444

References

1. Y. Xiong, A. Mahmood and M. Chopp, *Expert Opin. Emerg. Drugs* **14**, 67 (2009).
2. M. Kochanek *et al.*, *Semin. Neurol.* **35**, 83 (2015).
3. S. F. Carron, D. S. Alwis and R. Rajan, *Front. Syst. Neurosci.* **10**, 47 (2016).
4. Y. Xiong, A. Mahmood and M. Chopp, *Neural Regen. Res.* **12**, 19 (2017).
5. A. R. Harvey *et al.*, *Brain Res.* **1619**, 36 (2015).
6. O. Bondarenko and M. Saarma, *Front Cell Neurosci.* **15**, 682597 (2021).
7. C. Bjorkholm and L. M. Monteggia, *Neuropharmacology* **102**, 72 (2016).
8. C. Geral, A. Angelova and S. Lesieur, *Pharmaceutics* **5**, 127 (2013).
9. S. Kandalam *et al.*, *Acta Biomater.* **49**, 167 (2017).
10. S. Bathina and U. N. Das, *Arch. Med. Sci.* **11**, 1164 (2015).
11. A. Dekmak *et al.*, *Behav. Brain Res.* **340**, 49 (2018).
12. C. G. Song *et al.*, *Neural Regen. Res.* **13**, 1294 (2018).
13. E. Palasz *et al.*, *Int. J. Mol. Sci.* **21**, 1170 (2020).
14. Deng *et al.*, *Expert Opin. Biol. Ther.* **16**, 1025 (2016).
15. M. Wurzelmann, J. Romeika and D. Sun, *Neural Regen. Res.* **12**, 7 (2017).
16. I. Khalin *et al.*, *Int. J. Nanomed.* **10**, 3245 (2015).
17. T. K. Kim and J. H. Eberwine, *Anal. Bioanal. Chem.* **397**, 3173 (2010).
18. K. J. Lampe *et al.*, *J. Biomed. Mater. Res. A* **96**, 595 (2011).
19. I. Khalin *et al.*, *Drug. Deliv.* **23**, 3520 (2016).
20. J. Bertram *et al.*, *Pharm Res.* **27**, 82 (2010).
21. Y. Zhong and R. V. Bellamkonda, *J. R. Soc. Interface* **5**, 957 (2008).
22. P. Trucillo, *Processes* **9**, 470 (2021).
23. H. K. Makadia and S. J. Siegel, *Polymers (Basel)* **3**, 1377 (2011).
24. H. J. Byeon *et al.*, *Int. J. Nanomed.* **10**, 739 (2015).
25. J. Li and D. J. Mooney, *Nat. Rev. Mater.* **1**, 16071 (2016).
26. M. S. Davis *et al.*, *Osteoarthr. Cartilage Open* **2**, 100125 (2020).
27. A. Muheremu *et al.*, *Transl. Neurosci.* **12**, 494 (2021).
28. J. Sun and H. Tan, *Materials* **6**, 1285 (2013).
29. Q. Li *et al.*, *NPG Asia Mater.* **14**, 14 (2022).

30. S. Kumar *et al.*, *Nano LIFE* **5**, 1550004 (2015).
31. J. Barminko *et al.*, *Biotechnol. Bioeng.* **108**, 2747 (2011).
32. M. S. Davis *et al.*, *J. Mater. Sci. Nanotechnol.* **9**, 202 (2021).
33. M. S. Davis *et al.*, *Drug Deliv. Transl. Res.* **8**, 226 (2018).
34. Recombinant Human BDNF Protein, https://www.rndsystems.com/products/recombinant-human-bdnf-protein_248-bd.
35. T. Maguire, M. Davis, I. Marrero-Berrios, C. Zhu, C. Gaughan, J. Weinberg, D. Manchikalapati, J. Schianodi Cola, H. Kamath, R. Schloss and J. Yarmush, *Int. J. Anesthesiol. Pain Med.* **2**, 1 (2016).
36. J. Stetefeld, S. A. McKenna and T. R. Patel, *Biophys. Rev.* **8**, 409 (2016).
37. T. Li *et al.*, *Neuroreport* **20**, 295 (2009).
38. J. Yuan *et al.*, *Clin. Lab.* **63**, 1421 (2017).
39. S. Suzuki *et al.*, *Peptides* **89**, 42 (2017).
40. J. Xiong *et al.*, *Oncol. Rep.* **30**, 2719 (2013).
41. J. Houlton *et al.*, *Front. Neurosci.* **13**, 790 (2019).
42. M. Jahromi *et al.*, *J. Mol. Neurosci.* **71**, 746 (2021).
43. E. Vögelin *et al.*, *Exper. Neurol.* **199**, 348 (2006).
44. S. Senapati *et al.*, *Sig. Transd. Targeted Therapy* **3**, 7 (2018).
45. Y. Wu *et al.*, *Nanomaterials (Basel)* **12**, 904 (2022).
46. S. K. Sims *et al.*, *Neural. Plast.* **2022**, 3889300 (2022).
47. M. Xia *et al.*, *Iran. J. Pharm. Res.* **20**, 137 (2021).
48. B. Ghosh *et al.*, *J. Neurosci.* **38**, 5982 (2018).
49. D. J. Cook *et al.*, *J. Cereb. Blood Flow Metab.* **37**, 1030 (2017).
50. D. Santos *et al.*, *Brain Res.* **1636**, 93 (2016).
51. Y. Xu *et al.*, *J. Biomed. Mater. Res. B Appl. Biomater.* **105**, 1692 (2017).
52. A. Jarrahi *et al.*, *Biomedicines* **8**, 389 (2020).
53. M. Terashvili *et al.*, *Neuroscience* **223**, 68 (2012).
54. Y. R. Tsai *et al.*, *Int. J. Mole. Sci.* **19**, 3252 (2018).
55. N. Ismail *et al.*, *Oxidat. Med. Cellular Long.* **2016**, 1 (2016).
56. B. Morrison *et al.*, *Ann. Rev. Biomed. Eng.* **13**, 91 (2011).
57. U. Freudenberg *et al.*, *Biomaterials* **30**, 5049 (2009).
58. A. Angelova and B. Angelov, *Neural. Regen. Res.* **12**, 886 (2017).
59. S. J. Chan *et al.*, *Neurochem. Int.* **107**, 57 (2017).

https://doi.org/10.1142/9789819809028_0006

Chapter 6

A Review of Three Major Factors Controlling Carbon Nanotubes Synthesis from the Floating Catalyst Chemical Vapor Deposition*

Daniel Rui Chen[†,§], Megha Chitranshi[‡],
Mark Schulz[†] and Vesselin Shanov[†]

[†]*Department of Mechanical and Materials Engineering*
University of Cincinnati, OH 45221, USA
[‡]*Department of Electrical and Computer Engineering*
University of Cincinnati, OH 45212, USA
[§]*chenru@mail.uc.edu*

After the discovery of carbon nanotubes (CNTs) by Sumio Iijima in 1991, several methods have been developed to synthesize them. High-temperature techniques, such as laser ablation and arc discharge, are now replaced by a low-temperature technique like chemical vapor deposition (CVD). Floating catalyst chemical vapor deposition (FCCVD) method is extensively researched due to its ease of fabrication, mass production at low cost and high purity output. The motive of this paper is to discuss the influence of three major factors on the growth of CNTs using the FCCVD method, which can help us better understand the process of FCCVD as well as the potential challenges faced by this method.

Keywords: FCCVD; carbon nanotube synthesis; controlling factors.

---

*To cite this article, please refer to its earlier version published in the *Nano LIFE*, Vol. 9, No. 4 (2019) 1930002 (19 pages), DOI: 10.1142/S1793984419300024
§Corresponding author.

1. Introduction

Carbon nanotubes (CNTs) have been used in broad applications mainly due to their excellent electrical, mechanical and thermal properties.[1–4] The synthesis of CNTs also plays an important role in these applications because it dictates the chirality, porosity and other physical properties of the nanotubes. Earlier, three methods were used for CNTs synthesis: the arc discharge,[5] the laser ablation[6] and the chemical vapor deposition (CVD).[7–13] The arc discharge and the laser ablation methods are used mainly for single-walled nanotubes (SWNTs) synthesis and CVD method for multi-walled nanotubes (MWNTs). Synthesis methods like laser ablation and arc discharge have low yield and contain impurities as amorphous carbon, while CVD offers a controlled synthesis process for industrial applications. CVD is further divided into two categories: fixed catalyst CVD and substrate-based CVD, which involve catalyst deposition on the substrate and FCCVD which synthesizes nanotubes in the vapor phase.[14] In the substrate-based CVD technique, a thin layer of transition metal is deposited on to the support layer and then both layers will be deposited on the substrate. The reaction mixture containing a hydrocarbon source and inert gas is carried into the CVD furnace at temperatures ranging from 600°C to 1200°C. In the FCCVD technique, a catalyst, such as a ferrocene, is injected in the gas phase along with the carbon source. The comparison of these four methods is listed in Table 1. Basic floating catalyst chemical vapor deposition (FCCVD) method mainly consists of five steps, which are illustrated in Fig. 1: in step A, catalyst source decomposes into small nanoparticles, these small nanoparticles start to coalesce and form bigger particle size in step B, the significance of the sulfur is characterized by its ability to assist the growth of CNTs in steps C and D, and during step E, CNTs are macroscopically collected by a rotating drum. FCCVD overcomes all the problems by providing high yield at low temperature and low-cost.[9,15–17]

Many studies showed that sulfur improves the growth mechanism of CNTs by removing blocking groups and stabilizes the growing edge of CNTs.[10,19,20] The role of sulfur is associated with surface chemistry,

Table 1. The comparison of various CNTs synthesis techniques.

Synthesis method	Process	Operating temperature	Source	Advantages	Disadvantages	References
Arc-discharge	High purity graphite electrodes, high purity He and Ar gases,	Above 1700°C	Graphite	Simple, inexpensive	High temperature and energy, and less control over the alignment.	5,14
Laser ablation	High-power laser vaporization, Ar atmosphere	500–1000°C	Pure graphite	High yield and low metallic impurities.	Short reaction time, tangled nanotubes	6,14
CVD	Thin film deposition	700–1200°C	Hydrocarbon source	Simple process, controllable, scalable industrial production.	Batch processing, non-continuous production	7,12,14
Floating catalyst CVD	Gas-phase pyrolysis	1100–1400°C	Hydrocarbon source	High purity output, continuous process	Low efficiency, Low yield	9,14–16,18

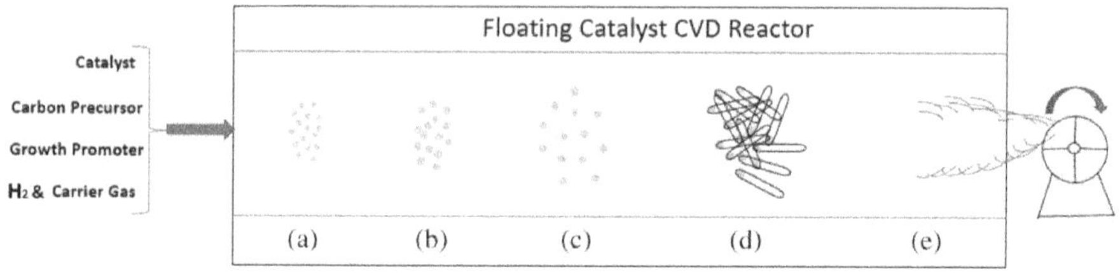

Fig. 1. Schematic diagram of CNTs growth in the FCCVD reactor: (a) The formation of the catalyst nanoparticles; (b) The collision of the nanoparticles to form bigger size particles; (c) The coating of the sulfur on catalyst particles; (d) The growth of the CNTs; (e) The CNTs collection process in the lab setting.

nucleation, renucleation and the aerogel formation of the catalyst nanoparticles. As CNTs grow, they bundle due to van der Waals force and these bundles link to form an aerogel which is later drawn from the reactor and winded onto winding drum.[20] The amount of sulfur in carbon feedstock can also result in single, double and multi-walled nanotubes.[12] However, the underlying mechanisms have solemnly been explored, both kinetically and thermodynamically, which are both very essential for us to unravel how sulfur actually "promotes" the synthesis process.

In FCCVD method, different hydrocarbon sources have been used to synthesize nanotubes. Different pyrolysis temperature and chemical structure affect the morphology of CNTs. The synthesis of CNTs using methane and toluene showed that the CNTs fibers synthesized by toluene were stronger and had fewer impurities compared to methane because toluene has a low break down temperature.[21] The flow rate of carrier gases, such as hydrogen[21] and nitrogen,[22] during synthesis process controls the retention time, or residence time in the reactor, where the formation of the catalyst nanoparticles collision to form bigger particles and growth of the CNTs occur. The low flow rate results in a larger diameter of catalyst particles, whereas higher flow rates result in smaller diameter particles due to the smaller collision probability of catalyst nanoparticles.[23,24] Although hydrocarbon and catalyst have a similar effect on the CNTs growth in substrate-based CVD, without the consideration of concepts, such as residence time, particles collision, or gas flow rate, a lack of continuous process and scale-up potential of substrated-based CVD has left researchers to explore more in FCCVD, the complexity of FCCVD also makes it as one of the very unique methods that require a three-dimensional parameter space rather than a linear correlation, in order to predict or have a better control of final product. On that account, we strive to collect the latest scientific publication, especially ones from credible sources, in order to present a better picture, try to build the connections between these three key factors (sulfur, hydrocarbon, catalyst), and pave the way for the future research in FCCVD method.

2. The role of sulfur

It has been known that sulfur is a crucial material in terms of successfully synthesizing CNTs through FCCVD and numerous evidences suggested that CNTs aerogel is simply not being formed without the presence of sulfur. Sulfur was being called "growth promoter" and was commonly used for 45 latest publications,[21,25,26] although one research group claimed the possibility of producing direct-spun products without the assistance of the sulfur, there was no valid approval from the people who attempted to replicate the experiment by using the same equipment setup.[21] The effect of sulfur as a growth promoter was also identified in other CNTs synthesis methods, such as arc discharge method, to increase the CNTs yield.[27] In majority of the publications, sulfur demonstrated the capability of controlling the product type and ratio (SWNTs versus MWNTs), increasing the diameter range of the CNTs, facilitation of the CNTs synthesis at a lower temperature as well as the ability to stabilize the nascent growth edge of CNTs.[7,8,15,28–30]

2.1. *Sulfur as growth promoter*

Various chemical compounds have been used in the recent literature, for the delivery of sulfur component to the CNTs synthesis, commonly used compounds are thiophene (C_4H_4S),[9,16,31] carbon disulfide (CS_2).[32] In the early stage of the FCCVD reaction, thiophane/carbon disulfide decomposes earlier than ferrocene (commonly used chemical compounds for catalyst) due to its low bonding energy between the sulfur atom and carbon atom, the resultant products are hydrocarbon species and liberated sulfur atoms, these liberated sulfur atoms form a thin layer of coating on the surface of the metallic catalyst,[33] which is the later decomposition product of ferrocene. This has dual purposes that are both beneficial to the growth of CNTs, first the sulfur surfactant prevents the encapsulation of carbon particle, which could lead to the early catalyst poisoning or the phenomenon called "carbon choking",[34] the sulfur-coated catalyst particles also prevent themselves from agglomerating with each other. However, the prevention of catalyst particle coarsening by collision is still under debate,[35] but the general conclusion is that the coarsening was not prevented completely, the coated particle may not coarsen as frequently as the noncoated one.[36]

The sulfur coating layer dissolves less amount of carbon, therefore serving as the barrier for carbon transport, the best example is that sufficient amount of sulfur is added into molten steel to prevent the oxidation and carbonization of the steel.[10]

According to the CVD process of CNTs growth mechanism suggested by Baker and Harris,[30] the whole process consists of four steps: in the first step, the carbon atoms are dissociated from hydrocarbon source as the result of the high temperature; in the second step, the carbon atoms dissolve into molten iron catalyst and precipitate to the rear end to form filament, due to the supply of carbon which is faster than the bulk diffusion, the majority of the carbon diffuses through surface rather than bulk diffusion to achieve the precipitation; therefore in the third step, the bulk diffusion becomes insignificant, and surface diffusion dominates the carbon transportation to form the CNTs; in the final step, the deactivation and termination of tubes growth occurs. Dai *et al.*[37] also proposed that carbon forms a hemispherical graphene cap (yarmulke) on the catalyst particle, CNTs grow from the cap, which is summarized as "Yarmulke mechanism". The Yarmulke mechanism can be used to explain the CNTs growth mechanism of CVD and HiPco (High-pressure carbon monoxide method) method,[38,39] note that HiPco has been demonstrated as a method to mass-produce high-purity SWNTs, by flowing CO on Fe catalyst clusters, it was introduced by a research group from the Rice University.[40]

In the FCCVD method, it is believed that sulfur enhances the bending of small-cap of nascent CNTs formation, which further validates the Yarmulke mechanism, sulfur is capable of stabilizing the unsaturated sp^2 orbitals of the edge of the graphene layer by overlapping with the metal orbitals,[46] the anchoring of the graphitic layers introduce defect, this defect will serve as the nucleation site for the growth, five member carbon rings start to form in the defect center and lead to the bending of the graphitic layers,[29] with the help of incoming carbon supply, tubular carbon filament keeps growing until the termination occurs or catalyst is being deactivated.

2.2. *Sulfur and island mechanism*

In order to understand the role of sulfur, two major viewpoints are pointed out: (1) the delay of the catalysts, which was explained in Sec. 2.1, before the reaction zone; as well as (2) the temperature gradient during the whole reaction, promote the growth of the catalyst particles by collision, from atomic nuclei to nano-size particles. In the closed-loop reactor which used the HiPco method, since small and stabilized catalyst particle can be obtained for the growth of SWNT without any delay, also in most of the substrate CNTs growth, catalysts are static and sufficient for the CNTs growth, therefore sulfur is not seen to be beneficial in these methods.[18]

Based on the surfactant nature of sulfur in liquid iron combined with the evidence from high solution TEM and EELS, sulfur liquid forms the outer shell of the catalyst particles.[42] This outer shell can be a series of dispersed islands, or complete coverage, which is dependent upon the S/Fe molar ratio as well as the temperature of the reaction, there were a number of publications which indicated the synthesis of SWNTs with notable smaller diameter, in comparison with the diameter of their active catalyst nanoparticle, with S/Fe molar ratios in the range of 0.002–0.4.[18,43–46] This phenomenon is further explained by the island mechanism proposed by Ren *et al.*[18] and

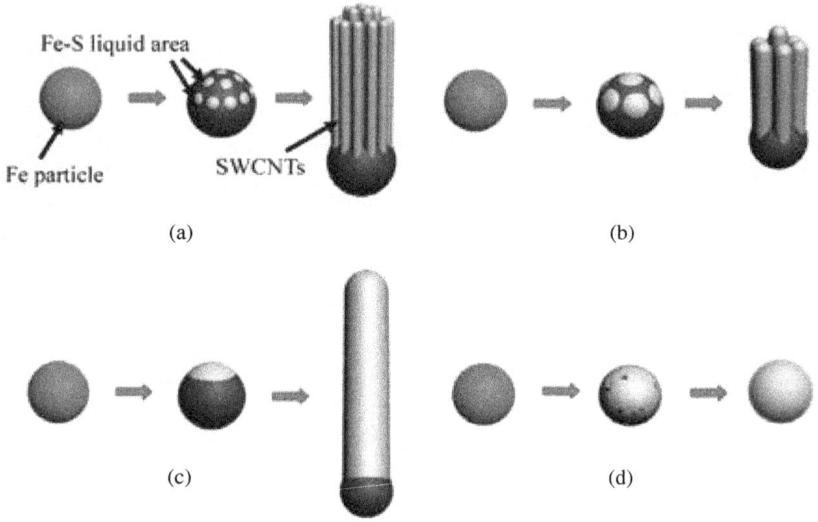

Fig. 2. Schematic of the growth mechanism by controlling the concentration of thiophane,[33] from (a)–(d), sulfur gradually increases its concentration on the surface of the catalyst particle, the low solubility of carbon in sulfur leads to the CNTs precipitation, bigger CNTs diameter formed as a result of ever-increasing sulfur concentration, the complete sulfur coverage eventually causes the catalyst poisoning. (Adapted with permission from Yu *et al.*[33] © 2012 Elsevier)

Yu *et al.*,[33] by adjusting the concentration of the sulfur, the diameter of SWNTs can be controlled from ~1.0 nm to ~5.8 nm.[34]

The island growth mechanism is illustrated in Fig. 2. From (a)–(d), with the increase of S/Fe molar ratio, the surface coverage of sulfur on catalyst particle is getting larger, from small dispersed island to full coverage, which causes the diameter change of the CNTs. Low solubility of carbon in sulfur, as well as the capability of sulfur stabilizing nascent CNTs growth edge, both promote the growth the CNTs, note that temperature gradient further assists the graphitic precipitation, keeping in mind that these nano-scale particles can have a lower melting point due to Gibbs–Thomas effect,[47] therefore the onset temperature of melting and immiscible formation of Fe and S is lower, compared with their bulk phase counterpart, which indicates the existent of the minimum critical operating temperature for CNTs aerogel formation.[26] Although some established theory stated that the diameter of the CNTs is correlated with the size of catalyst particle,[48,49] it is more likely that, in the FCCVD method, the synergistic interplay between sulfur concentration and catalytic particle size determines the final diameter of the CNTs. Note that there is a linear correlation between the wall number and the diameter of the CNTs.[11]

According to Yu *et al.*,[33] thiophene promotes the growth of MWNTs and restricts the formation of SWNTs, between the temperature range of 1000–1100°C, while the same concentration of thiophene did not show the same effect at higher temperature, with the only observation of SWNTs, however, this paper stated the general trend showing the addition of thiophene leads to the CNTs with large diameter or MWNTS. The formation of SWNTs and MWNTs are also dependent on the temperature of the reaction.[50] For instance, Li *et al.*[51] discovered that by increasing the furnace temperature, the corresponding tensile strength of the materials show major improvement, which correlates the increase in the number of MWNTs, compared with SWNTs. Similarly, Hou *et al.*[52] found the trend of CNTs morphology shift from SWNTs to MWNTs, from synthesis temperature 1150–1500°C, coupled with the increase rate in thermal pyrolysis and soot formation in the final products. Many physical properties of the CNTs have been related to the diameter of the tube, such as the electrical, thermal and mechanical properties of CNTs, by controlling the diameter of the CNTs, the physical properties of CNTs can be fine-tuned.[53,54]

2.3. *The role of sulfur in thermodynamics*

Sulfur has negligible carbon solubility and is capable of lowering the surface energy of the catalyst particle, the depression of the surface energy ($\Delta\sigma$) can be expressed as $\Delta\sigma = \mathrm{RT}\Gamma \ln(1 + \mathrm{K}\alpha_s)$ ($\Gamma = 1.16 \times 10^{-5}$ mole/m^2 is the maximum concentration of surface, which was first calculated by Halden and Kingery,[55] α_s is the chemical activity of the sulfur in the iron, $\mathrm{K}\alpha_s = \theta_s/(1 - \theta_s)$, where θ_s is the fractional of the sulfur in iron surface), the mathematic relationship between the percentage of sulfur and a decrease in surface energy is indicated in this equation, note that temperature plays another important role in the change of surface energy.

According to the statement from the classical nucleation theory (CNT),[56] the free energy barrier for the homogeneous nucleation ΔG is a summation of two terms, which are the bulk-free energy (=4/3 $\pi r^3 \Delta g$, "r" is the radius of embryo or nucleus, "Δg" is the volume free energy), and the interfacial free energy (=$4\pi r^2 \sigma$, "σ" is specific surface free energy). In the bulk-free energy term, Δg is defined by the volume-free energy difference between two-phases: namely, the nucleated phase (solid-phase) and the phase that nucleation occurs (liquid-phase), because Δg_{solid} is smaller than Δg_{liquid}, the bulk free energy is a negative term, while interface free energy term is a positive term and σ is the surface tension between the nucleus and its surroundings. During the nucleation process, the retarding energy from surface free energy change compensate the driving energy, which is from volume free energy change, when the size of the particle is smaller than critical nucleus size, retarding energy dominates and causes the particle shrinkage, however, when the particle size is bigger than the critical nucleus, the driving energy dominate and particles grow.

According to the effect of sulfur, lower the surface free energy, which is explained before, with the addition of sulfur, the retarding energy reduces correspondingly, as the result of this, based on the classical nucleation theory, the critical nucleus size shifts to a smaller size, the implication is that the population of the nuclei increases, the size distribution of nuclei becomes narrower, which means the growth of CNTs more likely occurs at an earlier stage and the morphology of CNT is more consistent.

According to Fig. 3, the energy barrier is decreases in the presence of sulfur, and the critical nucleus size has seen reduction both at a temperature of 750°C and 1250°C, which has been explained in the first and second paragraph of this section. The free energy nucleus curve is temperature-dependent, the size of the critical nucleus increases under the higher temperature, the nucleation rate decreases with the increase in the temperature because the increase of vapor pressure leads to the decrease of supersaturation ratio, therefore

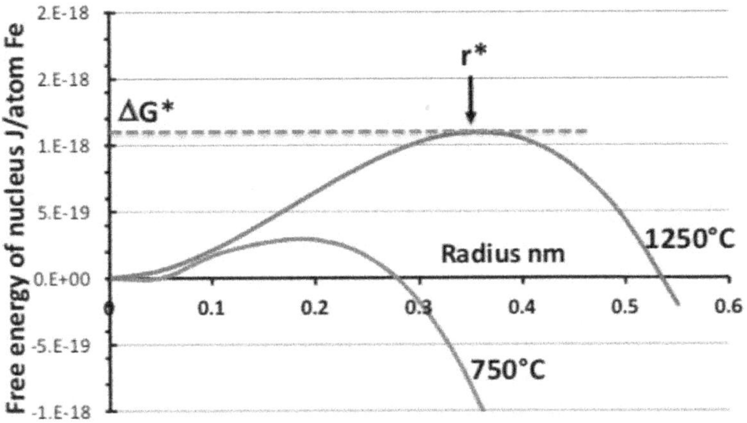

(a)

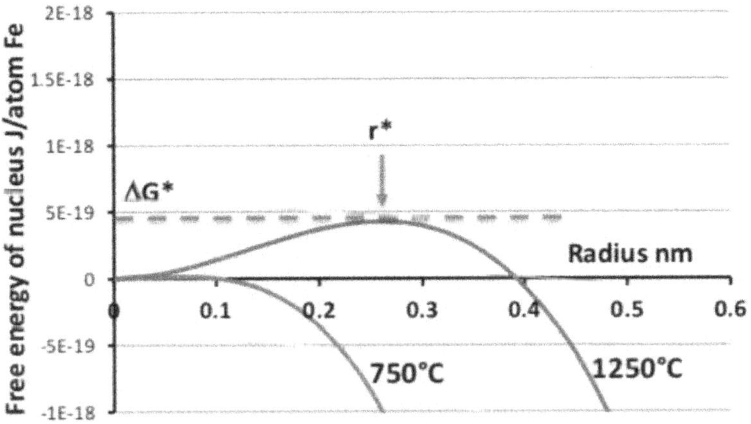

(b)

Fig. 3. Free energy plot for nucleation of iron particles without the presence of sulfur (a), and with the presence of sulfur (b).[58]

leading to the increase of the critical nucleus size, in order for the driving force to counterbalance the retarding force, which explains why the critical nucleation particle size at 1250°C is bigger than the particle size at 750°C.[57]

The graphs also hinted the importance of the reaction heating rate, if the reaction is instantly heated to 1250°C, the rate of iron particles nucleation is very small, since the probability of an initial collision of two atoms to form stable nucleus is very small theoretically under the fast heating rate, according to the Arrhenius equation. Also if increasing the temperature of the reaction from 750°C to 1250°C instantly, after slow heating to 750°C the stable formed nucleus at 750°C will reevaporate, however, if the growth of the nucleated particle can keep up with the rate of the temperature, one would expect larger diameter nuclei distribution. Overall, one can conjecture that if sufficient slow heating is provided, the nuclues with a larger diameter will be formed, thus the CNTs are formed with a large diameter.[58]

The significant drop of the activation energy proves the importance of the sulfur for helping the nucleation of Fe particles, especially in the temperature region above 1000°C, which is normally used as the temperature for FCCVD method.

2.4. *Hoecker's experiment*

In a paper published by Hoecker *et al.*,[19] a series of experiments conducted by one Cambridge research group show that the successful synthesis of direct-spun aerogel, which consists of interconnected CNTs, relies more on critical mass concentration (CMC), which is defined as the total mass input at the entrance of the FCCVD furnace, rather than critical particle number concentration and particle size, which is considered important in the substrate-based CVD process. The early catalyst particles nucleation within the hot zone before the evaporation, as well as the renucleation event at the outlet, are directly associated to the successful synthesis of CNTs, albeit the previous experiment shows that $d_{p,\text{mean}} \approx 15\,\text{nm}$ is ideal size and the major source for the CNTs nucleation and growth. The successful synthesis of much larger ($d_{p,\text{mean}} > 100\,\text{nm}$) catalyst particle size has been proven to be possible. This indicated the important role played by the CMC during the synthesis, this universally applied CMC decoupled with catalyst particle size/number that normally required for the successful synthesis of CNTs, which provides the paradigm shift for the CNT synthesis, more flexibility can be given to novel reactor design, morphology control, purity control as well as the improvement of the production yield.[19]

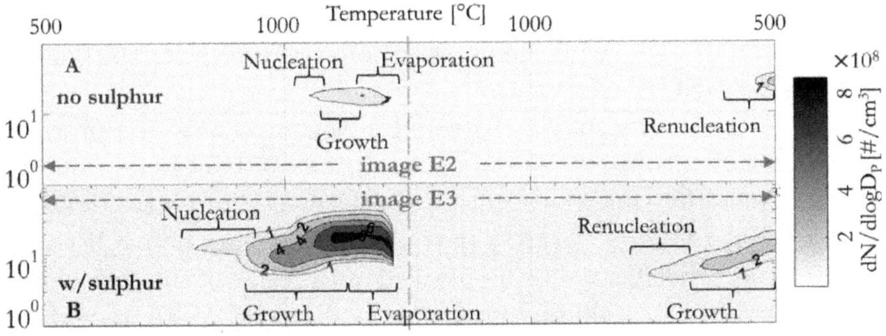

Fig. 4. The comparison of the catalyst particles distribution without the presence of sulfur (a) and with the presence of sulfur (b) along the axis of the reactor.[19] (Adapted with permission from Hoecker *et al.*[19] © 2017 Scientific Reports).

The experiment was conducted by the same group by using ceramic filter placed inside the furnace at different positions, they were able to track and map the particle concentration profile, it shows that with the help of sulfur, catalyst particles are able to nucleate as well as renucleate within the hot zone of the reactor in a relatively large quantity, as sulfur hastens the renucleation of catalyst particles at the downstream region of reactor, the onset point of renucleation starts to shift more toward the hotter zone (> 1200°C) of the reactor, where CNTs synthesis can occur rapidly due to the higher temperature, from Fig. 4, the catalyst particle concentration profile has shown significant discrepancy from A without sulfur to B with sulfur, sufficient concentration of catalyst particles provide the condition necessary for the forming of large quantity of long CNTs, which can not only lead to the spinnable CNTs aerogels, the mechanical and electrical properties of the CNTs, but can also be improved because of the longer individual CNTs.

2.5. *The other sources of growth promoter*

The major source of sulfur are thiophene and CS_2 rather than solid sulfur compounds such as pure sulfur or gaseous state such as H_2S, the reason being liquid solvent thiophene and CS_2 can be easily dissolved in other carbon-containing organic compounds, the concentration of sulfur in the fuel can be precisely adjusted.[59] Thiophene mainly decomposes between the temperature of 800°C and 900°C,[43] with the boiling point of 84°C, while CS_2 shows more volatility with the boiling point below 50°C.[59]

The difference is also demonstrated in the decomposition process, the sulfur radicals from CS_2 can cover the catalyst particles rapidly, which render the smaller catalyst particle inactive due to its small surface area, the large catalyst particles may remain active because not all the active sites are being blocked, as a result of this, the chiral selectivity of CNTs shifts toward large diameter, with regard to the decomposition of thiophane, in addition to the sulfur radicals, hydrogen is also a product of the decomposition, hydrogen reacts with sulfur, i.e., on the surface of the catalyst particles to form hydrogen sulfide, which is a gas form, thus active site (the place that being covered by sulfur before) can be survived and the chiral selective shifts to small diameter CNTs.[59]

In fact, another group 16 elements, such as Selenium (Se), Tellurium (Te) or even Oxygen (O), have the same properties as sulfur that can stabilize the edge of newly formed CNTs structure, according to the Gibbs–Langmuir model, for the isotherms and segregation of solutes, it has been shown that surface coverage of the catalyst particles for group 16 elements is below 0.03%.[60–63] The high interfacial energy of Fe-S-X alloy system helps the extrusion of the graphitic layer to form the tubular shape, the diameter and number of layers can also be controlled by increasing the ratio of X (Se, Te, O)/C, the X/C ratio is essential for the understanding of the FCCVD reaction and the optimization of the CNT morphology.[63] According to the principle based on the group 16 assisted CNTs growth, the incoming carbon is determined by the size of catalyst surface as well as the carbon solubility, which can be expressed as $C_{\text{incoming}} = (D^2 * \pi)^*\text{s}$ (D is the diameter of the catalyst particle), whereas the extruded C can be expressed as $C_{\text{extruded}} = (D * \pi) * n * L$ (n is the layer of the CNTs, L is the length of the tube), when the equilibrium is reached, C_{incoming} will be equal to C_{extruded}, therefore solubility is proportional to n/D because Se has half the solubility of S in C, therefore, the n/D of Se is half the n/D of S, this can be further validated by experimental results from Fig. 5.[63]

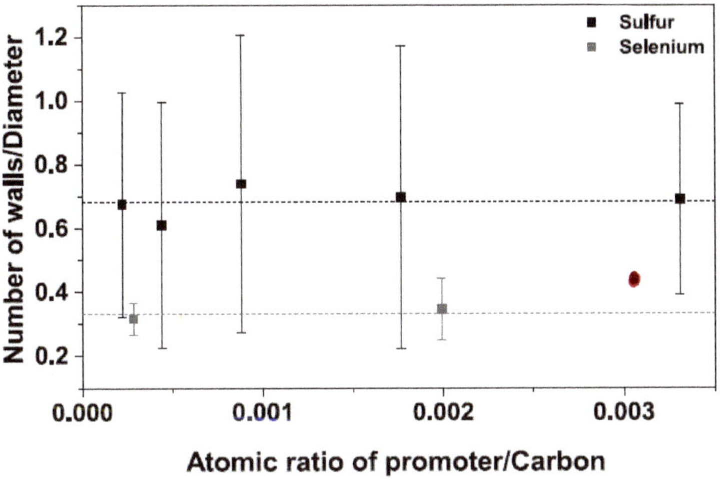

Fig. 5. The relationship between n/D and the atomic ratio of promoter/carbon of Sulfur and Selenium as a promotor, n/D of sulfur is shown twice of the value of n/D of selenium under the same atomic ratio.[63] (Adapted with permission from Mas *et al.*[63] © 2016 Carbon).

By replacing S with Se, the toughness of the CNTs can also potentially be enhanced due to the large interface between elements, which is explained by the data in Fig. 5, it shows that CNT with Se as promoter has larger diameter than one with S as promoter, larger diameter, in turn, increases the area of the overlapping surface, these large overlapping interfaces provide sufficient space for the shear stress transfer in the elastic regime, as well as CNTs sliding when shear strength is exceeded.[57] The potential applications include high tensile strength fiber or sheets.

3. The effect of hydrocarbon precursor

The source of hydrocarbon is another determining factor with respect to the type, morphology, as well as the crystallinity of CNTs synthesized, hydrocarbon precursor commonly can exist in two forms: namely, the liquid form as well as the gas form, and the decomposition products pertaining to the chemical structure of hydrocarbon precursor, therefore hydrogen-rich precursor generates more hydrogen

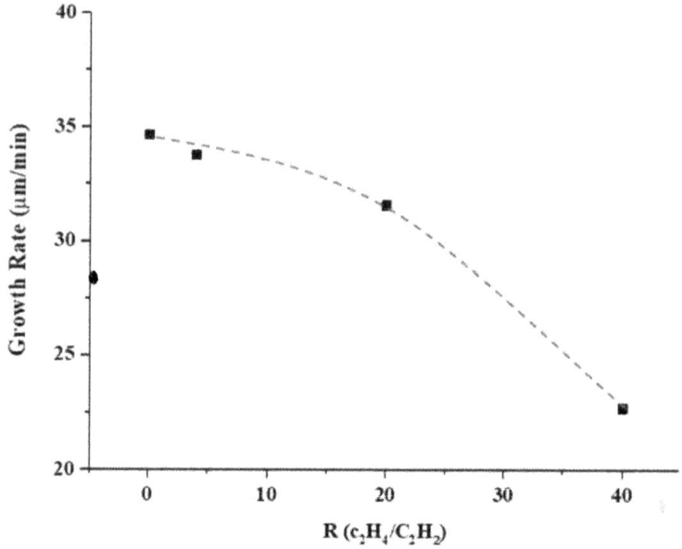

(a)

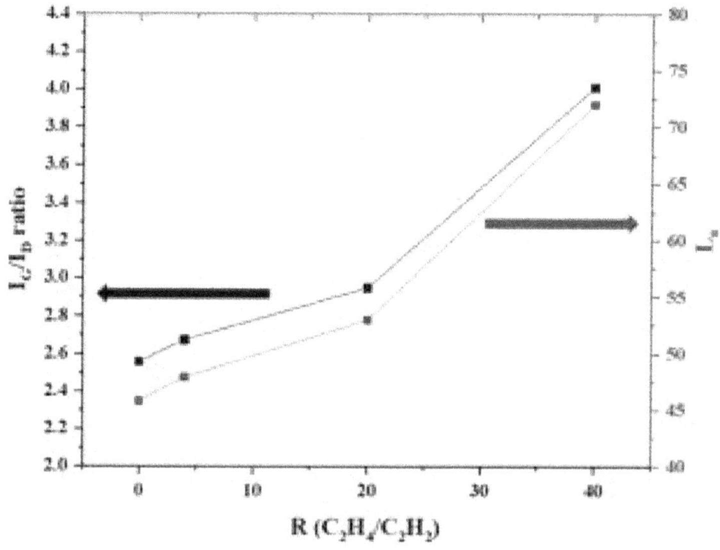

(b)

Fig. 6. The relationship between (a) CNT growth time and the ratio of C_2H_4/C_2H_2 used during the CNT synthesis; (b) I_G/I_D ratio and the ratio of C_2H_4/C_2H_2 used during the CNT synthesis.[64] (Adapted with permission from Moon *et al.*[64] © 2018 RSC Advances).

atoms, hydrogen atoms can break the unsaturated bonds on the surface of catalyst particles, the formation of C–H bonds can also cause the delay of CNTs growth, this structural transformation ultimately leads to the CNTs that have more crystallinity and high I_G/I_D ratio,[64] this principle can be applied in both CVD and FCCVD process.

3.1. *The effect on the chiral selectivity*

Among diverse types of carbon precursors, diameter and chiral angle distribution of CNTs can be influenced by the chemical structures of the precursors, which in fact determine the strength of C–C bonds as well as the decomposition temperatures of precursor. The chirality is one of the important characteristics of CNTs structure that depends on how the tube is rolled from a graphene sheet, a pair of integers (n, m) is used to describe how the tube of CNTs spans the circumference by using the two-dimensional-based lattice vectors, the chiral indices assuming the tube can extend indefinitely, which is only an ideal physical state.[65–67] Depending on the different chirality, CNTs exhibit both metallic and semiconducting characteristics, when the condition $n - m = 3i$ (where i is an integer) is satisfied, such as armchair CNTs, in which chiral indices n equal to m, behaves as metallic CNTs, however, zigzag CNTs can behave either metallic or semiconducting.[68] Based on the quantum mechanics, the bandgap is inversely proportional with the diameter of the tube,[69] large-diameter CNTs ($> 10\,\text{nm}$) therefore have small bandgap and exhibit metallic properties.

There are several ways to improve the chiral selectivity in the CVD process, such as by using high melting temperature catalyst to suppress the Ostwald ripening as well as using bi-metal catalyst approach,[70–72] basically there are two major mechanisms for particle size change, one is coalescence among catalyst particles, another one is Ostwald ripening,[73] the first one increases the catalyst particle size and decreases the number density, whereas the second one reduces the size of the small particles, but increases the size of the large particles. Because of Ostwald ripening, small catalyst particles disappear, while large particle gets larger and becomes inactive by suppressing the Ostwald ripening. The growth of the SWNTs with narrow chiral distribution can be preserved. CoMoCAT synthesis sets a new standard for synthesizing SWNTs with narrow and small chirality distribution.[74]

The strong temperature gradient of the reactor in FCCVD process leaves a narrow time window to the Ostwald ripening of the catalyst particles, the co-influence of the pyrolytic temperature of hydrocarbon precursor and the growth of the catalyst particles provide the condition for the CNTs nucleation with the narrow chiral distribution. According to Artyukov *et al.*, the hydrocarbon precursor that has low decomposition temperature, e.g., ethanol ($\sim 750^\circ$C) and toluene ($\sim 780^\circ$C), the interaction free energy between the CNTs and catalyst particles dictate the configuration or the arrangement of the CNTs nucleated, in this case, the near armchair or zig-zag chirality is preferred.[75] Other explanations according to Hedman *et al.* stress that the thermodynamic stability of the tube plays an important role in controlling the chirality.[76] Based on the model proposed by Artyukov *et al.*, the ratio of armchair/zig-zag for ethanol can be as large as 7, while the ratio is 3 for toluene, via the Boltzmann factor, the estimated contact energy difference is 90 meV determined for Ni and Co, Fe catalyst particle.[65–75] But this estimation method proposed by Artyukov has been criticized for ignoring the reactive influence of the hydroxyl radicals, hydroxyl radicals can help to increase the crystallinity by etching out the amorphous carbon.[77]

A different study has shown similar results that by using ethanol and toluene, the SWNTs synthesized have a narrower distribution of chirality, in which 90% are armchair. Although DWNTs have been rarely synthesized, the DWNTs synthesized by toluene have unusual narrow inter-tube distance. Compared with ethanol and toluene, methane produces mainly double-walled CNTs with broader chirality distribution, prioritized by the chirality that has the fastest kinetic growth rates in the kinetic-limited regime.[65] Another research group found different H_2 concentration could affect the collision frequency of catalyst particles to form different catalyst crystal structure, the epitaxial relationship between catalyst crystalline surface and carbon

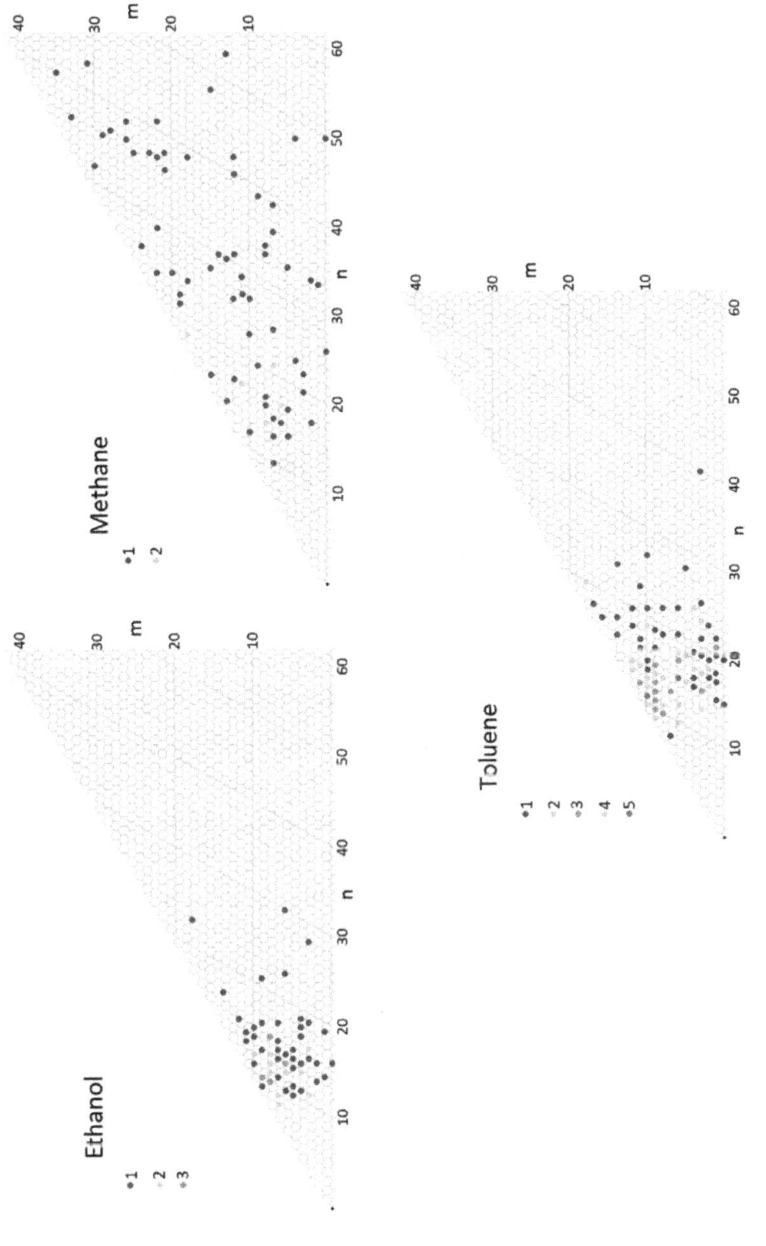

Fig. 7. Chirality distribution map of SWNTs by using Ethanol, Methane, and Toluene as carbon precursor, the sample size for each are 74 (ethanol), 77 (methane) and 152 (toluene), respectively.[65] (Adapted with permission from Barnard *et al.*[65] © Royal Society of Chemistry).

atoms determine the chiral selectivity of the CNTs.[78] Based on the first principle and density functional theory, it has been found that high concentration H_2 helps the transition of the iron catalytic particle from BCC to FCC structure,[79] this phase change plays a major role in the chirality transformation from semiconducting SWNTs to metallic SWNTs.

Overall, chiral selectivity in FCCVD method is a complex physical and chemical process, it is also the most challenging one, among various other parameters of CNTs, such as diameters, number of walls and length, although there are various established approaches in substrate-based CVD to control the chirality, in FCCVD, the scientific publication in this area has fallen short, the common consensus is that the interfacial energy between carbon atoms and catalyst particle dictates the formation of different chirality, however, many factors, such as the species of the hydrocarbon precursor, and their decomposition temperature, as well as the crystal structure of the catalyst particle, make the analysis and prediction more difficult.

3.2. *Critical hydrocarbon precursors*

The common notion is that when carbon precursors are absorbed on the surface of the catalyst, the precursor is dissociated and a closed carbon network transforms into the "CNT cap", then the continual growth of CNT is perpetuated by the formation of carbon precipitation from the catalyst underneath the "CNT cap", the growth stops when the catalyst termination occurs.[80] It has been found that preheating the carbonaceous feedstock before being delivered into the reactor can accelerate the rate of the CNTs formation by the factor of 20.[81,82] It is believed that the pre-thermal treatment can generate volatile organic compounds (VOCs), and some VOCs can enhance the CNTs formation while others degrade the CNTs quality.[83–85] The formation of VOCs are common both in substrate-based CVD and FCCVD. In the FCCVD method, VOCs are the by-products of hydrocarbon precursor breakdown, those that are not able to contribute to the growth of the CNTs, including carbon, encapsulated catalyst nanoparticle, amorphous carbon deposits, badly formed carbon tubules and soot,[25] these VOCs add more impurity to the CNTs product.

VOCs can also be in gas form, one of the most likely is carbon monoxide (CO), CO serves as a carbon sink along with compound like carbon dioxide (CO_2), theoretically, methane and methanol should perform equally as hydrocarbon precursor for CNT growth, since they contain the same amount of C per unit molecule, but only methane can produce direct-spun product, the reason is that 90% of C is released from the methanol decomposition forms CO, and rest converts to methane that contributes to the CNT growth, meanwhile methane has much higher C content to be used for CNT production.[86–88]

Acetylene is also one of the VOCs generated during the pyrolysis process, the study shows via the secondary decomposition of hydrocarbon, acetylene continues to decompose and produce one order of magnitude of CNTs more growth than propylene, acetylene can accomplish successful SWNTs growth without the assistance of plasma, however, the acetylene becomes more stable under the higher temperature, whereas other hydrocarbon species get unstable at the same temperature range, therefore critical temperature window is required in order for acetylene to proceed with the pyrolysis process.[44,89,90] Some other VOCs with O-containing species have an etchant role to preserve the catalytic activity, as a replacement for H_2, in Zhang *et al.*[91] research work, the deactivated iron catalyst nanoparticle can be reactivated after reacting with H_2 and water vapor, water vapor reactivates the catalyst nanoparticle by etching away amorphous carbon at high temperature.

It is also important to know what the "critical precursor" molecule is, by the "critical precursor" it means the hydrocarbon components can be fully utilized in the CNTs nucleation process, the importance of understanding of the "critical precursor" is demonstrated in the following three points:

(1) the avoidance of the preheat treatment could potentially reduce the total energy consumption of the CNTs synthesis,[92] (2) the conversion efficiency of carbon precursor to CNTs mass also needs

to be improved,[93] (3) the result can be the reduction in the formation of unintended by-products.[94]

According to Plata *et al.*,[80] it is possible to use many alkynes (e.g., acetylene, methyl acetylene, and vinyl acetylene) to accelerate the CNTs formation, furthermore the pre-thermal treatment of feedstock gases (e.g., C_2H_4/H_2) can also be avoided to prevent the generation of the VOCs that could degrade the CNTs quality, which brings forth not only the reduction in energy cost, but also the decrease in unwanted formation of byproducts (e.g., toxic and greenhouse gases). It is also reported that polycyclic aromatic hydrocarbons (PAHs), such as Naphthalene, Fluoranthenem and Pyrene, have the reduction of 20-, 60- and 40-fold, respectively.[95] Although fluoranthene is believed to be a very important carbon compound for the CNTs nucleation, based on the resemblance between fluoranthene and CNTs cap, most PAHs are toxic and highly flammable.[96]

3.3. *The importance of the hydrogen gas*

H_2 is considered as the most important and common gas used in FCCVD system, it plays various leading roles during the synthesis, these roles can be specified as preserving catalyst lifetime[97] helping breakdown of the hydrocarbon precursors,[51] not only H_2 acts as carrier gas, H_2 can also be generated during the synthesis, excess amount of H_2 cause concerns about the safe operation of the reactor,

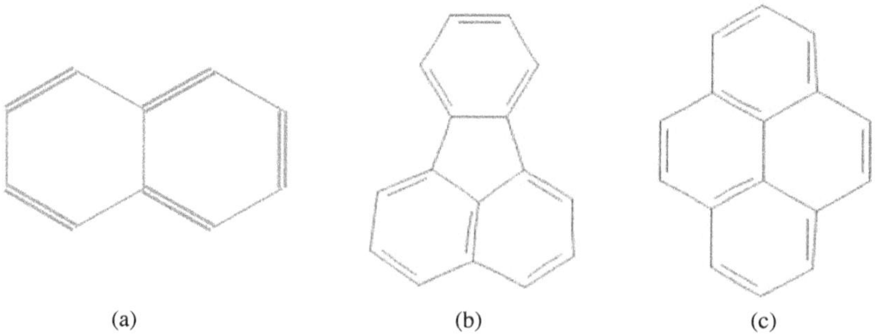

Fig. 8. The 2D chemical structure of resultant PAHs: (a) Naphthalene; (b) Fluoranthenem; (c) Pyrene.[96]

the exploration of using 100% inert gas (Ar,[98,99] N_2[100,101]) or the mixture of inert gas with H_2 has been realized by several groups.

It has been believed that pyrolysis products from the inert environment may be different from the H_2 environment, the formation of particular pyrolysis products may have assisted the formation of the direct-spun CNTs.[102] The mixture of H_2 with inert gas needs different C to H molar input to synthesize direct-spun

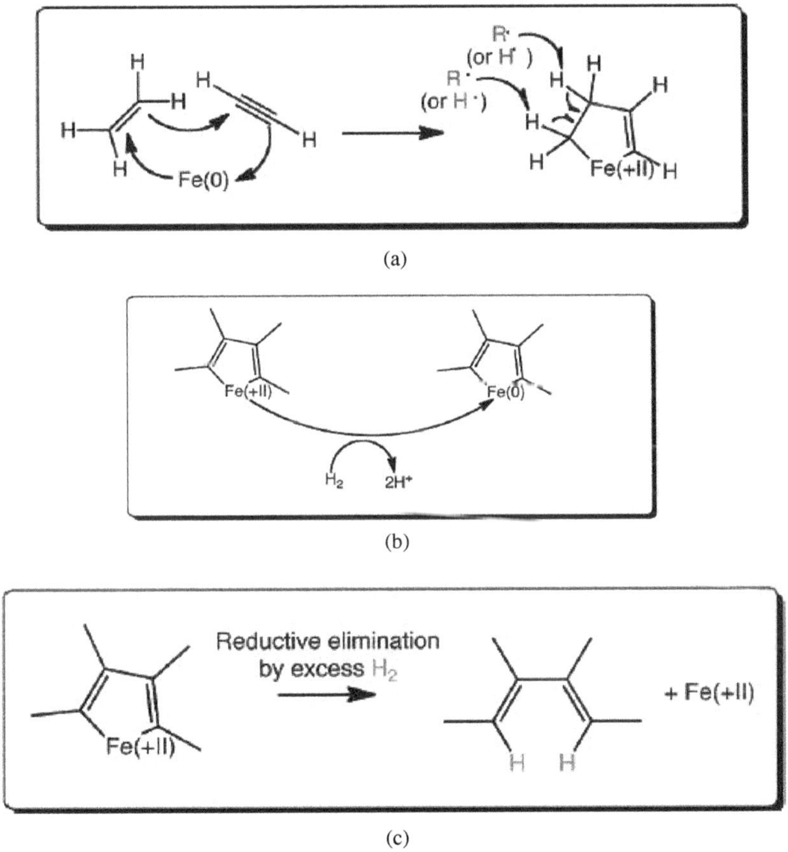

Fig. 9. (a) The diagram shows that ethylene reacts with acetylene to form a metallacycle intermediate; (b) The hydrogen acts as a reductive agent to regulate the lifetime of the catalyst; (c) An excessive amount of hydrogen terminates the chain propagation and deactivate the catalyst.[108] (Adapted with permission from Plata *et al.*[108] © 2010 American Chemical Society).

CNTs, the results are highly dependent on the ratio of the mixture, generally, the system with higher H_2 concentration needs higher C to H molar ratio input, therefore it is necessary to adjust the C to H molar ratio input in the corresponding carrier gas environment, in order to synthesize the direct-spun CNTs, the adjustment of C to H molar ratio can also be achieved by using different types of hydrocarbon as fuel.

The composition of carrier gas in the system has an effect on the CNTs diameter distribution as well, Liu *et al.*[103] have observed a decrease in the SWNTs diameter distribution with increasing Ar content, which reflects another advantage of using Ar as the carrier gas, small diameter distribution brings assurance to the CNT products for applications that require more stability and consistency.

In terms of the CNTs production efficiency, there are two popular ways to calculate the yield of CNTs: the first way to calculate the efficiency that can be expressed as "CNT yields is the Mass of the CNT products/Mass of the carbon precursor"; the other way is being expressed as "CNT yields is the Mass of the CNT products/Mass of the catalyst", improving the efficacy and lifetime of the catalyst has been seen as a direct approach to address the CNTs low yield production problem, multiple unsaturated hydrocarbon feedstock can form cyclic intermediates with catalyst, this metallacycle intermediate can be grown by principle feedstock into longer CNTs.[104]

Hydrogen as a reductive agent plays an important role to extend the lifetime of the catalyst, insufficient hydrogen can result in the formation of polyacetylene and possible soot production,[105] although certain amount of hydrogen is able to prolong the catalyst activity, excessive hydrogen can lead to the depreciation of catalyst capability, the similar effects can be found during the polymerization process, P_{H2} (partial pressure of hydrogen) is usually being used to tailor the length of the polymer,[106] additionally hydrogen can also be used to cleave the metal catalyst — CNTs contact.[107]

Hydrogen can also come from the decomposition of the hydrocarbon precursor, the synthesis process is hydrogen self-sustainable, but other reactants species can compensate H_2 (such as oxygen content),

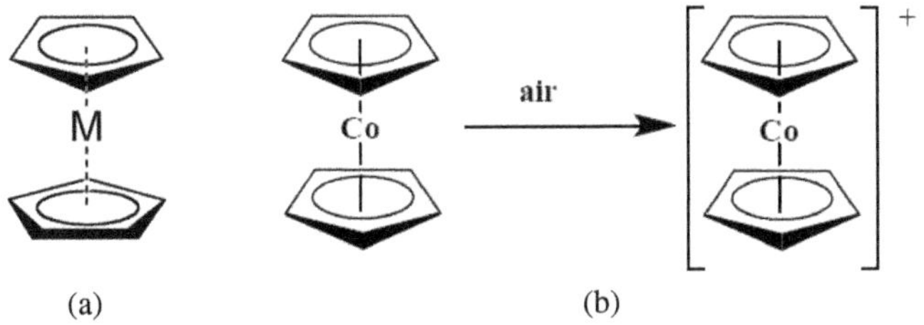

Fig. 10. (a) The structure of metallocene (M = Fe, Ni, Co, etc.,); (b) Cobaltocene can be easily oxidized to Cobaltocenium ion in air.

to ensure the quality of CNTs, the laboratory reactor set-up usually adopts the H_2 one-pass system for basic research purpose, while the cost of H_2 on scale-up makes the H_2 recycling a necessary approach to take, the recycling of H_2 can be achieved through the rearrangement of the reactor design, these steps can be fulfilled by fully taking advantage of the flexibility of FCCVD reactor.

4. Catalysts

The catalyst is indispensable for the growth of the CNTs, it not only reduces the energy needed for the synthesis, but also influences the morphology of the CNTs. Fe, Ni and Co are the most commonly used catalysts for CNT growth by CVD,[109] the reason being metals such as Fe, Ni, and Co, can become catalyst rooted in their atomic structure,[110] and have very few *d*-vacancies that make them have finite carbon solubility. Other transition metals, such as Ti and Mo, can form strong chemical bonds with carbon due to their many *d*-vacancies, the high solubility of Ti and Mo in carbon to form stable carbide prohibits the precipitation of carbon from the metals, therefore, more concentration of carbon is needed to exceed the solubility limit to form graphitic carbon,[111,112] the efficient size of the catalyst for the growth of SWNTs usually located in the range of 1–10 nm diameter, in the so-called volcano plot, which indicated the popular catalysts (Fe, Ni, Co) are capable of absorbing, and possibly dissolving carbon precursor molecules into the nanoparticles,[113] but their bulk form is reported to be non-zero, but limited-carbon solubility.

4.1. *Bi-metal and transition metal catalysts for substrate-based CVD*

In the CVD system, some other transition metals are also approved to be the catalysts for the CNT growth, mixture of different active catalysts are observed to possess higher efficiency than individual one,[114] non- or weakly active elements are often mixed with active catalyst to prevent the coarsening of the active catalyst, the notable example includes mixing Mo[115] and Mg[116] with Fe or Co. Other transition metals such as Cu, Pd show their capability of growing SWNTs and MWNTs on silicon and quartz substrate without the presence of the traditional catalysts (such as Fe, Ni, Co).[117]

Noble metals, such as Au, Ag, Pt, Pd, Rh, Os, are not capable of promoting CNTs growth due to their low solubility and negligible carbide formation[118]; however, when the particle size of metal particles is small enough ($< 5\,\text{nm}$), they are able to dissolve carbon effectively for CNTs growth. While Si and Ge semiconductor nanoparticles alone are not capable of being used as the catalyst for CNT synthesis, their oxidation and carbide state can be the suitable candidates, for instance, SiC has been demonstrated by Kusunoki *et al.* for the SWNTs production.[119]

The solubility of transition metal in carbon increases from right to left in the period table.[120] For instance, the solubility of carbon (700°C) is negligibly small in Zn and Cu, 0.3–0.5% at. in Ni and 1.2% at. in FCC–Co,[111] while Fe is able to form metastable carbide (Fe_3C) with carbon, the solubility of Fe in carbon, which is also dependent upon the composition, α-Fe, and γ-Fe have the solubility of ~ 0.1 at.% (700°C) and ~ 4 at.% (800°C), respectively.[121]

Although Fe, Ni, and Co are commonly used to catalyze the growth of the CNTs due to their intermediate carbon solubility, Cu that exhibits low carbon solubility, as well as Ti that has high affinity with carbon are also reported to display catalytic activities in promoting CNTs growth.[122]

4.2. *The catalysts for the FCCVD*

In the FCCVD system, metallocenes are commonly used for the major catalyst sources, metallocenes are organometallic compounds made up of a metal center which is connected to one or two cyclopentadienyl rings (Cp-ring), metallocenes were first discovered in the mid-1950s by Dunitz *et al.*[123] Ferrocene is one of the most important organometallic compounds, in fact, ferrocene was considered as the choice in all the latest 32 publications,[26] it has been favored due to its lower toxicity and low cost, it is an orange color solid with 18 valence electrons, it also has good stability under ambient condition, due to its sandwich structure as well as the satisfaction of 18 electrons rule, the vacancy *d*-orbital of Fe element enable Fe to form strong bond with cyclopentadienyl anion ring.[124] Besides ferrocene, other metallocenes, such as nickelocene, cobaltocene and ruthenocene, possess similar sandwich structure, but only cobaltocene was able to produce direct-spun in FCCVD system.[125]

These metallocenes (ferrocene, cobaltocene, and nickelocene) have similar decomposition temperatures, which are around 450°C under vacuum or inert condition, however, the decomposition mechanism of these metallocenes show disparities, in the case of ferrocene decomposition, which started with the loss of an H atom from Cp-ring, which form H_2 gas as the result, followed by breakage of remaining Cp-ring fragments from Fe atoms,[126,127] albeit cobaltocene and nickelocene decompose through direct and complete separation of bondage between metal and Cp-ring, without the initial H atom loss.

The disparities in their decomposition mechanism underly the differences in the kinetics of decomposition, with the presence of excessive H_2 as the carrier gas, H_2 gas could potentially disturb the equilibrium of ferrocene decomposition because H_2 is one of the products of the decomposition, as a result of shifting the reaction in a reverse direction according to the Le Châtelier's principle. Compared to ferrocene and cobaltocene, nickelocene is the least stable one, it can decompose at 50°C below its pyrolysis temperature under H_2 environment,[128] the instability of nickelocene could cause its early decomposition before reaching the hot zone, therefore losing its contribution for the CNT synthesis.

The very unique phenomenon in the floating catalyst method is that when nanoparticle is liberated from the metallocene, nanoparticles float along the tube by passing through different temperature zones, experience through nucleation, evaporation and renucleation steps, decoupling of critical particle number and particle size with the aerogel formation makes the aerogel formation more feasible.[19] The homogeneous nucleation of the nanoparticles requires Fe (if using ferrocene as catalyst) to reach critical cluster size of 9–12 atoms, according to some studies,[129,130] followed by coalescence and agglomeration, below the critical size, the reduction in bulk energy is not able to sustain the increase in surface energy, vaporization of the particles occurs. Temperature also is a big factor for the particle nucleation, although ferrocene decomposes at 450°C, below 1050°C, insufficient Fe atoms were present for the nuclei of critical cluster size to form.[19] Other factors like the materials of ceramic tubes, such as commonly used mullite, Alumina and quartz tube, the H_2 etching of the ceramic tube can create potential heterogeneous nucleation sites, which reduces the nucleation barrier of the nanoparticles.

4.3. *How catalysts affect the CNT morphology?*

In the substrate-based CVD system, when using Fe, Ni and Co as catalysts, the CNTs growth with Ni are more uniform and stable compared with using other catalysts, Co catalyst can give smaller diameter CNTs, the CNTs growth with Fe are not stable in term of the morphology distribution due to the formation of metastable carbide, the carbon diffusion in Fe can be increased by increasing the temperature to stabilize the synthesis process and improve the CNTs quality. Although the catalytic activity of Fe is the highest among the three, the produced CNTs have the lowest G/D ratio. Ni shows high activity even at a lower temperature (500–600°C), the catalytic activity can be improved by increasing the temperature, generally speaking, the catalytic activity follows order: Fe > Ni > Co, whereas the quality of as-synthesized CNTs follows the order of Ni > Co > Fe.[131] Note that in FCCVD method, only ferrocene and cobaltocene are able to produce the direct-spun product, which is discussed in Sec. 4.1, cobaltocene has been reported to produce nanofiber product with high selectivity (a concept defined as "the volume of nanotubes/the volume of deposit"), when cobaltocene and thiophene are both present, along with acetylene as hydrocarbon precursor, herringbone nanostructure fiber was synthesized, results also showed cobaltocene was more efficient as a catalyst to synthesize herringbone carbon nanofibers, which consist of layers of graphite platelets with metal catalyst at the top, than ferrocene in their system. The cobaltocene decomposes into clusters of cobalt particles, then reacts with thiophene to form cobalt sulfide clusters, these clusters interact with incoming hydrocarbon to form the nanostructures, the arrangement of the herringbone-like graphite layer from precipitated carbon, depends on the unique shape of cobalt metal catalyst surface.[132]

Some elements are also beneficial and acting as the promotors to extend the lifetime of the catalyst as well as to further improve the structural integrity of the CNTs, for instance in the case of synthesizing a large quantity of DWNTs, a trace amount of halide has been added in an iron sulfide catalyst, which resulting DWNTs have more uniform structure, this method has been demonstrated by using an arc discharge method.[133] While in FCCVD method, sulfur, as well as group 16 elements, have been the favorite choice for the "growth promoter", which is discussed in great detail in Sec. 1, therefore the morphology of the CNTs are dependent upon the S/Fe (if thiophene and ferrocene are used as S and Fe source) ratio, high S/Fe ratio usually leads to CNTs with larger diameter (MWNTs), whereas low S/Fe ratio produces the small diameter CNTs (SWNTs).[26]

Metals, such as Co, Ni, Pt, Pd, Mn, Mo, Cr, Sn, Au and even Mg and Al, can be used to grow SWNTs on quartz substrate,[134] some oxides including SiO_2[103] and ZrO_2[135] as well as diamond are also on the list. While in FCCVD method, the situation is more complicated and unpredictable sometimes, generally speaking, the balance of the ratio between Fe and C is required, in order for the successful formation of the direct-spun product, for instance, when the C/Fe ratio is larger than 2500, the oversupply of carbon leads to the soot and amorphous carbon formation, which can affect the quality and morphology of the CNTs, the D/G ratio (from the Raman characterization results) will increase, as well as the appearance of thicker amorphous layer around the CNTs, when the C/Fe ratio is smaller than 300, most of the CNTs will be deposited on the cold part of the tube wall, because the density of the CNTs is not sufficiently high enough, which makes them difficult to form bundles and creat direct-spun product, the thicker deposition that mostly is consisted of amorphous carbon prevents the further possible direct-spun aerogel formation. Note that the main drawback of FCCVD is that the inefficient use of the iron catalyst, Reguero *et al.*[28] calculated that less than 0.1% of Fe-based catalyst nanoparticles are able to survive and contribute to the CNTs aerogel formation, the rest of nanoparticles are either deactivated or plated on the inner wall of the reactor tube, another experiment showed that minimum catalyst mass concentration ($[Fe] = 0.2\,g/m^{-3}$), after the deduction from the catalyst that potentially will be deactivated, is required for the aerogel formation.

According to the publication from the research group of University of Cambridge, they have concluded that the optimal aerogel formation requires the corresponding C/Fe/S ratio is kept between 70 000:100:10 to 700:1:10.[26] However, it is not clear whether the researchers take other factors, such as the operating temperature, the injection rate of catalyst and hydrocarbon precursor, etc. into consideration. This window of molar ratio provides invaluable information. Besides S/Fe ratio, the residence time is another key factor associated with the morphology of the CNTs, an average of 20 s can be found in the most successful direct-spun process, whereas shorter residence time correlates with the formation of smaller diameter CNTs, due to smaller catalyst particle size, and vice versa, longer residence time results in larger diameter CNTs, shorter residence time also can decrease the percentage of amorphous carbon formation, because of the time window offered for the decomposition of hydrocarbon is shortened,[23,136] the residence time can be adjusted by changing the fuel injection rate or the carrier gas flow rate, however, the morphology change from the subsequent flow patterns shift, in other words, how the growth of the catalyst particle is affected, is not being fully explored, future work is needed in order to have a better understand this process.

5. Summary

In this paper, three major factors, namely, the role of sulfur, hydrocarbon as well as catalyst, are systematically reviewed based on the previous publications. Although all these factors play very important roles for the successful synthesis of CNTs in the FCCVD methods, due to the complex nature and synergistic interplay of these factors, more comprehensive study is needed to fully understand the whole process, and systematic improvement and mitigation need to be done in order to optimize the CNTs synthesis process.

Although FCCVD process has the scale-up potential for commercialization, in fact, couple of companies have been running successfully entirely based on this method, but the less efficiency and high production cost of this method has been the major bottleneck. The fewer efficiencies have been identified as high running temperature, less output/input ratio, etc. this problem can be solved by choosing the types of hydrocarbon gases, for instance, Butanol replaces Methanol as the hydrocarbon precursor could potentially increase the CNTs synthesis efficiency, twice number of carbon number in butanol molecule provides the sufficient carbon input, less amount of butanol molecule is needed therefore leading to high efficiency, but this is not necessarily always the truth, different hydrocarbon decompose followed different chemical routes, carefully utilize the carbon component into CNTs growth only happens when condition like critical time or temperature window is satisfied.

In the aspect of morphology control, long CNTs have been highly sought after, how to grow longer CNTs have met many obstacles, the growth of the CNT is controlled by factors such as the kinetics and catalyst activity, normally catalyst loses its efficacy after 1mm growth, the deactivation of catalyst particle can be caused by "carbon choking", thermal degradation and sintering, loss of internal surface area due to attrition/crushing, etc., therefore sufficient amount of sulfur is necessary to prevent the "carbon choking" and collisions of catalyst particles, keep adding the catalyst particles at various points of the reaction can also be helpful in terms of preserve the potency of the catalyst particles. There has been the hypothesis that longer tube with a smaller thermal gradient can prolong the growth window of the CNTs and increase its growth length.

The design of the reactor is important for the future commercialization of CNTs production, FCCVD has been notable for its flexible reactor design, which can be either horizontal or vertical arrangement, ceramic tubes can be made of quartz (SiO_2), mullite ($3Al_2O_3$-$2SiO_2$ or $2Al_2O_3SiO_2$) or alumina (Al_2O_3), empirical observations show that due to H_2 gas etching, element Si and Al can be detected in the final CNTs products, the type of tube has a correlation with catalyst lost (Fe plating) on the wall, additionally fuel injector arrays and position of the injection, as well as the flow rate all have synergistic influence on the flow pattern as well the CNTs aerogel formation, low Reynolds number has been proved to be advantageous in synthesizing anisotropic CNTs materials, while high Re indicating the onset of the turbulence and flow instability has not been fully explored.[137]

Furthermore, temperature profile and residence times are also the key parameters associated with the CNTs production, temperature steepness is limited by the temperature ranges and gradients, achieving the better control over the temperature is beneficial for the reaction control. Better adjustment of the temperature profile can be achieved by using furnace with the multi-temperature zone. Residence time can be reflected on the types of the CNTs, which is explained in Sec. 4.3, SWCNT dominated at lower residence time range, while MWCNTs are the result of long residence time, the residence time can be adjusted by controlling the gas flow rate.

Acknowledgments

This research was sponsored by the UC Accelerator for Commercialization Project, ONR Award N00014-15-1-2473, PM Dr. Ignacio Perez, the NSF ERC EEC-0812348; the UC TAC Seed Grant under ESP TECH 15-0160; and the UC ERC-TRT Program.

References

1. R. H. Baughman, A. A. Zakhidov and W. A. de Heer, *Science* **297**, 787 (2002).
2. M. F. L. De Volder, S. H. Tawfick, R. H. Baugman and A. J. Hart, *Science (80-.).* **339**, 535 (2013).
3. P. M. Ajayan and S. Lijima, *Nature* **361**, 333 (1993).
4. A. Eatemadi *et al.*, *Nanoscale Res. Lett.* **9**, 393 (2014).
5. T. W. Ebbesen and P. M. Ajayan, *Nature* **358**, 220 (1992).
6. D. S. Bethune *et al.*, *Nature* **363**, 605 (1993).
7. Y. Jung, J. Song, W. Huh, D. Cho and Y. Jeong, *Chem. Eng. J.* **228**, 1050 (2013).
8. S. Suzuki and S. Mori, *Diam. Relat. Mater.* **89**, 74 (2018).
9. S. Roy, M. David-Pur and Y. Hanein, *Carbon N. Y.* **116**, 40 (2017).
10. M. S. Motta, A. Moisala, I. A. Kinloch and A. H. Windle, *J. Nanosci. Nanotechnol.* **8**, 2442 (2008).
11. N. Chiodarelli *et al.*, *Carbon N. Y.* **50**, 1748 (2012).
12. Y. Yuan *et al.*, *J. Chem. Mater.* **3**, 3310 (2015).
13. K. A. Shah and B. A. Tali, *Mater. Sci. Semicond. Process.* **41**, 67 (2016).
14. O. Yaglioglu, A. Cao, A. J. Hart, R. Martens and A. H. Slocum, *Adv. Funct. Mater.* **22**, 5028 (2012).
15. H. M. Cheng *et al.*, *Appl. Phys. Lett.* **72**, 3282 (1998).
16. H. B. Abdullah, I. Ramli, I. Ismail and N. A. Yusof, *Bull. Mater. Sci.* **42**, 241 (2019).
17. W. Ren, F. Li and H. M. Cheng, *J. Phys. Chem. B* **110**, 16941 (2006).
18. W. Ren, F. Li and H.-M.Cheng (2006), doi: 10.1021/JP062526X.
19. C. Hoecker, F. Smail, M. Pick, L. Weller and A. M. Boies, *Sci. Rep.* **7**, 14519 (2017).
20. M. S. Kim, N. M. Rodriguez and R. T. K. Baker, *J. Catal.* **143**, 449 (1993).
21. T. S. Gspann, F. R. Smail and A. H. Windle, *Faraday Discuss* **173**, 47 (2014).
22. J. N. Wang, X. G. Luo, T. Wu and Y. Chen, *Nat. Commun.* **5**, 1 (2014).
23. D. Conroy, A. Moisala, S. Cardoso, A. Windle and J. Davidson, *Chem. Eng. Sci.* **65**, 2965 (2010).
24. M. Motta *et al.*, *Phys. E Low-dimensional Syst. Nanostructures* **37**, 40 (2007).
25. W. Ren, F. Li, S. Bai and H.-M. Cheng, *J. Nanosci. Nanotechnol.* **6**, 1339 (2006).
26. L. Weller *et al.*, *Carbon N. Y.* **146**, 789 (2019).
27. C.-H. Kiang, M. S. Dresselhaus, R. Beyers and D. S. Bethune, *Chem. Phys. Lett.* **259**, 41 (1996).
28. V. Reguero, B. Alemán, B. Mas and J. J. Vilatela, *Chem. Mater.* **26**, 3550 (2014).
29. Y. Li *et al.*, *J. Phys. Chem. B* **105**, 11424 (2001).
30. R. T. K. Baker, J. J. Chludzinski, N. S. Dudash and A. J. Simoens, *Carbon N. Y.* **21**, 463 (1983).
31. C. Hoecker, F. Smail, M. Pick and A. Boies, *Chem. Eng. J.* **314**, 388 (2017).
32. X. Devaux *et al.*, *Phys. E Low-dimens. Syst. Nanostruct.* **44**, 1028 (2012).
33. F. Yu *et al.*, *Phys. E Low-Dimens. Syst. Nanostruct.* **44**, 2032 (2012).

34. M. Scarselli, P. Castrucci and M. De Crescenzi, *J. Phys. Condens. Matter* **24**, 313202 (2012).
35. R. M. Sundaram, K. K. K. Koziol and A. H. Windle, *Adv. Mater.* **23**, 5064 (2011).
36. S. H. Lee *et al.*, *Chem. Eng. Sci.* **192**, 655 (2018).
37. H. Dai *et al.*, *Chem. Phys. Lett.* **260**, 471 (1996).
38. P. Nikolaev *et al.*, *Chem. Phys. Lett.* **313**, 91 (1999).
39. R. E. Smalley and B. I. Yakobson, *Solid State Commun.* **107**, 597 (1998).
40. M. J. Bronikowski, P. A. Willis, D. T. Colbert, K. A. Smith and R. E. Smalley, *J. Vac. Sci. Technol. A Vacuum, Surfaces, Film.* **19**, 1800 (2001).
41. D. Hedman, H. Reza Barzegar, A. Rosén, T. Wågberg and J. Andreas Larsson, *Sci. Rep.* **5**, 16850 (2015).
42. D. R. Poirier, H. Yin, M. Suzuki and T. Emi, *ISIJ Int.* **38**, 229 (1998).
43. S. H. Lee, J. Park, H.-R. Kim, J. Lee and K.-H. Lee, *RSC Adv.* **5**, 41894 (2015).
44. S.-H. Lee *et al.*, *Carbon N. Y.* **124**, 219 (2017).
45. J. Wei *et al.*, *Carbon N. Y.* **45**, 2152 (2007).
46. F. Tafwidli and Y.-B. Kang, *ISIJ Int.* **57**, 782 (2017).
47. D. Lide, *CRC Handbook of Chemistry and Physics* (CRC Press, LLC, 2005).
48. T. Murakami *et al.*, *J. Appl. Phys.* **100**, 094303 (2006).
49. A. G. Nasibulin, P. V. Pikhitsa, H. Jiang and E. I. Kauppinen, *Carbon N. Y.* **43**, 2251 (2005).
50. H. Dai, *Surf. Sci.* **500**, 218 (2002).
51. Y. Li, K. Ji, Y. Duan, G. Meng and Z. Dai, *Coatings* **7**, 221 (2017).
52. G. Hou *et al.*, *Mater. Des.* **132**, 112 (2017).
53. K. Mustonen *et al.*, *Beilstein J. Nanotechnol.* **3**, 692 (2012).
54. T. W. Odom, J.-L. Huang, P. Kim and C. M Lieber, *J. Phys. Chem.* B2000104132794-2809 (2000), https://doi.org/10.1021/jp993592k.
55. F. A. Halden and W. D. Kingery, *J. Phys. Chem.* **59**, 557 (1955).
56. F. F. Abraham, *Homogeneous Nucleation Theory the Pretransition Theory of Vapor Condensation* (Academic Press, 1974).
57. K. Y. Park and H. J. Jeong, *Korean J. Chem. Eng.* **16**, 64 (1999).
58. M. J. Schulz, V. N. Shanov, Z. Yin and M. Cahay, *Nanotube Superfiber Materials: Science, Manufacturing, Commercialization* (Elsevier).
59. Y. Yuan *et al.*, *J. Mater. Chem. A* **3**, 3310 (2015).
60. M. J. McNallan and T. Debroy, *Metall. Trans. B* **22**, 557 (1991).
61. K. Nakashima and K. Mori, *ISIJ Int.* **32**, 11 (1992).
62. S. Stølen and T. Grande, *Chemical Thermodynamics of Materials* (John Wiley & Sons Ltd., 2003), doi: 10.1002/0470092688.
63. I. Dopico, I. Martin-bragado, J. J. Vilatela, T. Naranjo and M. P. Emilio, *Carbon N. Y.* **101**, 458 (2016).
64. S. Y. Moon, W. S. Kim and C. S. Kim, *RSC Adv.* **8**, 25815 (2018).
65. J. S. Barnard, C. Paukner and K. K. Koziol, *Nanoscale* **8**, 17262 (2016).
66. M. S. Dresselhaus, G. Dresselhaus and P. C. Eklund, *Science of Fullerenes and Carbon Nanotubes* (Academic Press, 1996).
67. A. Hirsch and C. Backes, *Angew. Chemie Int. Ed.* **49**, 1722 (2010).

68. B. K. Kaushik and M. K. Majumder, *Springer Briefs Appl. Sci. Technol.* **2**, 17 (2015).
69. J. W. Mintmire and C. T. White, *Carbon N. Y.* **33**, 893 (1995).
70. R. Ouyang, J.-X. Liu and W.-X. Li, *J. Am. Chem. Soc.* **135**, 1760 (2013).
71. S. Forel *et al.*, *Nanoscale* **11**, 4091 (2019).
72. K. Hasegawa and S. Noda, *Carbon N. Y.* **49**, 4497 (2011).
73. P. Wynblatt and N. G.-P, *Supported Metal Crystallites* **11**, 121 (1975).
74. J. E. Herrera, L. Balzano, A. Borgna, W. E. Alvarez and D. E. Resasco, *J. Catal.* **204**, 129 (2001).
75. V. I. Artyukhov, E. S. Penev and B. I. Yakobson, *Nat. Commun.* **5**, 4892 (2014).
76. D. Hedman, H. Reza Barzegar, A. Rosén, T. Wågberg and J. Larsson, *Sci. Rep.* **5**, 1 (2015).
77. D. N. Futaba *et al.*, *Adv. Mater.* **21**, 4811 (2009).
78. M. D. Yadav, A. W. Patwardhan, J. B. Joshi and K. Dasgupta, *Diam. Relat. Mater.* **97**, 107432 (2019).
79. J. Sanchez, J. Fullea, C. Andrade and P. L. de Andres, *Phys. Rev. B* **78**, 014113 (2008).
80. L. Plata, E. R. Meshot, C. M. Reddy, A. J. Hart and P. M. Gschwend, *ACS Nano.* **4**, 7185 (2010).
81. A. J. Hart, L. van Laake and A. Slocum, *Small* **3**, 772 (2007).
82. E. R. Meshot *et al.*, *ACS Nano* **3**, 2477 (2009).
83. D. L. Plata, A. J. Hart, C. M. Reddy and P. M. Gschwend, *Environ. Sci. Technol.* **43**, 8367 (2009).
84. H. Ago *et al.*, *Carbon N. Y.* **44**, 2912 (2006).
85. S. Sobri *et al.*, *MATEC Web Conf.* **39**, 01006 (2016).
86. R. M. Sundaram and A. H. Windle, *Sci. Adv. Mater.* **7**, 643 (2015).
87. G. Ingram and S. M. H. Rizvi, *Microchem. J.* **20**, 324 (1975).
88. B. C. Capelin, G. Ingram and J. Kokolis, *Microchem. J.* **19**, 229 (1974).
89. G. Zhong *et al.*, *J. Phys. Chem. C* **113**, 17321 (2009).
90. A. Holmen, O. A. Rokstad and A. Solbakken, *Ind. Eng. Chem. Process Des. Dev.* **15**, 439 (1976).
91. Y. Zhang and S. Han, *Mater. Sci.* **23**, 15 (2017).
92. T. G. Gutowski *et al.*, *Environ. Sci. Technol.* **43**, 1584 (2009).
93. I. Vesselényi *et al.*, *React. Kinet. Catal. Lett.* **74**, 329 (2001).
94. W. Christen, G. Cunibert, E. R. Hilf and D. Tomanek, *ATO ASI Series B* **294**, 21 (2006).
95. C. Liu and H. M. Cheng, *Mater. Today* **16**, 19 (2013).
96. B. T. Sese, A. Grant and B. J. Reid, *Caenorhabditis Elegans. J. Toxicol. Environ. Heal. Part A* **72**, 1168 (2009).
97. Y. Ma, A. B. Dichiara, D. He, L. Zimmer and J. Bai, *Carbon N. Y.* **107**, 171 (2016).
98. J.-M. Feng *et al.*, *Carbon N. Y.* **48**, 3817 (2010).
99. Q. Zhang *et al.*, *Chinese Phys. B* **26**, 028802 (2017).
100. W. Xu, Y. Chen, H. Zhan and J. N. Wang, *Nano Lett.* **16**, 946 (2016).
101. T. Wu and J. N. Wang, *RSC Adv.* **6**, 38187 (2016).

102. R. I. Silsby and E. W. Sawyer, *J. Appl. Chem.* **6**, 347 (2007).
103. S. Huang, Q. Cai, J. Chen, Y. Qian and L. Zhang, *J. Am. Chem. Soc.* **131**, 2094 (2009).
104. D. Umadevi and G. N. Sastry, *Front. Chem.* **2**, 75 (2014).
105. B. Shukla, A. Miyoshi and M. Koshi, *J. American Society for Mass Spectrometry* **21**, 534 (2010).
106. K. Y. Choi and W. H. Ray, *J. Appl. Polym. Sci.* **30**, 1065 (1985).
107. T. Yamada *et al.*, *Nano Lett.* **8**, 4288 (2008).
108. D. L. Plata, E. R. Meshot, C. M. Reddy, A. J. Hart and P. M. Gschwend, *ACS Nano* **4**, 7185 (2010).
109. L. M. Hoyos-Palacio, A. G. García, J. F. Pérez-Robles, J. González and H. V. Martínez-Tejada, *IOP Conf. Ser. Mater. Sci. Eng.* **59**, 012005 (2014).
110. R. Purohit, K. Purohit, S. Rana, R. S. Rana and V. Patel, *MSPRO* **6**, 716 (2014).
111. V. Jourdain and C. Bichara, *Carbon* **58**, 2 (2013).
112. W. P. Leroy, C. Detavernier, Meirhaeghe, R. L. Van, A. J. Kellock and C. Lavoie, *J. Applied Phys.* **99**, 063704 (2006).
113. J.-M. Aguiar-Hualde, Y. Magnin, H. Amara and C. Bichara, *Carbon N. Y.* **120**, 226 (2017).
114. M. Fouquet *et al.*, *J. Phys. Chem. C* **118**, 5773 (2014).
115. Y. Li, J. Liu, Y. Wang and Z. L. Wang, *Chem. Mater.* **13**, 1008 (2001).
116. E. Flahaut *et al.*, *Chem. Phys. Lett.* **300**, 236 (1999).
117. M. Trojanowicz, *TrAC Trends Anal. Chem.* **25**, 480 (2006).
118. M. Valcárcel, S. Cárdenas and B. M. Simonet, *Anal. Chem.* **79**, 4788 (2007).
119. M. H. Rümmeli *et al.*, *Nanoscale Res. Lett.* **6**, 303 (2011).
120. N. I. Medvedeva, D. Aken Van and J. E. Medvedeva, *J. Phys. Condens. Matter* **22**, 7 (2010).
121. A. Mostafa and M. Medraj, Structure, Texture and Phases in 3D Printed IN718 Alloy Subjected to Homogenization and HIP Treatments, *Mater.*, Vol. 7 (Basel, Switzerland, 2017), p. 196.
122. N. Zhao and J. Kang, *Carbon Nanotubes — Synthesis, Characterization, Applications* (InTech, 2011), doi: 10.5772/19275.
123. N. Philile and D. Ngidi, *Application of Metallocenes for the Synthesis of Multiwalled Carbon Nanotubes* (University of KwaZulu-Natal Durban Westville, 2016).
124. *Chem. Elem.* 905 (1997), doi: 10.1016/B978-0-7506-3365-9.50025-0.
125. C. Hoecker, F. Smail, M. Pick, L. Weller and A. M. Boies, *Sci. Rep.* **7**, 1–11 (2017).
126. L. M. Dyagileva, V. P. Marin, E. I. Tsyganova and G. A. Razuvaev, *J. Organomet. Chem.* **175**, 63 (1979).
127. K. Elihn and K. Larsson, *Thin Solid Films* **458**, 325 (2004).
128. G. J. M. Dormans, *J. Cryst. Growth* **108**, 806 (1991).
129. S. L. Girshick and C.-P. Chiu, *Plasma Chem. Plasma Process.* **9**, 355 (1989).
130. D. E. Jensen, *J. Chem. Soc. Faraday Trans. 2* **76**, 1494 (1980).
131. G. Allaedini, S. Tasirin, P. Aminayi, Z. Yaakob and M. Z. Meow Talib, *Int. J. Nano Dimens.* **7**, 186 (2016).

132. C. Singh *et al.* *J. Phys. Chem. B.* **106**, 10915 (2002).
133. H. Qiu *et al.*, *Carbon N. Y.* **44**, 516 (2006).
134. Y. Li *et al.*, *Adv. Mater.* **22**, 1508 (2010).
135. S. A. Steiner *et al.*, *J. Am. Chem. Soc.* **131**, 12144 (2009).
136. Y. Li and I. Kinloch, Science, A. W., undefined. Direct spinning of carbon nanotube fibers from chemical vapor deposition synthesis. *science.sciencemag.org*.
137. Q. Liu *et al.*, *ACS Nano* **2**, 1722 (2008).

https://doi.org/10.1142/9789819809028_0007

Chapter 7

Gold Nanoparticles in Cancer Imaging and Therapeutics*

Huang-Chiao Huang, James Ramos, Taraka Sai Pavan Grandhi, Thrimoorthy Potta and Kaushal Rege†

Molecular and Nanoscale Bioengineering Laboratory
Arizona State University, Tempe, AZ 85287-6106, USA
†*kaushal.rege@asu.edu*

The use of nanomedicine in the war on cancer diseases has progressed significantly in the recent past. Liposomal- and albumin-based chemotherapeutic agents as well as tumor contrast agents (e.g. Gd-DTPA, ferumoxides) have received FDA approval for human clinical use, while many other agents are in different phases of pre-clinical investigation and clinical trials. Plasmonic gold nanoparticles hold great promise as potential theranostic devices for detection and ablation of cancer diseases. This review discusses recent progress in the imaging, photothermal therapy, and nucleic acid/drug delivery using gold nanoparticles (spheres, shells, rods, cages) *in vitro* and *in vivo*. Issues relating to toxicity, biocompatibility, biodistribution, cellular uptake, and targeting efficiency are also discussed.

Keywords: Theranostics; gold nanoparticles; cancer.

1. Introduction

Cancer diseases are among the leading causes of death worldwide and account for approximately one in every four deaths in the United States. Rapid developments in nanotechnology offer promising approaches in theranostics, which can facilitate simultaneous diagnosis and therapy of cancer diseases using nanoscale materials.

*To cite this article, please refer to its earlier version published in the *Nano LIFE*, Vol. 1, Nos. 3 & 4 (2010) 289–307, DOI: 10.1142/S1793984410000274

Gold nanoparticles (Fig. 1) have been extensively investigated as potential theranostics due to their plasmonic properties (e.g. localized surface plasmon resonance; LSPR), biocompatibility, multiple imaging modalities, and ease of surface functionalization.

LSPR of different shapes of gold nanoparticles, including nanorods, nanopheres, nanoclusters, and nanocages, involves the collective oscillation of free electrons on metallic nanoparticle surface upon light excitation. The scattering and absorption properties of gold nanoparticles depend on size and shape of the nanoparticle as well as the dielectric constant of the surrounding medium, and are greatly enhanced upon light excitation.[1]

The LSPR band of gold nanorods falls in two regions of the light absorption spectrum. A transverse band, due to the electron oscillations along the diameter, lies in the visible region at approximately 520 nm and is similar to that of gold nanospheres. A stronger longitudinal band in the near-infrared (NIR) and far-infrared region is due to electronic oscillations along the length of the rods and is tunable based on the aspect ratio of the gold nanorods. For gold nanoshells and nanocages, the plasmon band can be observed in the NIR and far-infrared region. Gold nanoparticles are excellent contrast agents for biological imaging applications due to strong Rayleigh (elastic) scattering properties. In addition, Raman (inelastic) scattering of molecules adsorbed on a gold surface can be greatly enhanced upon coupling of the gold plasmonic band and the electronic state of the molecule; enabling single molecule detection.[2]

Hyperthermia and chemotherapy have been widely explored as therapeutic approaches against cancer diseases. Absorption of NIR (700–1000 nm) light by certain shapes of gold nanoparticles (nanorods, nanoshells, and nanocages) can result in generation and dissipation of heat via electron– phonon and phonon–phonon interactions. This is promising for future work in photothermal therapies, especially since NIR light can penetrate deeper and causes less photodamage in tissues when compared to UV-vis irradiation.[3] Moreover, the surface of gold nanoparticles can be easily functionalized with therapeutic molecules and/or antibodies for systemic targeting of drugs to tumors.

Gold nanoparticles have therefore emerged as versatile platforms for various imaging modalities, photothermal therapy, and for delivery of therapeutic drugs. Here we review the latest developments in the use of gold nanoparticles in cancer imaging, therapeutics, and drug delivery.

2. Synthesis of gold nanoparticles

2.1. *Gold nanospheres*

Colloidal gold nanospheres are commonly prepared via citrate reduction of gold salt ($HAuCl_4$) in water, based on methods first introduced by Turkevich *et al.*[4] in 1951. The size of gold nanospheres can be tuned by controlling the gold/citrate ratio and temperature during synthesis. Typical size of gold nanospheres ranges from 2–100 nm, with a corresponding single LSPR band between 510–570 nm. Many other strategies, including the use of various reducing agents, ligands,[5,6] dendrimers,[7,8] and block copolymers,[9] have been reported for the generation of gold nanospheres.

2.2. *Gold nanorods*

Several methods have been developed for the synthesis of gold nanorods. The *template method*, introduced by Martin,[10] involves electrochemical and electroless deposition of gold within the nanopores of porous polycarbonate or alumina template membranes. We developed a high-throughput method in order to overcome yield limitations associated with traditional template methods.[11] In this method, gold nanorods and nanowires were prepared in a multilayer fashion with alternating layers of the desired metal (gold) and selectively dissolvable metal. This resulted in increased yields over traditional methods that use only one layer of gold in the synthesis; the method also reduced material costs and processing times. *Electrochemical synthesis* of gold nanorods, introduced by Yu *et al.*[12] and Chang *et al.*,[13] involves the reduction of gold anions at the cathode surface or within cetyltrimethyl ammonium bromide (CTAB) cylindrical templates. *Seed-mediated growth method*, introduced by Jana *et al.*[14–1516] and later modified by Nikoobakht and El-Sayed[17] is among the most widely used methods for the preparation of gold nanorods. This multistep seed-mediated growth method first involves the formation of gold seeds by reducing gold salt with a strong reducing agent (sodium borohydride) in the presence of CTAB. Next, gold seeds, acting as nucleation sites, are introduced into a growth solution of gold salt with a weak reducing agent (ascorbic acid) and CTAB surfactant. CTAB forms a bilayer[18] on the surface of the nanorods; repulsion between the cationic head groups of the surfactant results in stable aqueous dispersions of the gold nanorods. Different modification strategies have been investigated for replacing CTAB on nanorods for use in biological applications due to cytotoxicity of the surfactant.

2.3. *Gold nanoshells and gold nanocages*

Nanoshells consist of a composite metallic shell (e.g. gold) or dielectric core (e.g. silica) structure. The most well-known method for preparing a nanometer-thick gold nanoshell around silica core (~100 nm) was introduced by Oldenburg *et al.*[19–2021] Monodispersed silica cores were prepared via basic reduction (NH_4OH) of tetraethyl orthosilicate (TEOS) in ethanol, known as Stober method, and then followed by surface amination. The negatively charged gold colloid (2–4 nm in diameter) can be adsorbed on the silica surface in order to generate nucleation sites for the reduction of additional gold ions. Typically, gold nanoshells possess a single LSPR band in NIR region, which can be controlled based on the thickness of the gold shell; reducing shell thickness from 20 nm to 5 nm results in absorption peak red shift from 700 nm to 1000 nm due to increased coupling between plasmons. The ratio between scattering and absorbing events of gold nanoshells depends on the size of the silica core; smaller silica cores show higher absorption of energy, while larger silica cores are more effective at scattering incident light energy. Introduced by Sun *et al.*,[22] Chen *et al.*,[23] and Skrabalak *et al.*,[24] hollow and porous gold nanocages are formed via galvanic replacement reaction between silver nanocubes and $HAuCl_4$ solution. Deposition of gold atoms and removal of silver atoms on silver nanocubes results in the formation of Au/Ag alloy shell around partially hollow silver nanocubes. Different degrees of galvanic replacement reaction first result in the formation of corner-reconstructed Au/Ag nanoboxes, followed by Au nanocages with pores in the wall. Hollow and porous gold nanocages possessing single LSPR band around 800 nm have been reported.

2.4. *Gold nanorings and gold nanodisks*

Aizpurua *et al.*[25] used colloidal lithography on a soda-glass substrate for the generation of gold nanorings and nanodisks. Colloidal polystyrene particles of 110-nm-diameter were electrostatically deposited onto a glass substrate followed by a 30-nm gold film coating. Next, an argon ion beam was used as an etchant to create nanorings around the polystyrene particles via secondary sputtering and removing unwanted gold atoms. This was followed by a UV-ozone treatment to remove the reminder of the polystyrene particles, leaving the gold nanorings in place. A slight modification in the sequence of synthesis steps gave rise to nanodisks. Tseng *et al.*[26] used silica-deposited sapphire substrate for the electrostatic deposition of the colloidal polystyrene followed by trifluromethane as the etchant and ozone treatment.

2.5. *Surface modification of gold nanoparticles influences stability, efficacy and toxicity*

Gold nanoparticles are unstable in physiological conditions and have a propensity to form large aggregates due to their high surface energy. Surface modification of gold nanoparticles using appropriate chemistries can improve their colloidal stability, increase their persistence in circulation by slowing their removal by the reticuloendothelial system, and improve targeting to desired tissues.[27–29] Furthermore, functionalized gold nanoparticles have several applications in the fields of therapeutics, diagnostics, and imaging. Several chemistries have been investigated for the surface modification of gold nanoparticles in order to improve their colloidal stability and biocompatibility.

Strong interactions between gold and various functional groups (thiol/amine/phosphine)-containing molecules make it easy to functionalize gold nanoparticles with various small molecules, DNA, and proteins. Ding *et al.*[30] exploited electrostatic interactions between gold surfaces and amines in order to bind thionine to gold nanoparticles. In another study, Porta *et al.*[31] successfully capped aminoalcohols on gold surfaces through ionic bonds between the protonated amine group and the gold nanoparticle surface. Phosphine-stabilized gold nanoparticles were developed by Shem *et al.*[32] by using the mild reducing agent, 9-borabicyclononane (9-BBN). The size of the nanoparticles was in the rage of 1.2–2.8 nm, depending on the type of phosphine ligand used.

Thiol-containing ligands have emerged as the most effective functional group for modifying surfaces of gold nanoparticles because of the strong conjugation through S-Au covalent bonding. Aryal *et al.*[33] generated stable gold nanoparticles through cysteine capping on the gold particle surface. Chechik and Crooks[34] synthesized poly(amidoamine) (PAMAM) dendrimers with terminal groups partially or fully functionalized with thiol groups. X-ray photoelectron spectroscopy showed that most thiol groups on dendrimers directly interacted with the gold surface and formed stable monolayers. The size of the nanoparticles was in the range of 1.5–2.1 nm in diameter; stable gold nanoparticles were obtained at gold (Au)/dendrimer ratios as large as 120:1. Zhou *et al.*[35] synthesized gold nanoparticles coated with thyminethiol derivatives containing long hydrocarbon chains; the thymine moieties of thyminethiol derivatives were used to link gold nanoparticles surface. Particle size ranges from 2–7 nm in diameter with a relatively narrow size distribution. The colloidal stability of the functionalized gold nanoparticles was studied as a function of salt concentration in aqueous dispersions. Gold nanoparticles were found to be stable in concentrated sodium chloride (NaCl), potassium chloride (KCl) solutions, while they demonstrated low stability in lithium chloride (LiCl) and cesium chloride (CsCl) solutions. Coagulation of gold nanoparticles in the presence of LiCl and CsCl was attributed to van der Waals attraction and reduced hydration repulsion.

Liao and Hafner[36] replaced the stabilizing surfactant bilayer on gold nanorods with thiol-terminated methoxypoly (ethylene glycol). This surface modification facilitated subsequent conjugation with anti-rabbit IgG through a long-chain, hetero-bifunctional cross-linker.

Poly(ethylene glycol) (PEG)-coated gold nanoparticles possess a higher degree of biocompatibility compared to unmodified gold nanoparticles.[37] Furthermore, PEG coatings on gold nanoparticles prevent the aggregation of gold nanoparticles and support longer circulation *in vivo*, resulting in passive accumulation at tumor sites.[38,39] PEG (5 kDa)-grafted gold nanospheres exhibited prolonged blood circulation and lowest uptake by reticuloendothelial cells in tumor-bearing mice.[40] Radioactive-labeled gold nanoparticles of 5 nm inorganic core diameters were intravenously injected to rats, and their biodistribution profiles in different tissues, organs, and excretion were monitored after 1 h and 24 h of administration.[41] Gold nanoparticles coated with 10 kDa PEG exhibited slower clearance from the body compared to those coated with 750 Da PEG and unmodified gold nanoparticles. These studies correlated well with other investigations in which, 5 kDa and 10 kDa PEG-grafted gold nanorods exhibited higher stability in the blood circulation compared to GNRs coated with 2 kDa and 20 kDa PEG.[42]

Thiol-based functionalization can also be employed to functionalize gold nanoparticles with proteins or oligonucleotides.[43,44] Verma *et al.*[45] functionalized gold nanoparticles with cationic tetra alkyl ammonium groups via gold-thiol bonds. These mixed monolayer protected clusters recognize anionic proteins (e.g. bovine serum albumin, human growth hormone and beta-galactosidase) via complementary electrostatic interaction and inhibit their activity. The inhibition of activity was recovered by treating the protein–particle complex with glutathione (GSH), which results in release of free protein. In another protein release study Bhumkar *et al.*[46] demonstrated insulin release from chitosan-functionalized gold nanoparticles; chitosan-coated gold nanoparticles effectively delivered loaded insulin across the mucosa. The small size of the functionalized gold nanoparticles is attractive for nonviral transgene delivery since high surface-to-volume ratios can help maximize the payload (DNA)/carrier ratio. Furthermore, the monolayer coverage of the gold nanoparticles allows easy tuning of hydrophobicity and charge, which helps in improving the transfection efficiency while minimizing the toxicity. Several studies evaluated the use of cationic group

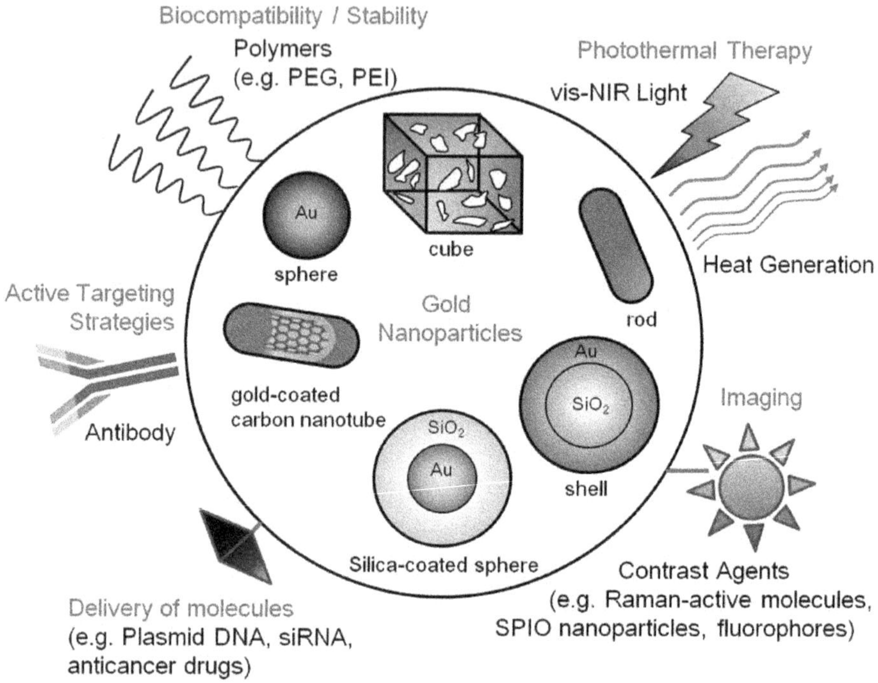

Fig. 1. Gold nanoparticles for nanomedicine applications.

functionalized gold nanoparticles for nucleic acid delivery (discussed later in the article).[47,48]

Imparting multifunctionality to gold nanoparticles[49,50] can be crucial in several applications, including biosensing, diagnostics, and therapy; Fig. 1 shows a schematic representation of multifunctional gold nanoparticles. Generally, biocompatible polymers can be used to stabilize gold nanoparticles and subsequently conjugated to targeting ligands. Monoclonal antibodies, aptamers, and peptides can be used as targeting ligands. The targeting ligands help in selective uptake of gold nanoparticles at disease sites. Cell-penetrating peptides (CPPs) can augment intracellular penetration of the conjugated cargo. Furthermore, stimulus-sensitive agents and magnetic nanoparticles can be added for imparting additional functionality in diagnosis and treatment.

3. Biomedical imaging using gold nanoparticles

The following sections discuss various different imaging modalities that are suitable for imaging of gold nanoparticles (Table 1).

3.1. *Dark field microscopy imaging*

Gold nanoparticles have been investigated as contrast agents for *in vitro* dark field imaging based on their light resonant scattering property. Dark field microscopy works by illuminating the sample with light at an angle and collecting only the scattered light from the target. Loo *et al.* demonstrated *in vitro* targeting, imaging as well as ablation of human epidermal growth factor receptor 2 (HER2) positive cancer cells using antibody-targeted gold nanoshells.[51,52] El-Sayed *et al.* successfully performed *in vitro* dark field imaging of cancer cells using antibody-conjugated gold nanospheres[53] and nanorods.[54] The light scattering properties of gold nanoparticles can facilitate their use as contrast agents for imaging, while their light absorption properties allow for cancer cell ablation due to hyperthermia.

3.2. *Optical coherence tomography*

Optical Coherence Tomography (OCT) is a real-time sub-cellular imaging technique introduced by Huang *et al.*[55] in 1991. This non-invasive interferometric-based imaging modality uses NIR and far-IR light to achieve maximal tissue penetration. OCT measures the reflected light off the optical scattering media after filtering out the scattered light and is capable of providing optical contrast for a target 2–3 cm deep in biological tissue with micrometer range resolution.[56]

The potential of gold nanoshells for *in vivo* backscattering OCT imaging applications was demonstrated by Loo *et al.*[52] A cuvette (1-mm path length) containing gold nanoshells solutions (10^9 nanoshells/ml) scattered light more intensely than a polystyrene microsphere-based scattering solution or saline. Kirillin *et al.*[57] and Zagaynova *et al.*[58] demonstrated the efficiency of the gold nanoshells as contrasting agents for OCT imaging and correlated

Table 1. Depth of penetration and resolution of gold nanoparticle-based imaging modalities.

	Penetration depth [reference]	Resolution/detection limit [reference]	Disadvantage	Advantage
OCT	2–3 mm[56]	Micrometer range[56]		
TPL	40–75 μm[65,156]	0.32∼1.25 μm[65,156]		
PAT	1∼5 cm[70,71]	∼0.2 mm[70,71]		
SERS	1–2 cm[89]	Single molecule detection[157] (e.g. 0.3 nm[91])	Limited penetration depth	Contact-free and noninvasive operation
DOS	Few millimeters (∼6 mm)[158]	Millimeter range[159]		
X-Ray CT	Not limited[95]	∼100 μm[160]	High-dose radiation increases the risk of cancer and allergic reaction.	

their experimental findings with Monte Carlo simulations in pig skin and rabbit skin. Skala *et al.*[59] generated monoclonal EGFR antibody-conjugated gold nanospheres to target and differentiate cells over-expressing EGFR from EGFR underexpressing cells with a 300% OCT signal difference. The use of PEGylated gold nanoshells as OCT contrast enhancers in mouse xenograft colon tumor model was reported by Gobin *et al.*[60] The brightness of the tumor in OCT image was enhanced due to accumulation of tail vein-injected gold nanoshells. Kah *et al.*[61] reported the use of anti-EGFR functionalized PEGylated gold nanoshells as OCT imaging contrast agents. Improved nanoparticle accumulation in epidermoid tumors of xenograft mouse models was observed. The time required for delivery of nanoshells to the tumor site was reduced from 6 h to 2 h, with antibody-functionalized particles compared to nonfunctionalized gold nanoshells. Delivery of antibody-conjugated gold nanospheres via microneedles and ultrasound to oral tumor in hamster model for OCT contrast enhancement was reported by Kim *et al.*[62] Microneedles provided passages for the deep penetration of nanospheres and the ultrasonic force generated by the ultrasound caused improved distribution of the nanospheres into the tumor model. This multimodal approach increased the mean intensity of OCT images to around 177% for the tumor tissue over the untreated segments.

3.3. *Two-photon luminescence*

Two-photon luminescence (TPL) involves two low-energy photonic excitation of electrons from the occupied d band to the unoccupied sp bands of a noble metal atom, producing an electron–hole in the respective bands. Subsequently, some amount of energy is lost to heat scattering and the rest is given out as a measurable luminescent signal due to electron–hole recombination.[63] Gold nanomaterials are capable of enhanced luminescent signal following resonance coupling of these electrons due to their surface plasmon properties.[64]

Durr *et al.*[65] reported TPL imaging of gold nanorod labeled skin cancer cells in three-dimensional (3D) tissue phantom deep down up to 75 μm, with a TPL intensity three times stronger than unlabeled cancer cells. Park *et al.*[66] used TPL to determine cellular level/intra-organ biodistribution of gold nanoparticles. Multiplexed imaging was demonstrated by simultaneously imaging nuclei, cytoplasm, and gold nanoparticles distributed within the subcutaneous xenograft tumor model (tumor slices) of colorectal cancer. Liu *et al.*[67] studied the two-photon absorption imaging properties of dextran-coated 11-mercaptoundecanoic acid functionalized gold nanospheres (diameter 1.33 ± 0.12 nm) by imaging their internalization and localization around the nucleus in human mesenchymal stem cells *in vitro* by two-photon and confocal microscopy. Huff *et al.*[68] used TPL to track the trafficking of single gold nanorods inside the oral epithelium-derivate KB cells. Higher nonspecific uptake of CTAB-coated gold nanorods in KB cells was observed compared to PEGylated gold nanorods. *In vivo* TPL imaging of gold nanorods in mouse earlobe vessels was demonstrated by Wang *et al.*[69] Picomolar concentrations of gold nanorods were injected via the tail vein in mice followed by real-time TPL imaging. TPL intensities generated by nanorods were approximately three times higher than that of the background.[40]

3.4. *Photoacoustic tomography*

Photoacoustic effect is the production of acoustic waves by the target when irradiated by a short electromagnetic pulse beam. A portion of this incident light is absorbed by the target, causing localized thermal excitation. This thermal excitation causes a buildup of pressure difference between the target and the surrounding body producing a detectable ultrasonic wave. In the context of biological media, this ultrasonic wave is dependent on the thermal and mechanical properties of tissues, which determine the initial optical absorption and the transmission of this ultrasonic wave to the transducer above. Photoacoustic tomography (PAT) imaging affords a spatial resolution around 0.2 mm, with a penetration depth up to 5 cm.[70,71] Passive and active targeting of cancer cells using gold nanoparticles to enhance tumor photoacoustic signal intensity have been demonstrated.

Photoacoustic imaging of breast tumor in the abdominal wall of xenograft mouse model has been investigated using PEGylated gold nanospheres.[72] Wang *et al.*[73] demonstrated noninvasive PAT of rat brain vasculature using with a maximal 63% enhancement in optical absorption using PEGylated gold nanoshells compared to that observed before administration of the nanoparticles. The nanoshells were cleared in 6 h after 3 sequential administrations. Intravenously injected PEGylated gold nanocages gradually enhanced the optical absorption in the cerebral cortex of rats; measurements were taken up to 5 h after the final injection of the nanoshells. The images were compared to the absorption profile of the cortex prior to nanocage injections.[74] Photoacoustic imaging and mapping of a sentinel lymph node using gold nanocages as contrast agent was reported by Song *et al.*[75] with a penetration depth up to approximately 3 cm. Hollow gold nanospheres and gold nanobeacons have also been investigated as photoacoustic imaging contrast agents for imaging brain vasculature and sentinel lymph node in mouse models.[76,77] The use of degradable gold nanoclusters for photoacoustic imaging has also been investigated recently.[78]

Mallidi *et al.*[79] demonstrated multiwavelength photoacoustic imaging in subcutaneous gelatin implants in mouse tissue *ex vivo* containing anti-EGFR gold nanoparticles targeted toward human epithelial carcinoma cells. It was possible to differentiate cancerous cells from nonmalignant cells based on the multiwavelength photoacoustic signal and optical absorption properties of the cancer cells. Cancer cells showed a characteristic red-shifted peak on the extinction spectra, while nontargeted Au-NPs showed green peak due to the aggregation of anti-EGFR labeled gold nanoparticles around the cancer cells, which is absent in the cells incubated nontargeted NPs. Olafsson *et al.*[80] reported 10–18 dB contrast enhancement of human prostate tumors in severe combined immunodeficient (SCID) mice using intratumorally injected gold nanorods. Tail vein injected antibody-conjugated gold nanorods enhanced optical contrast of xenograft squamous tumor by 3.5 dB (Cal27) in mice compared to control group (untargeted-gold nanorods treated mice).[81] Kim *et al.*[82] reported imaging of melanomas *in vivo* using Nle4, D-Phe7-melanocyte-stimulating hormone-modified gold nanocages. Following tail-vein injectioin, targeted gold nanocages accumulated at the B16 melanoma tumor site at levels that were

3.6 times greater than PEGylated gold nanocages, resulting in three-fold enhancement in optical contrast. In addition to gold nanoparticles, Kim *et al.*[83] introduced novel light-absorbing gold carbon nanotubes, which are single-wall carbon nanotubes with a thin layer of gold coating, and successfully employed them for *in vivo* mapping of the lymphatic endothelial receptor. Gold-coated carbon nanotubes demonstrated higher photoacoustic signals and lower bubble-formation thresholds than carbon nanotubes and gold nanospheres alone (individual treatments). Antibody-conjugated gold-coated carbon nanotubes were investigated as contrast agents for photoacoustic imaging for improving detection sensitivity and specificity of circulating tumor cells *in vivo*.[84,85]

3.5. *Surface-enhanced Raman scattering*

Raman spectroscopy and surface-enhanced Raman scattering (SERS) can be employed for bioimaging and biodiagnostics of cancer cells. Raman spectroscopy measures the inelastic scattering of monochromatic light by materials. Surface enhancement, which involves an enhancement of Raman scattering by molecules adsorbed on a rough metal surface, pushes the detection limit to single molecules.

Laurent *et al.*[86] reported the *in vitro* Raman imaging and Raman spectra of methylene blue molecule adsorbed as a single layer on gold nanospheres. Huang *et al.*[87] presented the enhanced, sharpened, and polarized Raman spectrum of antibody-conjugated gold nanorods as potential diagnostic signatures for cancer cells. Free prostate-specific antigen (PSA) in femtomolar concentration in human serum was detected using gold nanoparticles coated with a Raman reporter molecule (5, 5′-Dithiobis(succinimidyl-2-nitrobenzoate)) and mouse anti-PSA monoclonal antibody.[88]

Tumor detection and imaging in live animals based on SERS gold nanoparticles and Raman spectroscopy have also been reported. Active targeted SERS nanoparticles demonstrated optical enhancement of Raman spectra that were 10 times more efficient than nontargeted SERS nanoparticles.[89] Keren *et al.*[90] demonstrated multiplexed Raman imaging using four different SERS nanoparticles (gold core covered with Raman-active material and coated with silica) (Nanoplex Biotag, Oxonica) in mice and demonstrated a detection limit of 8.125 pM. von Maltzahn *et al.*[91] synthesized Raman-active molecules-functionalized PEGylated gold nanorods (SERS-coded PEG-NRs) for multiplexed Raman detection and photothermal heating (Fig. 2). SERS-coded PEG-NRs can be detected and to

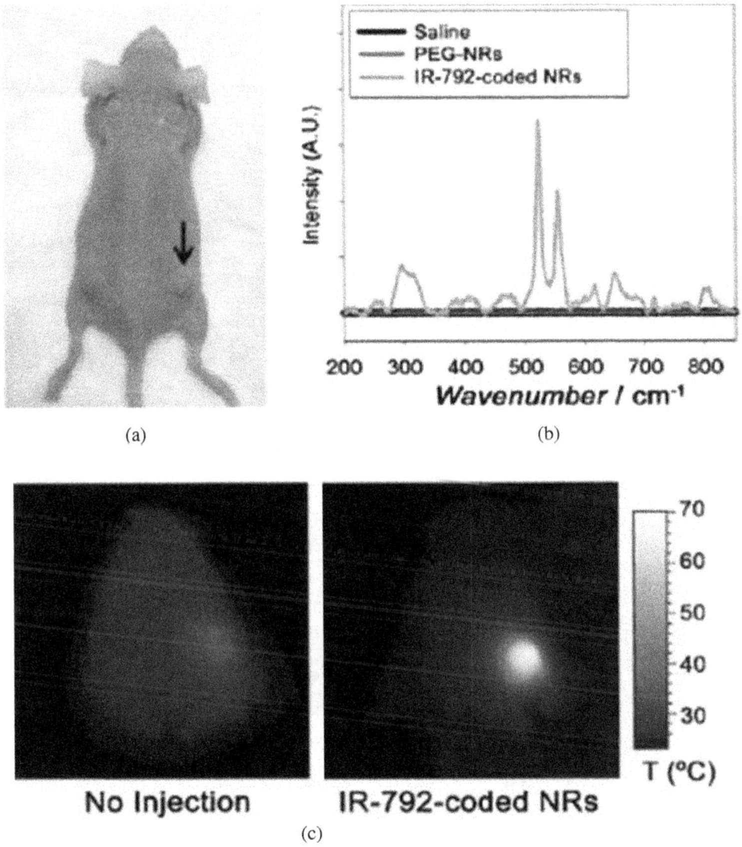

Fig. 2. *In vivo* Raman detection and photothermal heating using Raman-active molecules (IR-792)-functionalized PEGylated gold nanorods (IR-792-coded-GNRs). (a) IR-792-coded-GNRs, Pegylated GNRs, or saline were intratumorally injected into bilateral human MDA-MB-435 tumors-bearing mice. (b) Raman spectra of IR-792-coded-GNRs, and two controls. (c) Photothermal heating of tumor with or without IR-792-coded-GNRs using laser light (810 nm, 2 W/cm^2, 3 min) (Reproduced with permission from Ref. 91; Copyright Wiley-VCH Verlag GmbH & Co. KGaA).

provide Raman spectra after subcutaneous injection into athymic (nu/nu) mice. The minimum detection limit of the SERS-coded PEG-NRs was reported between 2×10^{-12} and 4×10^{-16} M.

3.6. *Diffuse optical spectroscopy*

An alternative method for noninvasive detection of gold nanoshell concentrations in tumors of live mice was reported by Zaman *et al.*[92] using diffuse optical spectroscopy (DOS). *In vitro* estimations of gold nanoshell concentrations were first carried out on tissue phantoms with concentration measurement error less than 12.6%. *In vivo* studies were performed using a mouse xenograft tumor model, which demonstrated the sensitivity of DOS for detecting nanoshells localized within the tumor. These concentrations showed agreement to within 20% with neutron activation analysis (NAA), a current standard method to measure gold nanoshell concentrations in tissue.

3.7. *X-ray computed tomography and magnetic resonance imaging*

Optical or acoustic scattering-based imaging techniques listed above with limited tissue penetration depths are challenging for deep tissue imaging. X-ray computed tomography (CT) and magnetic resonance (MR) imaging are common clinical imaging modalities with micrometer spatial resolution and are better suited for *in vivo* imaging of deep-suited tissues. The 3D sections of X-ray CT images are created by a computer which adds up two-dimensional (2D) slices taken along a single circular axis in the area of interest.

Gold nanoparticles were introduced as an X-ray contrast agent with the potential to address the limitations of iodine-based agents by Hainfeld *et al.*[93] in 2006. In this study, 2-nm gold nanospheres were injected via the tail vein in mice in order to provide contrast of EMT-6 syngeneic mammary tumor in xenograft mouse model and blood vessels. Accumulation of gold nanospheres was first observed in liver and spleen after injection; nanoparticles were cleared via the kidney and bladder after 1 h. The use of PEGylated gold nanoparticles for *in vivo* CT imaging of heart/great vessels[94] and antibody-coated gold nanorods for *in vitro* cancer targeting/imaging[95] demonstrated the use of gold nanoparticles promising as X-ray contrast agents. Alric *et al.*[96] successfully showed *in vitro* and *in vivo* X-ray CT and MR imaging using gadolinium chelate coated gold nanoparticles as contrast agents. Gold nanoparticles at 50.7 mM concentration (10 mg of Au per ml) resulted in an equivalent X-ray absorption as that demonstrated by 280 mM iodine (35 mg of I per ml). The presence of gadolinium in the nanoparticles, behaved as positive contrast agents for MRI, appeared brighter than the negative controls. von Maltzahn *et al.*[97] demonstrated *in vivo* X-ray CT of intratumorally injected PEGylated gold nanorods (GNRs) in MDA-MB-435 human tumor-bearing mice. Detailed 3D distribution of nanorods demonstrated two-fold higher X-ray absorption over iodine. Computational predictions of photothermal treatments were employed to better guide surgical irradiation (Fig. 3).

Magnetic gold nanoparticles/nanoshells provide a platform for both magnetic and optical imaging as well as hyperthermia via the tunable plasmonic photothermal properties of gold. Ji *et al.*[98] described the use

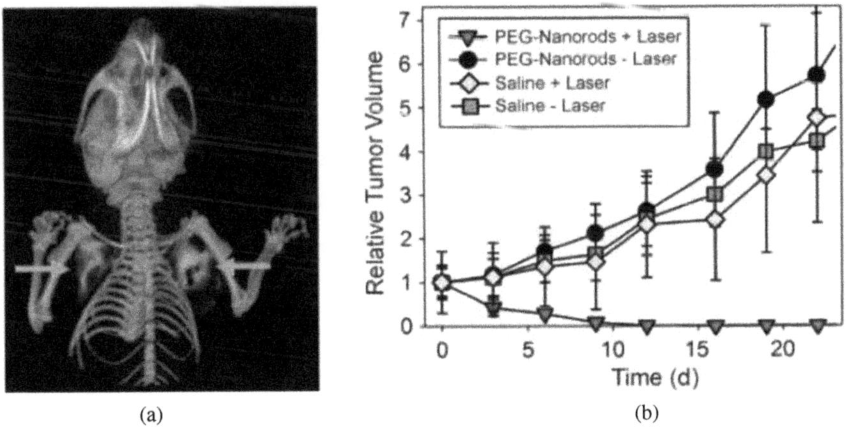

Fig. 3. (a) Three-dimensional X-ray CT of PEGylated gold nanorods (green arrows) enable computational prediction to better guide photothermal therapy. (b) Computationally determined laser parameters (810 nm, 2 W/cm^2, 5 min) were employed at tumor sites 72 h following systemic injection of nanorods. Tumor volumes were monitored as a function of time (Ref. 97; Adapted and reprinted with permission from the American Association for Cancer Research) (color online).

of a novel hybrid molecule consisting of superparamagnetic iron oxide (SPIO)-silica core and a gold nanoshell for MRI imaging, NIR-induced hyperthermia and postulated magnetic field driven accumulation of the nanoparticles for enhanced hyperthermia effects. Chen *et al.*[99] developed a magnetoplasmonic assembly containing inner $Fe_3O_4@SiO_2$ core coated with gold nanoparticles, which were further loaded with biocompatible PEG-SH and anticancer drug curcumin and tested against HL60 cancer cells for uptake followed by cellular

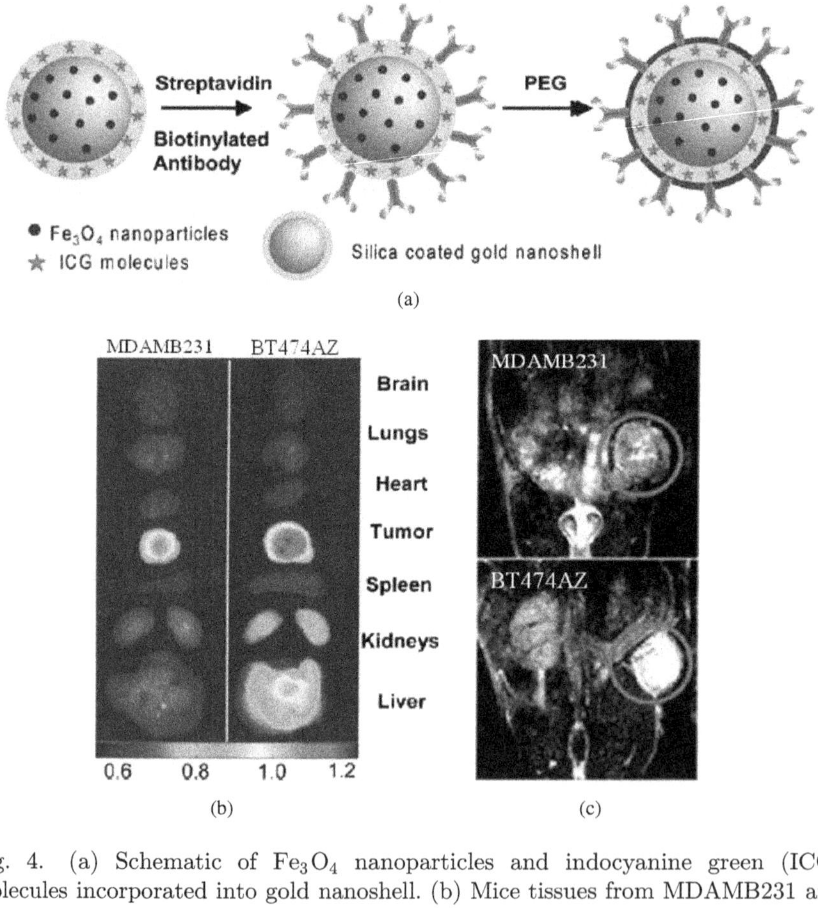

Fig. 4. (a) Schematic of Fe_3O_4 nanoparticles and indocyanine green (ICG) molecules incorporated into gold nanoshell. (b) Mice tissues from MDAMB231 and BT474AZ tumor-bearing mice were harvested 72 h post-injection of nanoshells for optical fluorescence imaging. (c) The BT474AZ tumor showed higher intensity of MRI contrast than MDAMB231 24 h post-injection of nanoshells (Reprinted with permission from Ref. 101. Copyright 2010, American Chemical Society).

apoptosis. Su *et al.*[100] demonstrated the use of Au_3Cu_1 nanocapsules as contrast agents in mice for MR imaging; Au_3Cu_1 nanocontrast agents enhanced the contrast of blood vessels of mice at a dose of 20 mg/kg with 83% viability rate, suggestig their potential use in MR angiography as blood-pool agents. Bardhan *et al.*[101] synthesized gold nanoshell-based nanocomplexes, where Fe_3O_4 nanoparticles and indocyanine green (ICG) molecules are incorporated in the silica epilayer coated around the gold nanoshell, for fluorescence optical imaging (FOI) and MR imaging. Nanocomplexes were conjugated with PEG and HER2 antibody prior to intravenous injection into HER2 overexpressing and underexpressing human breast tumors (BT474AZ, and MDAMB231)-bearing female nude mice. FOI and MRI demonstrated highest imaging contrast in both BT474AZ and MDAMB231 tumors at 4 h and 24 h, respectively, following injection *in vivo*. The BT474AZ tumor showed a maximal 71.5% increase in florescence intensity and 50% increase in dark T2-weighted MR image contrast compared to the MDAMB231 tumor in the presence of nanocomplexes (Fig. 4.)

4. Photothermal cancer therapy using gold nanoparticles

High conversion of absorbed light to heat, photostability, and biocompatibility make gold nanoparticles attractive candidates for photothermal therapy, an adjunctive therapeutic modality for cancer diseases. As opposed to traditional whole-body hyperthermia, site-specific generation of mild or moderate hyperthermic temperatures (40–46 °C) holds significant promise for cancer therapy. Studies of photothermal treatments using immunotargeted gold nanoparticles of various shapes including spheres,[53,102] clusters,[103] rods,[54] shells[51] and cages,[104] have demonstrated the ability to selectively induce cancer cell damage via hyperthermia, while causing minimal damage to nontargeted cells.

4.1. *Gold nanospheres and clusters*

LSPR absorption of gold nanospheres is in the visible region (~520 nm) and therefore suitable mainly for superficial cancers due to strong absorption of light in this wavelength region by tissue. Both pulsed and continuous-visible wavelength lasers have been employed for cancer cell ablation *in vitro*.[53,105] Clustering of antibody-conjugated gold nanoparticles results in red-shifting of light absorption and formation of microbubbles around clusters upon pulsed near-IR lasers irradiation, which can result in effective *in vitro* and[103,106] and *in vivo* cell damage.[107] Lukianova-Hleb *et al.*[108] generated a multistage tunable plasmonic nanobubble and used it for selective disruption of cancer cells. Antibody-conjugated gold nanoparticles formed aggregated clusters after receptor-mediated internalization by cancer cells. Plasmonic nanobubbles were generated when anti-EGFR-conjugated gold nanoparticles were subjected to pulsed-laser irradiation. Rapid expanse and collapse of nanobubbles resulted in disruption of the cell membrane, leading to death of EGFR-positive lung carcinoma cells.

4.2. *Gold nanoshells and gold nanocubes*

Unlike gold nanospheres, LSPR absorption of gold nanoshells[21] and gold nanocubes[109] is in the NIR region, which is better suited for photon-based noninvasive applications. *In vivo* destruction of canine transmissible venereal tumor in female nonobese diabetic mice was carried out by Hirsch *et al.*[110] using interstitially injected PEGylated gold nanoshells. Exposure of nanoshells to NIR laser (820 nm, 4 W/cm^2) resulted in significant temperature increase and irreversible thermal damage of tissue. O'Neal *et al.*[111] demonstrated murine colon carcinoma tumor regression in female albino mice with intravenously injected PEGylated gold nanoshells (20 μl/g) and laser irradiation (3 min, 820 nm, 4 W/cm^2). Tumor-bearing mice, treated with nanoshells and laser, were tumor free up to few months, while control animals, treated with laser irradiation alone, showed growth in tumor size. Stern *et al.*[112] demonstrated a high degree (93%) regression of tumors at high doses of nanoshells (8.5 μl/g) in PC-3-bearing male athymic (nu/nu) mice; a slightly lower nanoshell dose (7.0 μl/g) did not result cancer cell ablation. Recently, Schwartz *et al.*[113] successfully demonstrated passive delivery of PEGylated gold nanoshells to brain tumors in an orthotopic canine model. Accumulation of the nanoshells facilitated the selective elevation of tumor tissue temperature to 66°C.

Specific molecular targeting strategies have also been investigated in order to further increase the efficiency of *in vivo* photothermal ablation using gold nanoshells.[51,114] Melancon *et al.*[114] employed epidermal growth factor receptor-targeted hollow gold nanoshells (30 nm average diameter) for *in vitro* photothermal ablation. Targeted gold nanoshells showed higher delivery efficacies to tumors compared to nontargeted nanoshells (6.8% ID/g versus 4.6% ID/g; ID/g: Injected dose per gram of tissue); however, the majority of gold nanoshells were found in spleen, liver, and kidney (~65% ID/g). Anti-HER2 antibodies conjugated to PEGylated silica core gold nanoshells and nanocubes have been shown to selectively bind and photothermally ablate HER2 overexpressing tumor cell lines *in vitro*, including HER2 positive Daoy medulloblastoma cells and HER2 overexpressing SK-BR-3 breast carcinoma cells.[104,115,116]

4.3. *Gold nanorods*

Cylindrical gold nanorods (GNRs) also absorb light in the NIR region similar to gold nanoshells and nanocages. Moreover, the absorption cross-section of GNRs absorption is reported to be 50% and 30% higher than of the gold nanoshells and cubes, respectively.[117] This advantage over gold nanospheres, nanoshells, and nanocubes makes nanorods attractive candidates for biological photothermal applications. Huang *et al.*[54] employed gold nanorods conjugated to an anti-EGFR antibody in order to target malignant oral epithelial cell cancer cells. The targeted nanorods were subjected to laser irradiation from an external source, leading to the selective localization of hyperthermic treatment to the malignant cells. Black *et al.*[118] demonstrated selective ablation of colon cancer cell-expressing delta-opiod receptor using deltorphin peptide-modified PEGylated gold nanorods. We have recently developed GNR–elastin-like polypeptide (GNR-ELP) matrices for simultaneous administration of hyperthermia and chemotherapy to human prostate cancer cells *in vitro*.[119]

PEGylation of gold nanorods reduced cytotoxicity and maintained the stability of GNRs in mice. Approximately half of injected

PEGylated GNRs remained in blood 30 min after intravenous injection, while unmodified GNRs accumulated largely in the liver.[120] Dickerson *et al.*[121] demonstrated *in vivo* photothermal therapy of subcutaneous squamous cell carcinoma xenografts grown in nude (nu/nu) mice using nontargeted PEGylated gold nanorods irradiated by NIR laser. Laser irradiation of intratumorally and intravenously delivered nanorods demonstrated 96% and more than 74% regression in tumor volume regression after two weeks, respectively. Goodrich *et al.*[122] demonstrated photothermal therapy using tail vein injection of PEGylated GNRs in a murine colon cancer model. The survival percentage of photothermally treated mice was approximately 44% at 60 days, while the mean survival time of mice for control groups (nanorod alone and laser irradiation) was less than 10 days. Substantial accumulation of GNRs was observed in the liver, spleen, and lymph nodes 30 days post injection. Intravenously injected PEGylated GNRs showed long circulation times ($t_{1/2}$ of 17 h).[97] Systemically injected PEGylated GNRs, coupled with a computationally designed irradiation regimen ($2\,W/cm^2$, 5 min), completely inhibited human xenografted tumors regrowth in mice within 20 days of photothermal therapy. In addition, a photothermal comparison of PEGylated GNRs to gold nanoshells showed that GNRs exhibited less than one-third of the spectral bandwidth, more than six times the heat generation and up to three times higher extinction coefficient per gram gold than PEGylated gold nanoshells.

4.4. *Delivery of bioactive/therapeutic molecules*

There is great need and interest in developing delivery systems in which biological activities of the bionanomaterial conjugates can be inducibly controlled via applied electronic, optical, ultrasonic, or magnetic signals. Light irradiation is a simple technique to execute in cells and organisms and can be used to trigger the biological activity of delivered biomolecules. Delivery of small molecules (e.g. anticancer drugs) and nucleic acids (e.g. plasmid DNA, small interfering RNA, and small hairpin RNA) to cancer cells have been successfully demonstrated using surface-modified gold nanoparticles via several controlled release mechanisms, including cleavage of gold-thiol bonds via pulsed laser irradiation,[123,124] facilitated molecule release in acidic environments,[125] diffusion,[126] and NIR-induced surface coating shrinkage.[127] It has also been observed that gold nanoparticles can undergo a shape transformation to nanospheres after the absorption of NIR to IR photons.[128–130] This property of GNRs can affect the binding of conjugated molecules on their surface and can be used as a triggered release control of biomolecules at specific sites in the body. This is aided by the enhanced permeability and retention (EPR) effect facilitates the passive accumulation of nanoparticles (< 100 nm) in tumor tissue due to the highly permeable and poorly organized vascular network.[131]

4.5. *Anticancer drugs*

Two analogues, P1 and P2, of the antitumorial drug candidate Kahalalide F, conjugated to gold nanoparticles (20 and 40 nm) demonstrated enhanced cytotoxic effect in HeLa tumor cells[132] while exhibiting 5 to 40 times less activity in nonmalignant cell lines. Nanoparticle conjugates for the 40-nm diameter nanoparticle showed higher cytotoxicity for the P1 and P2 peptides when compared to the free peptides, presumably due to higher uptake efficacy. *In vivo* delivery of dihydrofolate reductase inhibitor, methotrexate (MTX) using gold nanospheres, was reported by Chen *et al.*[133] MTX-loaded nanospheres inhibited proliferation of Lewis lung carcinoma tumor in mouse and demonstrated greater effect than direct delivery of MTX. Delivery of tumor necrosis factor alpha (TNF-α)-modified gold nanospheres to murine fibrosarcoma tumor in combination hyperthermia resulted in increased tumor recession compared to the individual treatments acting alone.[134,135]

Receptor-mediated delivery of drug-loaded gold nanoparticles has been employed to actively target tumor tissue in order to enhance treatment efficacy due to increased retention at the tumor tissue. Dreaden *et al.*[136] delivered increased amounts of tamoxifen to breast cancer cells using GNRs conjugated with PEGylated tamoxifen derivative, which competes with 17-estradiol for binding to the estrogen receptor. Enhanced endocytosis of nanorods into the estrogen receptor-positive cell lines increased the potency of the drug up to

2.7 times over the passive diffusion-based drug delivery. Brown *et al.*[123] synthesized PEGylated-gold nanoparticles with the active component of the platinum drug oxaliplatin, [Pt(1*R*, 2*R*-diaminocyclohexane]c2+ ([Pt(*R*, *R*-dach)]), tethered to PEG linker molecules on the surface of the gold nanoparticles. Platinum-tethered nanoparticles were found to be up to 6-fold and 5.6-fold more cytotoxic than oxaliplatin alone in a human lung epithelial and 4 colon cancer cell lines, respectively. PEGylated gold nanoparticles did not induce cytotoxicity in all cell lines investigated up to a dose of 10 nm. Platinum-tethered gold nanoparticles were observed in contact and inside the plasma membrane as well as inside the nucleus of the A549 lung cells. Unfunctionalized nanoparticles did not enter cell nuclei, implying that the [Pt(*R*, *R*-dach)] mediated transport into the nuclei. Amphiphilic gold nanoparticles conjugated with folate containing a poly(L-aspartate-doxorubicin)-b-poly(ethylene glycol) monolayer were synthesized for tumor-targeted drug delivery.[137] pH-sensitive hydrazine linkages were used to conjugate the doxorubicin (DOX) molecules to the hydrophobic poly(L-aspartate) for purposes of inducible release upon folate receptor-mediated endocytosis. Nanoparticles conjugated with folate and DOX molecules showed enhanced toxicity in 4T1 mouse mammary cancer cells that overexpress the folate receptor, compared to NIH-3T3 mouse embryonic fibroblasts, which do not overexpress the receptor.

A novel combination delivery system consisting of SERS-active molecule functionalized gold nanorods and DOX-encapsulated thermosensitive liposomes was reported by Park *et al.*[138] SERS-active GNRs provided Raman imaging and photothermal heating. Drug-encapsulated thermosensitive liposome delivered 12 times more DOX to MDA-MB-435 human tumors in mice in response to the thermal stimulus by the nanorods compared to nonheated vesicles. Gold nanoparticles were investigated as both a cage as well as a carrier for the anticancer drug, 5-fluorouracil (5-FU).[139] Exposure to UV radiation at 365 nm resulted in photolytic cleavage of ligands for the controlled release of 5-FU. MCF-7 cells, treated with fluorouracil-conjugated gold nanoparticles and 20 min of 365 nm UV-A radiation, resulted in an IC_{50} value of 0.7 μM on a per particle basis, corresponding to 11.9 μM on a per drug basis. Cells treated with only light, only Au-PCFUs, and light followed by incubation with the fluorouracil-conjugated gold nanoparticles exhibited negligible cell death.

4.6. *Nucleic acid delivery*

Gene therapy is based on the idea that a disease can be corrected by compensating for abnormal genes at the genetic level. This can be done by the delivery of exogenous DNA or RNA. However, due to the low efficacy of passive transport of nucleic acids through the cellular membrane, an appropriate delivery vehicle is needed. Viruses have emerged as some of the most efficient delivery vectors that are known at present. Despite their efficacy as gene delivery vectors, concerns pertaining to the safety, immunogenicity, degradation, and production scale-up persist with the use of viral vectors. This has resulted in an investigation into nonviral approaches to delivery of exogenous nucleic acids for gene therapy.[140] Recently, functionalized gold nanoparticles have been investigated for the delivery of nucleic acids, including DNA and RNA.[141]

4.7. *DNA delivery*

Photoinducible shape change of gold nanorods was employed to control the release of two independent DNA oligionucleotides.[142] A mixture of 6-carboxyfluorescein-labeled DNA 40 mers (FAM-DNA) conjugated short nanorods ($\lambda_{max} \sim 800$ nm) and tetramethylrhodamine-labeled DNA 40 mers (TMR-DNA) conjugated long nanorods ($\lambda_{max} \sim 1100$ nm) was used for the selective release of DNA via laser irradiation at two different wavelengths. Wu *et al.*[128] self-assembled DNA, encoding enhanced green fluorescent protein (EGFP) onto gold nanorods for the study of gene expression using HeLa cells upon femto-second NIR laser irradiation. DNA-nanorod conjugates were able to enter the cell; laser irradiation was capable of triggering the shape transformation resulting in release of the DNA for subsequent EGFP expression in localized regions in culture. The Oh group[143] synthesized cationic photocleaveable gold nanoparticles for temporal and spatial release of DNA by light. Positively charged gold nanoparticles were generated with a photoactive o-nitrobenzyl ester linkage and were then complexed with DNA through electrostatic interactions. Near-UV irradiation leads to cleavage of the nitrobenzyl linkage and resulted in a release of positively charged alkyl amines, leaving behind anionic carboxylate groups. Effective DNA delivery of fluorescein (FAM)-labeled 37 mer DNA and release into mouse embryonic fibroblast cells was observed with significant nuclear localization after UV irradiation.

Bifunctional Au/Ni nanorods ware fabricated by Leong and and Searson for transgene delivery.[144] Rhodamine-tagged transferrins were bound to the gold segment (100 nm in length) via a thiolate linkage for receptor-mediated endocytosis. Plasmid DNAs, encode for either firefly luciferase or GFPmut1 variant, were compacted with $CaCl_2$ and attached to the nickel segment (100 nm in length) of the nanorod in the form of $CaPO_4$ complexes. Red fluorescence of the rhodamine tag, transmission electron microscope (TEM) images, and electron dispersive X-ray (EDX) analysis confirmed that the nanorods were located in vesicles or the cytoplasm of HEK293 cells after 1 and 4 h incubation. Nanorods conjugated with transferrin increased green fluorescent protein (GFP) expression by a factor of 2 and luciferase expression by a factor of 3.4 compared to nanorods without transferrin. A 4-fold increase and 255-fold higher transfection efficiency for GFP and luciferase expression, respectively, were observed compared to naked DNA. *In vivo* luciferase expression in the skin of mice was 830 times higher than background (skin with no nanorod delivery) 1 day after injection, the luciferase expression decreased by approximately 10 times after 3 weeks. In addition, intramuscular delivery of the nanorods to mice demonstrated 17 times higher transgene expression compared to background levels.

Cationic polymer-mediated gene delivery has emerged as a promising alternative to virus-mediated gene therapy and there has been a recent push in combining this method with gold nanoparticles.[145] Our group[146] synthesized stable polyelectrolyte gold nanorods (PE-GNRs) for delivery of exogenous plasmid DNA. Nanorods were first modified with negatively charged polystyrene sulfonate (PSS) followed by coating with a cationic polymer assembled by means of electrostatic interactions; EDGE-3, 3′, a polymer synthesized in our laboratory,[140,147] or polyethyleneimine (PEI, 25 kDa) (PEI25) were used as cationic polymers. Photothermally stable EDGE-3,3′-PSS-GNRs were able to induce significant cell death in PC3-PSMA human prostate cancer cells on laser irradiation and exhibited lower cytotoxicity than PEI25-PSS-GNRs. In addition, PC3-PSMA cells treated with EDGE-3, 3′-PSS-GNRs containing 350 ng pGL3 plasmid, encoding for the firefly luciferase protein, had a maximal 10-fold increase in gene expression compared to the PEI25-PSS-GNRs for similar loadings of the pGL3 plasmid [Fig. 5(a)].

4.8. *RNA delivery*

RNA interference (RNAi)-mediated gene silencing has emerged as a powerful therapeutic approach for gene silencing treatment against several human diseases.[148] RNAi has high sequence specificity and potency in silencing gene expression for genes with known sequences.

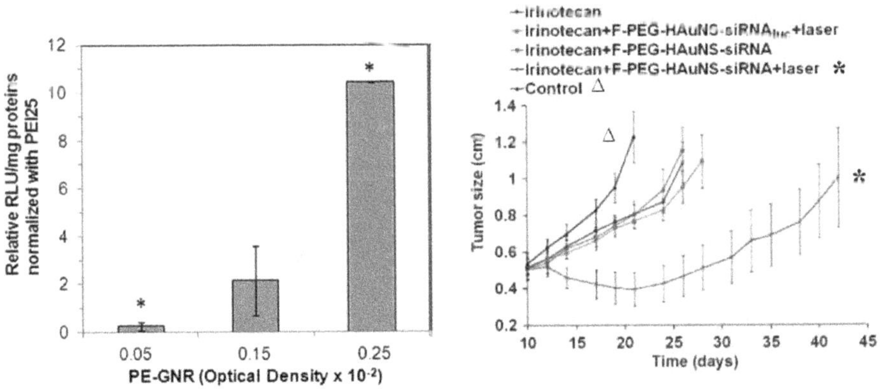

(a) (b)

Fig. 5. (a) Transfection of PC3-PSMA human prostate cancer cells using EDGE-3, 3′-PSS-GNR and pEI25-PSS-GNR. Asterisks indicate p values < 0.02 (two tailed t-test) (Reprinted with permission from Ref. 146. Copyright 2009, American Chemical Society). (b) Delivery of p65 siRNA (down regulate NF-kB) and irinotecan using folate receptor-targeted nanoshells (F-PEG-HAuNS) to tumor-bearing mice resulted in inhibition of tumor growth (Ref. 154; Adapted and reprinted by permission from the American Association for Cancer Research).

Short interfering RNA (siRNA) are short double-stranded nucleic acids that mediate RNAi in the cytoplasm of cells via post-transcriptional silencing.[149] However, naked siRNAs have a short half-life and demonstrate low efficacies for cell entry when exposed to physiological conditions due to their susceptibility for endogenous nuclease degradation.[150] Therefore, it is necessary to develop effective delivery strategies for carrying siRNA into cancer cells for achieving high levels of therapeutic efficacy.[151]

Bonoiu *et al.*[151] synthesized nanoplexes consisting of GNRs with multilayers of cationic polymers, and functionalized with siRNA molecules specific for adenosine 3, 5-monophosphate-regulated phosphoprotein (DARPP-32) silencing; more than 80% of DARPP-32 expression was silenced up to 1 week following the transfection. PEI-capped gold nanoparticles were recently generated by incubating a mixture of aqueous HAuCl4 with PEI followed by reduction of the gold.[152] The nanoparticles bound siRNA via electrostatic interactions without a significant increase in particle size. For silencing studies, MDA-MB-432 cells were pre-transfected with pEGFP-N2 plasmid allowing 60%–70% of the cells to express green fluorescent protein (GFP). Transfected cells were treated with the PEI gold nanoparticles complexed with anti-GFP siRNA; significant reduction in GFP fluorescence was observed 48 h after incubation due to silencing of GFP.

Braun *et al.*[153] used gold nanoshells demonstrated *in vivo* controlled silencing of GFP-expressing C166-GFP mouse endothelial cell line at lower laser powers in a nonthermodestructive manner. *In vivo* and *in vitro* NIR-induced silencing of NF-κB p65 via folate receptor-targeted hollow gold nanospheres carrying siRNA was demonstrated in HeLa cervical cancer xenograft-bearing mice.[154] Intravenously injected nanospheres carrying p65 siRNA were allowed to circulate for 6 h prior to 1-min laser irradiation (50 mW/cm^2). Gold nanoparticles irradiated with NIR light resulted in shape transformation, leading to siRNA release to the cytosol for downregulation of NF-κB. NF-κB silencing induced the sensitization of tumors to a chemotherapeutic drug, irinotecan, leading to inhibition of tumor growth [Fig. 5(b)]. Shim *et al.*[155] mimicked the mildly acidic environment of the tumor tissue as the stimulus to cleave ketal linkages (Ketalized Linear Polyethylenimine) that connected the Au NPs to the siRNA. Both, OCT imaging of AuNPs, and silencing of eGFP-expressing NIH 3T3 cells were demonstrated. While these recent advances are very promising, detailed validation of their targeted delivery *in vivo* to myriad tumors, biodistribution profiles, and toxicity need to be characterized before extensive use.

5. Conclusions

Gold nanoparticles have been successfully employed for improvement of tumor imaging and enhancement of therapeutic efficacy against cancer diseases. Stealth PEGylated gold particles with prolonged circulation periods allowed passive accumulation of nanoparticles at the tumor site. Various optical and acoustic scattering-based imaging modalities have been developed to determine biodistribution of nanoparticles; some of these, however, are limited by low penetration depths *in vivo*. Actively targeted gold nanoparticles have demonstrated enhanced controllable delivery of chemotherapeutic drugs and nucleic acids to cancer cells, both *in vitro* and *in vivo*. Further preclinical investigations in stability, biodistribution, imaging capabilities, and enhancement of therapeutic efficacies are critical for the development of safe and efficient clinical theranostic platforms based on gold nanoparticles.

Acknowledgments

This work was supported by the National Science Foundation (CBET-0829128), National Institutes of Health (5R21CA133618-02).

References

1. M. A. El-Sayed, *Accounts of Chem. Res.* **34**, 257 (2001).
2. S. Link and M. A. El-Sayed, *J. Phys. Chem. B* **103**, 8410 (1999).
3. R. Weissleder, *Nat. Biotech.* **19**, 316 (2001).
4. J. Turkevich, P. C. Stevenson and J. Hillier, *Discuss. Faraday Soc.* **11**, 55 (1951).

5. D. V. Leff, L. Brandt and J. R. Heath, *Langmuir* **12**, 4723 (1996).
6. W. W. Weare, S. M. Reed, M. G. Warner and J. E. Hutchison, *J. Am. Chem. Soc.* **122**, 12890 (2000).
7. R. W. J. Scott, O. M. Wilson and R. M. Crooks, *J. Phys. Chem. B* **109**, 692 (2005).
8. X. G. Shi, S. H. Wang, S. Meshinchi, M. E. van Antwerp, X. D. Bi, I. H. Lee and J. R. Baker, *Small* **3**, 1245 (2007).
9. J. J. Yuan, A. Schmid, S. P. Armes and A. L. Lewis, *Langmuir* **22**, 11022 (2006).
10. C. R. Martin, *Science* **266**, 1961 (1994).
11. J. Burdick, E. Alonas, H. C. Huang, K. Rege and J. Wang, *Nanotechnology* **20**, 065306 (2009).
12. Y. Y. Yu, S. S. Chang, C. L. Lee and C. R. C. Wang, *J. Phys. Chem. B* **101**, 6661 (1997).
13. S. S. Chang, C. W. Shih, C. D. Chen, W. C. Lai and C. R. C. Wang, *Langmuir* **15**, 701 (1999).
14. N. R. Jana, L. Gearheart and C. J. Murphy, *Adv. Mater.* **13**, 1389 (2001).
15. N. R. Jana, L. Gearheart and C. J. Murphy, *J. Phys. Chem. B* **105**, 4065 (2001).
16. N. R. Jana, L. Gearheart, S. O. Obare and C. J. Murphy, *Langmuir* **18**, 922 (2002).
17. B. Nikoobakht and M. A. El-Sayed, *Chem. Mater.* **15**, 1957 (2003).
18. B. Nikoobakht and M. A. El-Sayed, *Langmuir* **17**, 6368 (2001).
19. S. J. Oldenburg, R. D. Averitt, S. L. Westcott and N. J. Halas, *Chem. Phys. Lett.* **288**, 243 (1998).
20. S. J. Oldenburg, J. B. Jackson, S. L. Westcott and N. J. Halas, *Appl. Phys. Lett.* **75**, 2897 (1999).
21. S. J. Oldenburg, S. L. Westcott, R. D. Averitt and N. J. Halas, *J. Chem. Phys.* **111**, 4729 (1999).
22. Y. G. Sun, B. T. Mayers and Y. N. Xia, *Nano Lett.* **2**, 481 (2002).
23. J. Y. Chen, J. M. McLellan, A. Siekkinen, Y. J. Xiong, Z. Y. Li and Y. N. Xia, *J. Am. Chem. Soc.* **128**, 14776 (2006).
24. S. E. Skrabalak, L. Au, X. D. Li and Y. Xia, *Nat. Protocols* **2**, 2182 (2007).
25. J. Aizpurua, P. Hanarp, D. S. Sutherland, M. Käll, G. W. Bryant and F. J. G. de Abajo, *Phys. Rev. Lett.* **90**, 057401 (2003).
26. H. Y. Tseng, C. K. Lee, S. Y. Wu, T. T. Chi, K. M. Yang, J. Y. Wang, Y. W. Kiang, C. C. Yang, M. T. Tsai, Y. C. Wu, H. Y. E. Chou and C. P. Chiang, *Nanotechnology* **21**, 295102 (2010).
27. H. Takahashi, T. Niidome, T. Kawano, S. Yamada and Y. Niidome, *J. Nanopart. Res.* **10**, 221 (2008).
28. A. Gole and C. J. Murphy, *Chem. Mater.* **17**, 1325 (2005).
29. S. Srivastava, A. Verma, B. L. Frankamp and V. M. Rotello, *Adv. Mater.* **17**, 617 (2005).
30. Y. H. Ding, X. M. Zhang, X. X. Liu and R. Guo, *Langmuir* **23**, 11342 (2007).
31. F. Porta, Z. Krpetic, L. Prati, A. Gaiassi and G. Scari, *Langmuir* **24**, 7061 (2008).

32. P. M. Shem, R. Sardar and J. S. Shumaker-Parry, *Langmuir* **25**, 13279 (2009).
33. S. Aryal, B. K. C. Remant, N. Dharmaraj, N. Bhattarai, C. H. Kim and H. Y. Kim, *Spectrochim. Acta Part A — Mol. Biomol. Spectrosc.* **63**, 160 (2006).
34. V. Chechik and R. M. Crooks, *Langmuir* **15**, 6364 (1999).
35. J. F. Zhou, D. A. Beattie, J. Ralston and R. Sedev, *Langmuir* **23**, 12096 (2007).
36. H. W. Liao and J. H. Hafner, *Chem. Mater.* **17**, 4636 (2005).
37. S. W. Choi, W. S. Kim and J. H. Kim, *J. Dispersion Sci. Technol.* **24**, 475 (2003).
38. S. Kommareddy and M. Amiji, *Nanomed. Nanotechnol. Biol. Med.* **3**, 32 (2007).
39. D. Shenoy, W. Fu, J. Li, C. Crasto, G. Jones, C. DiMarzio, S. Sridhar and M. Amiji, *Int. J. Nanomed.* **1**, 51 (2006).
40. G. D. Zhang, Z. Yang, W. Lu, R. Zhang, Q. Huang, M. Tian, L. Li, D. Liang and C. Li, *Biomaterials* **30**, 1928 (2009).
41. J. Lipka, M. Semmler-Behnke, R. A. Sperling, A. Wenk, S. Takenaka, C. Schleh, T. Kissel, W. J. Parak and W. G. Kreyline, *Biomaterials* **31**, 6574 (2010).
42. T. Niidome, Y. Akiyama, M. Yamagata, T. Kawano, T. Mori, Y. Niidome and Y. Katayama, *J. Biomater. Sci.* **20**, 1203 (2009).
43. J. M. Nam, K. J. Jang and J. T. Groves, *Nat. Protocols* **2**, 1438 (2007).
44. H. D. Hill and C. A. Mirkin, *Nat. Protocols* **1**, 324 (2006).
45. A. Verma, J. M. Simard, J. W. E. Worrall and V. M. Rotello, *J. Am. Chem. Soc.* **126**, 13987 (2004).
46. D. R. Bhumkar, H. M. Joshi, M. Sastry and V. B. Pokharkar, *Pharm. Res.* **24**, 1415 (2007).
47. K. K. Sandhu, C. M. McIntosh, J. M. Simard, S. W. Smith and V. M. Rotello, *Bioconj. Chem.* **13**, 3 (2002).
48. M. Thomas and A. M. Klibanov, *Proc. Natl. Acad. Sci. USA* **100**, 9138 (2003).
49. J. F. Zhou, J. Ralston, R. Sedev and D. A. Beattie, *J. Coll. Interf. Sci.* **331**, 251 (2009).
50. D. X. Li, Q. A. He and J. B. Li, *Adv. Coll. Interf. Sci.* **149**, 28 (2009).
51. C. Loo, A. Lowery, N. Halas, J. West and R. Drezek, *Nano Lett.* **5**, 709 (2005).
52. C. Loo, A. Lin, L. Hirsch, M. H. Lee, J. Barton, N. Halas, J. West and R. Drezek, *Technol. Cancer Res. Treatment* **3**, 33 (2004).
53. I. H. El-Sayed, X. H. Huang and M. A. El-Sayed, *Cancer Lett.* **239**, 129 (2006).
54. X. H. Huang, I. H. El-Sayed, W. Qian and M. A. El-Sayed, *J. Am. Chem. Soc.* **128**, 2115 (2006).
55. D. Huang, E. A. Swanson, C. P. Lin, J. S. Schuman, W. G. Stinson, W. Chang, M. R. Hee, T. Flotte, K. Gregory, C. A. Puliafito and J. G. Fujimoto, *Science* **254**, 1178 (1991).
56. A. F. Fercher, W. Drexler, C. K. Hitzenberger and T. Lasser, *Rep. Prog. Phys.* **66**, 239 (2003).
57. M. Kirillin, M. Shirmanova, M. Sirotkina, M. Bugrova, E. Zagaynova and B. Khlebtsov, *J. Biomed. Opt.* **14**, 021017 (2009).

58. E. V. Zagaynova, M. V. Shirmanova, M. Y. Kirillin, B. N. Khlebtsov, A. G. Orlova, I. V. Balalaeva, M. A. Sirotkina, M. L. Bugrova, P. D. Agrba and V. A. Kamensky, *Phys. Med. Biol.* **53**, 4995 (2008).
59. M. C. Skala, M. J. Crow, A. Wax and J. A. Izatt, *Nano Lett.* **8**, 3461 (2008).
60. A. M. Gobin, M. H. Lee, N. J. Halas, W. D. James, R. A. Drezek and J. L. West, *Nano Lett.* **7**, 1929 (2007).
61. J. C. Y. Kah, M. Olivo, T. H. Chow, K. S. Song, K. Z. Y. Koh, S. Mhaisalkar and C. J. R. Sheppard, *J. Biomed. Opt.* **14**, 054015 (2009).
62. C. S. Kim, P. Wilder-Smith, Y. C. Ahn, L. H. L. Liaw, Z. P. Chen and Y. J. Kwon, *J. Biomed. Opt.* **14**, 034008 (2009).
63. G. T. Boyd, Z. H. Yu and Y. R. Shen, *Phys. Rev. B* **33**, 7923 (1986).
64. A. Bouhelier, R. Bachelot, G. Lerondel, S. Kostcheev, P. Royer and G. P. Wiederrecht, *Phys. Rev. Lett.* **95**, 267405 (2005).
65. N. J. Durr, T. Larson, D. K. Smith, B. A. Korgel, K. Sokolov and A. Ben-Yakar, *Nano Lett.* **7**, 941 (2007).
66. J. Park, A. Estrada, J. A. Schwartz, P. Diagaradjane, S. Krishnan, A. K. Dunn and J. W. Tunnell, *Lasers Surg. Med.* **42**, 630 (2010).
67. C. L. Liu, M. L. Ho, Y. C. Chen, C. C. Hsieh, Y. C. Lin, Y. H. Wang, M. J. Yang, H. S. Duan, B. S. Chen, J. F. Lee, J. K. Hsiao and P. T. Chou, *J. Phys. Chem. C* **113**, 21082 (2009).
68. T. B. Huff, M. N. Hansen, Y. Zhao, J. X. Cheng and A. Wei, *Langmuir* **23**, 1596 (2007).
69. H. F. Wang, T. B. Huff, D. A. Zweifel, W. He, P. S. Low, A. Wei and J. X. Cheng, *Proc. Natl. Acad. Sci. USA* **102**, 15752 (2005).
70. X. D. Wang, Y. J. Pang, G. Ku, X. Y. Xie, G. Stoica and L. H. V. Wang, *Nat. Biotechnol.* **21**, 803 (2003).
71. G. Ku and L. H. V. Wang, *Opt. Lett.* **30**, 507 (2005).
72. Q. Zhang, N. Iwakuma, P. Sharma, B. M. Moudgil, C. Wu, J. McNeill, H. Jiang and S. R. Grobmyer, *Nanotechnology* **20**, 395102 (2009).
73. Y. W. Wang, X. Y. Xie, X. D. Wang, G. Ku, K. L. Gill, D. P. O'Neal, G. Stoica and L. V. Wang, *Nano Lett.* **4**, 1689 (2004).
74. X. M. Yang, S. E. Skrabalak, Z. Y. Li, Y. N. Xia and L. H. V. Wang, *Nano Lett.* **7**, 3798 (2007).
75. K. H. Song, C. H. Kim, C. M. Cobley, Y. N. Xia and L. V. Wang, *Nano Lett.* **9**, 183 (2009).
76. W. Lu, Q. Huang, G. Ku, X. X. Wen, M. Zhou, D. Guzatov, P. Brecht, R. Su, A. Oraevsky, L. V. Wang and C. Li, *Biomaterials* **31**, 2617 (2010).
77. D. P. J. Pan, M. Pramanik, A. Senpan, S. Ghosh, S. A. Wickline, L. V. Wang and G. M. Lanza, *Biomaterials* **31**, 4088 (2010).
78. S. J. Yoon, S. Mallidi, J. M. Tam, J. O. Tam, A. Murthy, K. P. Johnston, K. V. Sokolov and S. Y. Emelianov, *Opt. Lett.* **35**, 3751 (2010).
79. S. Mallidi, T. Larson, J. Tam, P. P. Joshi, A. Karpiouk, K. Sokolov and S. Emelianov, *Nano Lett.* **9**, 2825 (2009).
80. R. Olafsson, D. R. Bauer, L. G. Montilla and R. S. Witte, *Opt. Exp.* **18**, 18625 (2010).

81. P. C. Li, C. R. C. Wang, D. B. Shieh, C. W. Wei, C. K. Liao, C. Poe, S. Jhan, A. A. Ding and Y. N. Wu, *Opt. Exp.* **16**, 18605 (2008).
82. C. Kim, E. C. Cho, J. Y. Chen, K. H. Song, L. Au, C. Favazza, Q. Zhang, C. M. Cobley, F. Gao, Y. N. Xia and L. H. V. Wang, *ACS Nano* **4**, 4559 (2010).
83. J. W. Kim, E. I. Galanzha, E. V. Shashkov, H. M. Moon and V. P. Zharov, *Nat. Nanotechnol.* **4**, 688 (2009).
84. E. I. Galanzha, J. W. Kim and V. P. Zharov, *J. Biophotonics* **2**, 725 (2009).
85. E. I. Galanzha, E. V. Shashkov, T. Kelly, J. W. Kim, L. L. Yang and V. P. Zharov, *Nat. Nanotechnol.* **4**, 855 (2009).
86. G. Laurent, N. Felidj, S. L. Truong, J. Aubard, G. Levi, J. R. Krenn, A. Hohenau, A. Leitner and F. R. Aussenegg, *Nano Lett.* **5**, 253 (2005).
87. X. H. Huang, I. H. El-Sayed, W. Qian and M. A. El-Sayed, *Nano Lett.* **7**, 1591 (2007).
88. D. S. Grubisha, R. J. Lipert, H. Y. Park, J. Driskell and M. D. Porter, *Anal. Chem.* **75**, 5936 (2003).
89. X. M. Qian, X. H. Peng, D. O. Ansari, Q. Yin-Goen, G. Z. Chen, D. M. Shin, L. Yang, A. N. Young, M. D. Wang and S. M. Nie, *Nat. Biotechnol.* **26**, 83 (2008).
90. S. Keren, C. Zavaleta, Z. Cheng, A. de la Zerda, O. Gheysens and S. S. Gambhir, *Proc. Natl. Acad. Sci. USA* **105**, 5844 (2008).
91. G. von Maltzahn, A. Centrone, J. H. Park, R. Ramanathan, M. J. Sailor, T. A. Hatton and S. N. Bhatia, *Adv. Mater.* **21**, 3175 (2009).
92. R. T. Zaman, P. Diagaradjane, J. C. Wang, J. Schwartz, N. Rajaram, K. L. Gill-Sharp, S. H. Cho, H. G. Rylander, J. D. Payne, S. Krishnan and J. W. Tunnell, *IEEE J. Selected Topics Quantum Electron.* **13**, 1715 (2007).
93. J. F. Hainfeld, D. N. Slatkin, T. M. Focella and H. M. Smilowitz, *Brit. J. Radiol.* **80**, 65 (2007).
94. D. Kim, S. Park, J. H. Lee, Y. Y. Jeong and S. Jon, *J. Am. Chem. Soc.* **129**, 7661 (2007).
95. R. Popovtzer, A. Agrawal, N. A. Kotov, A. Popovtzer, J. Balter, T. E. Carey and R. Kopelman, *Nano Lett.* **8**, 4593 (2008).
96. C. Alric, J. Taleb, G. Le Duc, C. Mandon, C. Billotey, A. Le Meur-Herland, T. Brochard, F. Vocanson, M. Janier, P. Perriat, S. Roux and O. Tillement, *J. Am. Chem. Soc.* **130**, 5908 (2008).
97. G. von Maltzahn, J. H. Park, A. Agrawal, N. K. Bandaru, S. K. Das, M. J. Sailor and S. N. Bhatia, *Cancer Res.* **69**, 3892 (2009).
98. X. J. Ji, R. P. Shao, A. M. Elliott, R. J. Stafford, E. Esparza-Coss, J. A. Bankson, G. Liang, Z. P. Luo, K. Park, J. T. Markert and C. Li, *J. Phys. Chem. C* **111**, 6245 (2007).
99. W. Chen, N. F. Xu, L. G. Xu, L. B. Wang, Z. K. Li, W. Ma, Y. Y. Zhu, C. L. Xu and N. A. Kotov, *Macromol. Rapid Commun.* **31**, 228 (2010).
100. C. H. Su, H. S. Sheu, C. Y. Lin, C. C. Huang, Y. W. Lo, Y. C. Pu, J. C. Weng, D. B. Shieh, J. H. Chen and C. S. Yeh, *J. Am. Chem. Soc.* **129**, 2139 (2007).
101. R. Bardhan, W. X. Chen, M. Bartels, C. Perez-Torres, M. F. Botero, R. W. McAninch, A. Contreras, R. Schiff, R. G. Pautler, N. J. Halas and A. Joshi, *Nano Lett.* **10**, 4920 (2010).

102. I. H. El-Sayed, X. H. Huang and M. A. El-Sayed, *Nano Lett.* **5**, 829 (2005).
103. L. L. Ma, M. D. Feldman, J. M. Tam, A. S. Paranjape, K. K. Cheruku, T. A. Larson, J. O. Tam, D. R. Ingram, V. Paramita, J. W. Villard, J. T. Jenkins, T. Wang, G. D. Clarke, R. Asmis, K. Sokolov, B. Chandrasekar, T. E. Milner and K. P. Johnston, *ACS Nano* **3**, 2686 (2009).
104. J. Y. Chen, D. L. Wang, J. F. Xi, L. Au, A. Siekkinen, A. Warsen, Z. Y. Li, H. Zhang, Y. N. Xia and X. D. Li, *Nano Lett.* **7**, 1318 (2007).
105. C. M. Pitsillides, E. K. Joe, X. B. Wei, R. R. Anderson and C. P. Lin, *Biophys. J.* **84**, 4023 (2003).
106. V. P. Zharov, E. N. Galitovskaya, C. Johnson and T. Kelly, *Lasers Surg. Med.* **37**, 219 (2005).
107. E. Y. Hleb, J. H. Hafner, J. N. Myers, E. Y. Hanna, B. C. Rostro, S. A. Zhdanok and D. O. Lapotko, *Nanomedicine* **3**, 647 (2008).
108. E. Y. Lukianova-Hleb, E. Y. Hanna, J. H. Hafner and D. O. Lapotko, *Nanotechnology* **21**, 085102 (2010).
109. S. E. Skrabalak, J. Y. Chen, Y. G. Sun, X. M. Lu, L. Au, C. M. Cobley and Y. N. Xia, *Accounts Chem. Res.* **41**, 1587 (2008).
110. L. R. Hirsch, R. J. Stafford, J. A. Bankson, S. R. Sershen, B. Rivera, R. E. Price, J. D. Hazle, N. J. Halas and J. L. West, *Proc. Natl. Acad. Sci. USA* **100**, 13549 (2003).
111. D. P. O'Neal, L. R. Hirsch, N. J. Halas, J. D. Payne and J. L. West, *Cancer Lett.* **209**, 171 (2004).
112. J. M. Stern, J. Stanfield, W. Kabbani, J. T. Hsieh and J. R. A. Cadeddu, *J. Urol.* **179**, 748 (2008).
113. J. A. Schwartz, A. M. Shetty, R. E. Price, R. J. Stafford, J. C. Wang, R. K. Uthamanthil, K. Pham, R. J. McNichols, C. L. Coleman and J. D. Payne, *Cancer Res.* **69**, 1659 (2009).
114. M. P. Melancon, W. Lu, Z. Yang, R. Zhang, Z. Cheng, A. M. Elliot, J. Stafford, T. Olson, J. Z. Zhang and C. Li, *Mol. Cancer Therap.* **7**, 1730 (2008).
115. A. R. Lowery, A. M. Gobin, E. S. Day, N. J. Halas and J. L. West, *Int. J. Nanomed.* **1**, 149 (2006).
116. R. J. Bernardi, A. R. Lowery, P. A. Thompson, S. M. Blaney and J. L. West, *J. Neuro-Oncol.* **86**, 165 (2008).
117. M. Hu, J. Y. Chen, Z. Y. Li, L. Au, G. V. Hartland, X. D. Li, M. Marquez and Y. N. Xia, *Chem. Soc. Rev.* **35**, 1084 (1094).
118. K. C. Black, N. D. Kirkpatrick, T. S. Troutman, L. P. Xu, J. Vagner, R. J. Gillies, J. K. Barton, U. Utzinger and M. Romanowski, *Mol. Imag.* **7**, 50 (2008).
119. H. C. Huang, Y. Yang, A. Nanda, P. Koria and K. Rege, *Nanomedicine* **6**, 459 (2011).
120. T. Niidome, M. Yamagata, Y. Okamoto, Y. Akiyama, H. Takahashi, T. Kawano, Y. Katayama and Y. Niidome, *J. Control. Release* **114**, 343 (2006).
121. E. B. Dickerson, E. C. Dreaden, X. H. Huang, I. H. El-Sayed, H. H. Chu, S. Pushpanketh, J. F. McDonald and M. A. El-Sayed, *Cancer Lett.* **269**, 57 (2008).
122. G. P. Goodrich, L. L. Bao, K. Gill-Sharp, K. L. Sang, J. Wang and J. D. Payne, *J. Biomed. Opt.* **15**, 018001 (2010).

123. S. Brown, P. Nativo, J. Smith, D. Stirling, P. Edwards, B. Venugopal, D. Flint, J. Plumb, D. Graham and N. Wheate, *J. Am. Chem. Soc.* **132**, 4678 (2010).
124. J. You, G. D. Zhang and C. Li, *ACS Nano* **4**, 1033 (2010).
125. W. T. Wu, T. Zhou, A. Berliner, P. Banerjee and S. Q. Zhou, *Chem. Mater.* **22**, 1966 (2010).
126. Y. Cheng, A. C. Samia, J. Li, M. E. Kenney, A. Resnick and C. Burda, *Langmuir* **26**, 2248 (2010).
127. S. R. Sershen, S. L. Westcott, N. J. Halas and J. L. West, *J. Biomed. Mater. Res.* **51**, 293 (2000).
128. C. Chen, Y. Lin, C. Wang, H. Tzeng, C. Wu, Y. Chen, C. Chen, L. Chen and Y. Wu, *J. Am. Chem. Soc.* **128**, 3709 (2006).
129. S. Link, C. Burda, M. B. Mohamed, B. Nikoobakht and M. A. El-Sayed, *J. Phys. Chem. A* **103**, 1165 (1999).
130. S. Inasawa, M. Sugiyama and Y. Yamaguchi, *J. Phys. Chem. B* **109**, 3104 (2005).
131. H. Maeda, J. Wu, T. Sawa, Y. Matsumura and K. Hori, *J. Control. Release* **65**, 271 (2000).
132. L. Hosta, M. Pla-Roca, J. Arbiol, C. Lopez-Inglesias, J. Samitier, L. Cruz, M. Kogan and F. Albericio, *Bioconjug. Chem.* **20**, 138 (2009).
133. Y. H. Chen, C. Y. Tsai, P. Y. Huang, M. Y. Chang, P. C. Cheng, C. H. Chou, D. H. Chen, C. R. Wang, A. L. Shiau and C. L. Wu, *Mol. Pharm.* **4**, 713 (2007).
134. R. K. Visaria, R. J. Griffin, B. W. Williams, E. S. Ebbini, G. F. Paciotti, C. W. Song and J. C. Bischof, *Mol. Cancer Therap.* **5**, 1014 (2006).
135. R. Visaria, J. C. Bischof, M. Loren, B. Williams, E. Ebbini, G. Paciotti and R. Griffin, *Int. J. Hyperthermia* **23**, 501 (2007).
136. E. C. Dreaden, S. C. Mwakwari, Q. H. Sodji, A. K. Oyelere and M. A. El-Sayed, *Bioconj. Chem.* **20**, 2247 (2009).
137. M. Prabaharan, J. Grailer, S. Pilla, D. Steeber and S. Gong, *Biomaterials* **30**, 6065 (2009).
138. J. H. Park, G. von Maltzahn, L. L. Ong, A. Centrone, T. A. Hatton, E. Ruoslahti, S. N. Bhatia and M. J. Sailor, *Adv. Mater.* **22**, 880 (2010).
139. S. Agasti, A. Chompoosor, C. You, P. Ghosh, C. Kim and V. Rotello, *J. Am. Chem. Soc.* **131**, 5728 (2009).
140. S. Barua, A. Joshi, A. Banerjee, D. Matthews, S. Sharfstein, S. Cramer, R. Kane and K. Rege, *Mol. Pharm.* **6**, 86 (2009).
141. X. Huang, S. Neretina and M. El-Sayed, *Adv. Biomater.* **21**, 4480 (2009).
142. A. Wijaya, S. Schaffer, I. Pallares and K. Hamad-Schifferli, *ACS Nano* **3**, 80 (2009).
143. G. Han, C.-C. You, B.-J. Kim, R. S. Turingan, N. S. Forbes, C. T. Martin and V. M. Rotello, *Angew. Chem. Int. Ed. Engl.* **45**, 3165 (2006).
144. A. K. Salem, P. C. Searson and K. W. Leong, *Nat. Mater.* **2**, 668 (2003).
145. C. Hu, Q. Peng, F. Chen, Z. Zhong and R. Zhuo, *Bioconjug. Chem.* **20**, 836 (2010).
146. H.-C. Huang, S. Barua, D. B. Kay and K. Rege, *ACS Nano* **3**, 2941 (2009).
147. L. Kasman, S. Barua, P. Lu, K. Rege and C. Voelkel-Johnson, *Mol. Pharm.* **6**, 1612 (2009).

148. D. Kim and J. Rossi, *Current Protocols in Nucleic Acid Chemistry* (John Wiley & Sons, Inc., 2009).
149. A. J. Hamilton and D. C. Baulcombe, *Science* **286**, 950 (1999).
150. D. W. Bartlett, H. Su, I. J. Hildebrandt, W. A. Weber and M. E. Davis, *Proc. Natl. Acad. Sci. USA* **104**, 15546 (2007).
151. A. C. Bonoiu, S. D. Mahajan, H. Ding, I. Roy, K.-T. Yong, R. Kumar, R. Hu, E. J. Bergey, S. A. Schwartz and P. N. Prasad, *Proc. Natl. Acad. Sci. USA* **106**, 5546 (2009).
152. W. J. Song, J. Z. Du, T. M. Sun, P. Z. Zhang and J. Wang, *Small* **6**, 239 (2010).
153. G. B. Braun, A. Pallaoro, G. Wu, D. Missirlis, J. A. Zasadzinski, M. Tirrell and N. O. Reich, *ACS Nano* **3**, 2007 (2009).
154. W. Lu, G. D. Zhang, R. Zhang, L. G. Flores, Q. Huang, J. G. Gelovani and C. Li, *Cancer Res.* **70**, 3177 (2010).
155. M. S. Shim, C. S. Kim, Y. C. Ahn, Z. P. Chen and Y. J. Kwon, *J. Am. Chem. Soc.* **132**, 8316 (2010).
156. M. C. Skala, J. M. Squirrell, K. M. Vrotsos, V. C. Eickhoff, A. Gendron-Fitzpatrick, K. W. Eliceiri and N. Ramanujam, *Cancer Res.* **65**, 1180 (2005).
157. A. Campion and P. Kambhampati, *Chem. Soc. Rev.* **27**, 241 (1998).
158. S. P. Poplack, T. D. Tosteson, W. A. Wells, B. W. Pogue, P. M. Meaney, A. Hartov, C. A. Kogel, S. K. Soho, J. J. Gibson and K. D. Paulsen, *Radiology* **243**, 350 (2007).
159. H. Soliman, A. Gunasekara, M. Rycroft, J. Zubovits, R. Dent, J. Spayne, M. J. Yaffe and G. J. Czarnota, *Clinical Cancer Res.* **16**, 2605 (2010).
160. J. F. Hainfeld, D. N. Slatkin, T. M. Focella and H. M. Smilowitz, *Brit. J. Radiol.* **79**, 248 (2006).

https://doi.org/10.1142/9789819809028_0008

Chapter 8

Magnetic Nanoparticle Hyperthermia in Cancer Treatment*

Andrew J. Giustini

Dartmouth Medical School and the Thayer School of Engineering, Dartmouth College, Hanover, New Hampshire 03755, USA
andrew.j.giustini@dartmouth.edu

Alicia A. Petryk[†], Shiraz M. Cassim[‡], Jennifer A. Tate[§] and Ian Baker[¶]

Thayer School of Engineering, Dartmouth College, Hanover, New Hampshire 03755, USA
[†]*alicia.a.petryk@dartmouth.edu*
[‡]*shiraz.m.cassim@dartmouth.edu*
[§]*jennifer.a.tate@dartmouth.edu*
[¶]*ian.baker@dartmouth.edu*

P. Jack Hoopes

Dartmouth Medical School and the Thayer School of Engineering, Dartmouth College, Hanover, New Hampshire 03755, USA
p.jack.hoopes@dartmouth.edu

The activation of magnetic nanoparticles (mNPs) by an alternating magnetic field (AMF) is currently being explored as technique for targeted therapeutic heating of tumors. Various types of superparamagnetic and ferromagnetic particles, with different coatings and targeting agents, allow for tumor site and type specificity. Magnetic nanoparticle hyperthermia is also being studied as an adjuvant to conventional chemotherapy and radiation therapy. This review provides an introduction to some of the relevant biology and materials science involved in the technical

*To cite this article, please refer to its earlier version published in the *Nano LIFE*, Vol. 1, Nos. 1 & 2 (2010) 17–32, DOI: 10.1142/S1793984410000067

development and current and future use of mNP hyperthermia as clinical cancer therapy.

Keywords: Magnetic nanoparticle; hyperthermia; cancer; tumor.

1. Background

After decades of intense study and numerous clinical trials, most forms of human cancer are still not curable. The reasons for this are multifactorial. "Cancer" has multiple etiologies and manifestations. Each of these is distinct and responds differently to therapies. The primary limiting factors are the lack of understanding of the mechanisms of tumor development and of therapeutic intervention. While there have been some successes in treating certain types of neoplasms,[1,2] many tumor types are refractory to modern therapies.[3]

Over the past several decades, the principle types of cancer therapies have been chemotherapy, radiation therapy and surgery. Additional modalities, such as therapeutic hyperthermia, have achieved some success but are not yet considered standard-of-care therapies.

The primary reasons for hyperthermia's inability to enter mainstream cancer therapy have been: lack of differential normal tissue: cancer cytotoxicity, inability to target hyperthermia directly to tumors and an insufficient understanding of the mechanism of hyperthermia cytotoxicity.[4] In 1991, Roizin-Towle and Pirro studied the sensitivity of various cell types to hyperthermia. The authors compared the survival of normal and neoplastic human and rodent cell types, *in vitro*, as they were exposed to different thermal doses. The authors showed that, while all cell types could be killed by specific thermal doses, tumor cells did not display increased sensitivity to the treatment compared to normal cells.[4] This lack of inherent difference in normal versus tumor tissue sensitivity (therapeutic ratio) is unlike the differential responses of normal and cancerous tissue to radiation and chemotherapy. Their work showed that in order for hyperthermia to succeed as a cancer therapy, its mode of delivery must compensate for the lack of differential toxicity by localizing heat specifically to tumor cells. The implication of this finding was that, for hyperthermia to be therapeutically effective, it would have to be localized specifically to tumor tissue. Although cancerous tissues may be more sensitive to heat damage *in vivo* due to an insufficient blood supply, clinically available technologies (RF, microwave, ultrasound, conductive) have not been able to target heat specifically to tumors — especially metastatic tumors — in a clinically effect manner.

Recently, hyperthermia directed specifically to cancer cells through the use of magnetic nanoparticles heated with alternating magnetic fields has been used as a novel cancer therapy. This paper will explore this new application of magnetically-induced hyperthermia in cancer therapy.

2. Therapeutic Index (TI)

The challenge of cancer therapy is to control the tumor without unacceptable normal tissue toxicity. The terms "therapeutic index" (TI) or "therapeutic ratio" are used to quantify the ratio of a therapy's treatment potential in relation to its normal tissue toxicities. This measure can be used for populations of people or of cells to examine the relative effectiveness of a therapy. Therapies with high therapeutic index are essential for clinical success and can be achieved by exploiting differences in diseased tissue and normal tissue.

The similarity between normal and neoplastic tissue makes it difficult to develop therapies which will specifically kill tumor cells. This limitation explains many of the side effects seen with traditional anti-neoplastic chemotherapeutics. Unfortunately, many first line-chemotherapeutics do not have enough inherent selectivity. For example, Cisplatin — the most commonly used anti-neoplastic agent in the United States — can cause significant toxicity in bone marrow, gastrointestinal, and peripheral nerve cells.[5]

Currently there are three major types of anti-neoplastic therapy: (1) Surgical oncology relies on imaging techniques to delineate tumor tissue from normal tissue and then relies on the judgment of the surgeon and pathologist to determine which tissue to actually remove. Surgical oncology can be successful at controlling local neoplastic disease; it is, however, often challenged in the metastatic environment. (2) Use of chemotherapy has largely relied on exploitation of rapid cell division to kill cells, since most neoplasms divide rapidly.[6] Chemotherapy is also able to address tumor cells at virtually any site in the body. As noted previously, this approach can lead to severe toxicities in normal tissue and often with insufficient TI. (3) Radiation therapy has maximized TI by exploiting the suboptimal DNA damage repair mechanisms in tumor tissue, which causes neoplastic tissue to be more radiation-sensitive than normal tissue. None of these therapies, alone or in concert, has led to reliably curative therapy for most neoplasms. Combining different types of therapies, however, can improve the therapeutic index of the treatments by having nonadditive normal tissue side effects but additive or synergistic therapeutic effects.[7,8]

3. Magnetic Nanoparticle Hyperthermia (mNPH)

In 1957, Gilchrist *et al.* demonstrated that lymph nodes could be inductively heated to kill lymphatic metastases after the administration of magnetic particles.[9] In these experiments, 5 mg of 20–100 nm diameter Fe_2O_3 particles were delivered to lymph nodes (47 mg of Fe_2O_3 per gram of tissue). A temperature rise of 14°C was seen following an exposure to an alternating magnetic field (AMF) of 200–240 Oe (16–19.2 kA/m) at 1.2 MHz.[9] Because no control experiments were reported, there remains the distinct possibility that, because of the high frequency used, much of the temperature rise was produced directly by the induced electric field rather than through nanoparticle heating. Subsequently, various methods of heat delivery were tested as cancer treatment modalities.[10,11] Generally, these techniques achieved limited success.

In the mid-1990s, the idea of using nanoparticle hyperthermia to treat tumors was revisited.[12] This method involved the injection of magnetic nanoparticles directly into tumors and exciting these nanoparticles with alternating magnetic fields (AMFs) to produce heat. Further progress has been made in directing nanoparticles to tumors with targeting agents such as antibodies.[13–16] Nanoparticle hyperthermia appears well-suited as an effective tumor therapy if (1) the concentration of particles in the tumor is both sufficiently high and significantly higher than in surrounding, normal tissue, and (2) the particles possess a high enough specific absorption rate (SAR, in Watts per gram)

$$\mathrm{SAR} = \frac{c\Delta T}{\Delta t}, \tag{1}$$

where c is the specific heat capacity, and ΔT is the temperature rise during the time interval (Δt) to deliver significant intratumoral doses of heat with AMFs that are well-tolerated by the normal tissues.

Currently, three different nanoparticle heating technologies for therapeutic purposes are being explored: (1) optical heating using lasers;[17] (2) ultrasound heating of small bubbles;[18] and (3) iron oxide heating due to AMF, using one of a variety of physical mechanisms generally termed hysteresis heating.[14,16,19–21] Each method has certain strengths and limitations. Optical methods heat particles effectively, but are severely limited by the attenuation of the laser light by tissue. Ultrasound heating may ultimately be promising, as the energy is focused to a selected location; it, however, suffers from speed of sound variation in most tissues and, in many applications, from the limited aperture of the applicator. Magnetic particle heating can be accomplished at depths necessary for treatment of tumors located virtually anywhere in the human body. The same particles used for heating may also be sufficient for medical imaging uses.

4. Hyperthermia as an adjuvant to radiation and chemotherapy

It is well-known that exposing tumor cells to even mildly elevated temperatures sensitizes them to chemotherapy and radiation and may decrease their viability.[22,23] Although the combination of hyperthermia with chemotherapeutics and radiation has shown great promise, to date the clinical impact has been modest.

One of the most successful uses of hyperthermia as an antineoplastic agent is as a treatment for intraperitoneal metastases from ovarian tumors. In this technology hyperthermia is used as a way of increasing the efficacy of certain chemotherapeutics.[11,24] While the nonfocused nature of this heating is beneficial in this case, the inability to deliver a uniform, sufficient thermal dose to all metastases has limited its clinical efficacy.

The lack of selective deposition of chemotherapeutic agents to cancer cells has limited the TI of traditional chemotherapeutics. Therefore, to date, chemotherapy for solid tumors has been used most effectively as an adjuvant to radiotherapy and/or surgery.[25] The ability to localize hyperthermia (magnetic nanoparticle hyperthermia, mNP) to cancer cells may greatly enhance the use of chemotherapy by reducing the necessary dose, thereby sparing normal tissue toxicity.[26]

A significant amount of effort has been dedicated to directing chemotherapeutics and controlling their release at the tumor site. Nanoparticle (both iron oxide-based and others) constructs which act as chemotherapeutic "carriers" are under development for both sustained and stimuli-activated release (by pH, electric fields, ultrasound, UV-light, radiation, and temperature).[27,28] These technologies have not yet been extensively tested *in vivo*.

Optimizing the pairing of chemotherapy and hyperthermia is dependent on tumor type, dose, clinical site and temperature. Studies have suggested that alkylating agents such as cyclophosphamide, ifosfamide and melphalan, may be most effective at 41.5°C,[29] while other therapeutics such as cisplatinum appear to be also effective at lower temperatures. The temporal optimization of hyperthermia-chemotherapeutic administration has yet to be achieved. Temperatures as low as 2–3°C above basal temperature have been shown to increase blood flow during, and for some time after, removal of the heat source from tumors. Studies suggest that this localized increase in blood flow assists in depositing chemotherapy within the heated tissue.[30,31]

The enhancement of radiotherapy with hyperthermia is well-documented.[32] The proposed mechanism for hyperthermia enhancement of therapeutic radiation is two-fold: (1) Ionizing radiation damages DNA and hyperthermia damages the proteins responsible for DNA repair.[33] (2) Hyperthermia is also able to kill cells in hypoxic regions of tumors which are more radio-resistant than cells in well-oxygenated areas.[23] The interaction of radiation and hyperthermia is influenced by a number of factors including temperature, duration of hyperthermia and the temporal relationship between hyperthermia and radiation. Optimization of the combination of hyperthermia and ionizing radiation has not yet been achieved due to these complex relationships.[23] MNP-based hyperthermia in combination with radiotherapy has shown early promise.[34] The combined use of magnetic nanoparticle-delivered radionucleotides in combination with nanoparticle hyperthermia is potentially attractive.[35]

5. Biological heat dose equation

Cumulative Equivalent Minutes (CEMs) is a technique for determining and normalizing the total thermal dose (thermal history) of a heated tissue. The equation is:

$$\text{CEM43}^\circ\text{C} = tR^{(43-T)}, \tag{2}$$

where CEM43°C is the heat dose normalized to number of minutes at 43°C, t is the time at a given temperature in minutes, T is the average temperature during t, the time interval. R represents how many minutes would be required to account for a 1°C change in temperature above or below 43°C.[36] For human (rodent) cells, a typical value of R above the breakpoint is 0.45 (0.43) and value of R below the breakpoint is 0.25 (0.23).[36]

Thus, a population of rodent cells subjected to a temperature of 45°C for one minute would result in cytotoxicity equal to that of cells treated at 43°C for 5 min (CEM43°C = 5). A CEM43°C of 60 min yields approximately 50% cytotoxicity in CHO-10 B cells.[36]

6. Magnetic nanoparticle heating mechanisms

Given the overall goal of producing localized hyperthermia in a tumor, the primary objective of nanoparticle design is to maximize the power deposition. This will enable the nanoparticles to be heated using an AMF to result in direct cytotoxicity, or to sensitize the tumor to radiation treatment or chemotherapy. Magnetic nanoparticles have also been used as MRI contrast agents.[37] The nanoparticles that are most easily imaged *in vivo*, however, are not necessarily the same as the ones that provide the greatest heating effect. It is also possible that mNP with the highest SAR values may have biocompatibility limitations.

The SAR is the parameter of magnetic nanoparticles that must be maximized to optimize the heating. Heating of a material in an AMF can occur by four mechanisms: (1) dielectric losses in a material of low electrical conductivity; (2) eddy currents losses in a material of high electrical conductivity; (3) frictional heating due to the physical rotation of an anisotropic magnetic particle and; (4) hysteresis losses in a magnetic material.

Dielectric and eddy current losses may lead to unacceptable normal tissue heating. Below, we discuss the use of the three other types of heating for nanoparticles. The heating effect in each case depends on the size, shape and coercivity of the particles, and the frequency and magnitude of the applied AMF.

6.1. *Eddy current heating*

Ivkov *et al.* examined the effects of induction from the application of an alternating pulsed magnetic field, at 153 kHz, on nude mice. They found that for field strengths below 700 Oe (20 min exposure), no adverse effects were observed. Field strengths greater than 950 Oe resulted in significant morbidity.[38] They also found that fields up to 1300 Oe could be applied with no observable adverse effects on the mice as long as the off/on time of the applied field was adjusted to limit the tissue heating.

The power density for eddy current heating is given by:

$$\mathrm{PE} = Ef^2 H_{\mathrm{max}} d^2, \tag{3}$$

where E is the eddy current coefficient, f is the frequency, H_{max} is the maximum flux density, and d is the particle size.[9] The complication of eddy current heating of human tissue was first identified by Gilchrist *et al.* during their lymph node nanoparticle experiment.[9] Since PE increases as d^2, the eddy current heating becomes negligible on the nanoscale. While PE also increases as f^2, increasing the frequency beyond a few hundred kHz is not an attractive option, because it leads to the previously mentioned eddy current tissue heating.

6.2. *Frictional heating*

In a low-viscosity liquid, a magnetically anisotropic particle will physically rotate in an AMF. This effect has been used to mechanically damage cells.[39] The induced rotation leads to frictional heating of the surrounding medium, and as a result, energy losses, which are referred to as Brownian losses. A good theoretical understanding of the associated frictional forces does not yet exist. A first-order empirical approximation is that the force is proportional to the velocity squared. Therefore, the energy would be given by the dot product between this force and the displacement of the particle. The power would be given by this energy divided by the frequency of the magnetic field. However, this approximation does not account for collective effects, or how the size and shape of the particle, as well as the viscosity of the liquid in which the nanoparticles are dispersed, affect the power dissipation. It is important to note that if the particle is immobilized, for example by being bound to a cell, this type of heating is unlikely to occur.[40,41]

6.3. *Hysteresis heating*

The fact that disparate categories of magnetic materials behave differently in magnetic fields is integral to understanding why some magnetic nanoparticles heat better than others. The relevant categories of materials in this case are paramagnetic, superparamagnetic and ferromagnetic. The simplest way of describing the responses of these materials to different magnetic fields is by plotting their magnetizations against applied magnetic fields (Fig. 1).

As can be seen in Fig. 1, the magnetizations (M) of paramagnetic and superparamagnetic materials have no remnant magnetization when there is no applied magnetic field. When either of these materials is exposed to an increasing applied magnetic field (H), the dipoles within the material become more likely to be aligned with the field and the magnetization (M) of the material increases. M will continue to increase until all the dipoles within the material have completely aligned with H. Saturation is reached when M is maximized and the magnetization of the material at that point is termed the saturation magnetization (M_S). Once M_S has been reached within the material, M will not continue to increase with increasing H.

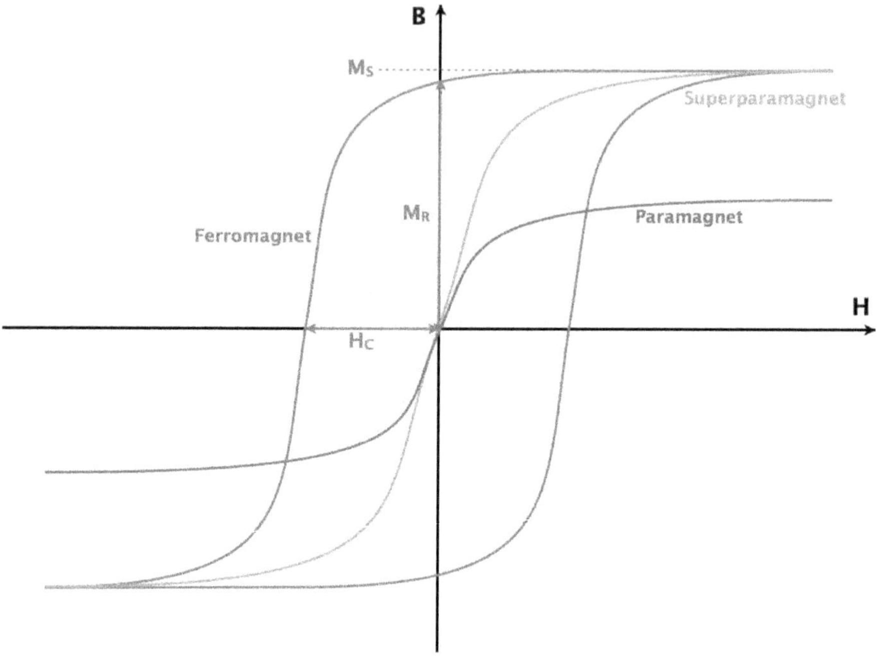

Fig. 1. B is the total magnetic field and H is the applied magnetic field in a sample. The hysteresis curves of various types of bulk materials are shown here. For the ferromagnetic material (blue), the saturation magnetization (M_S), coercivity (H_C) and remnant magnetization (M_R) are indicated. The B–H curves of super-paramagnetic (green) and paramagnetic (red) materials are also shown; these two types of materials demonstrate no magnetic hysteresis (no area enclosed by B–H the curve) (color online).

In ferromagnetic material, the magnetic dipoles actually have magnetic "memory". When ferromagnetic materials are raised above their Curie temperature ($T_C = 770°\text{C}$ for iron), they act as paramagnets and the dipoles within the material become randomly aligned.[42] When a ferromagnet is cooled below T_C, the material abruptly becomes ferromagnetic but the dipoles are still moderately aligned and the material possesses no net magnetization. When a magnetic field is first applied the dipoles within the ferromagnet align with the field. As the polarity of the applied field is reversed, the net magnetization of the dipoles decreases. At $H = 0$, there is still a net magnetization within the ferromagnet, known as the remnant magnetization (M_R). As an increasingly negative H is applied, the M of the material decreases until it is 0. The absolute value of this H is known as the coercivity (H_C) of the material.

The areas enclosed by the hysteresis loop, as can be seen in Fig. 1, are defined by M_S, H_C and M_R. These represent the amount of energy lost to the environment when H goes from $H(M_S)$ to $H(-M_S)$ and back. Theoretically, the total power lost to heat is given by the frequency times the integral of the B–H curve over a closed loop. Thus, when a ferromagnetic material is put into an oscillating/alternating magnetic field (AMF), energy will be released as heat. The larger the magnetic hysteresis curve of the ferromagnet, the "harder" that ferromagnet is said to be. "Hard" ferromagnets are used to create nanoparticles which will heat or particles which require a large H to switch their M from $+M_S$ to $-M_S$ (as is desirable in magnetic data storage) while "soft" ferromagnets used applications like electric power girds to minimize energy loss. The difference in H_C between a soft and a hard ferromagnetic material can be as great as a factor of 10 000. The greater the coercivity, the higher the SAR of the nanoparticles.[43]

For hysteresis heating, there two practical limits are the frequency and magnitude of the AMF that can be applied to live animal subjects. Andrä *et al.*[44] performed calculations on whether it would be possible to use mNP hyperthermia, with a SAR value of 365 W/g, to treat small breast carcinomas while sparing the surrounding normal tissue. The estimates are also applicable to other regions of the body where blood perfusion is low. Their computational models demonstrated agreement with their experimental data, in terms of the effects of an applied magnetic field of 82 Oe (6.56 kA/m) at 400 kHz on extended cow muscle tissue. They found that for tissues with low blood perfusion, in order to avoid significant heat dose to surrounding tissue, hyperthermia should be administered as rapidly as possible and with accurate dose control.

6.4. *Superparamagnetic particles*

There have been a number of studies where ($\sim$2–20 nm) superparamagnetic — typically Fe_2O_3 — nanoparticles have been used to demonstrate magnetic hyperthermia either *in vitro* or *in vivo*.[45]

In several instances where the AMF was applied with and without the presence of nanoparticles, experimental controls have been lacking. Therefore, it has not always been clear whether the temperature rise observed in the tissue was resulted from the presence of the nanoparticles or through eddy current heating. The *B–H* curve for superparamagnetic particles displays no magnetic hysteresis (Fig. 1), thus it seems unlikely that significant hysteresis heating occurs when using superparamagnetic nanoparticles.

Using appropriate controls, a commercial ferrofluid consisting of 3–15 nm Fe_2O_3 superparamagnetic nanoparticles and AMF exposure, Chan and Chou[10] found SAR values ranging from 60–370 mW per mg of Fe, at a frequency of 1.1 MHz and an applied field of 86 Oe (6.8 kA/m). For the highest-SAR nanoparticles, they found that, at 1 MHz and an output power density of 1 MW/m^3, a temperature rise of 5°C/min could be obtained with a concentration of nanoparticles of 1 mg Fe per cm^3 of body tissue. They concluded, based on several different experiments, that Néel relaxation (rotation of the magnetization vector in the particle) was the dominant mechanism of heat generation. This type of heating occurred because it is more energetically favorable for magnetic dipoles to be aligned with crystal planes in a material than to be aligned otherwise. Thus, in an alternating magnetic field when the dipoles are rapidly realigning with the applied magnetic field, there can be "magnetic friction" of the dipoles aligning against the crystal planes which generates heat.[46]

Hilger *et al.* completed an *in vivo* study using breast adenocaricinoma cells implanted into immunodeficient mice. They injected superparamagnetic nanoparticles (referred to as "ferrofluid") into the tumors and applied 6.5 kA/m magnetic fields at a frequency of 400 kHz and demonstrated temperature increases up to 73°C in regions within the tumors. This temperature increased resulted in significant tumor necrosis.[47]

Maier-Hauff *et al.* successfully demonstrated the tolerability of superparamagnetic iron oxide nanoparticle hyperthermia in human brain tumors. They accrued fourteen patients with glioblastoma muliforme (GBM), which is an extremely aggressive form of brain cancer. These patients received multiple treatments consisting of aminosilane-coated superparamagnetic nanoparticles injected directly into the tumor. The nanoparticles were heated by an externally applied AMF. The maximum temperature within each tumor during each treatment was between 42.4 and 49.5°C. During the course of the hyperthermia treatment, the patients also received fractionated radiation therapy. No significant toxicities were observed.[48]

Very recently, DeNardo *et al.*[15] demonstrated decreased tumor growth rates after applying AMFs to nude mice injected with antibody tagged, dextran- and PEG-coated, 20 nm diameter, superparamagnetic, iron oxide particles. It is worth noting that the applied fields used were quite large at 700, 1000 or 1300 Oe (56, 80, 104 kA/m). The study also demonstrated that the nanoparticles had no observable toxicity.

6.5. *Domain walls*

In bulk ferromagnetic materials, magnetic dipoles do not just aligned with one another. Over great enough distances (typically less than 100 nm), there exist independent magnetic domains. Within each domain the dipoles of adjacent atoms are oriented in the same direction but the magnetization of each domain is randomly aligned with respect to its neighbor domains. When a ferromagnet is heated above its T_C and then cooled, magnetic domains form within the material in orientations such that the net magnetization of the material is zero while each domain still maintains its own net magnetization.

When a H is applied to a ferromagnet with no net magnetization, dipoles do not randomly align with the H throughout the material. In reality, domain walls move with respect to one another and change in size.[49] The domain whose magnetization is parallel to H steadily grows in size until, at M_S, this is the only remaining domain within the material.[42] As the magnitude of H decreases, the other domains within the material will increase in size until there is no net M within the material at $-H_C$.

6.6. *Single-domain ferromagnetic particles*

Single-domain particles are typically 20–100 nm in size, depending on the material and particle shape. In these particles, the magnetic moments either rotate together, or in a complicated manner in which domain wall motion is not involved. The classification of a single-domain particle into superparamagnetic or ferromagnetic category has almost no meaning, because at low frequencies, a particle may behave superparamagnetically, while at higher frequencies it behaves ferromagnetically. The maximum possible size for a particle to contain a single-domain depends (for a particular material) on the ratio of major to minor axis for a lenticular particle, with the smallest size corresponding to equiaxed particles. Butler and Banerjee[50] estimated the maximum possible particle size for a cube-shaped particle of Fe_3O_4 is 80 nm.

Table 1 shows some of the work completed in biological systems evaluating the efficacy of nanoparticle hyperthermia created with superparamagnetic and single-domain ferromagnetic nanoparticles.

6.7. *Multi-domain ferromagnetic particles*

Bulk materials or particles larger than the single-domain limit contain multiple domains. In this case, reversal of magnetization occurs by flipping of the magnetic moments in domains where the magnetic moment vector is antiparallel to the applied field. It also occurs by domain growth in other domains, which occurs at lower fields. If the applied AMF can fully saturate the magnetization, then the energy losses in multi-domain materials depend on the coercivity. The latter decreases as the reciprocal of the domain size, which, in bulk materials, is related to the grain size. Thus, for fully saturated magnetic materials, the power loss decreases with increasing domain size. As a result, multi-domain particles should be avoided if the power loss is to be maximized. Jordan *et al.* demonstrated experimentally that the power loss in single-domain ferrite particles was significantly greater than that in multi-domain nanoparticles, at all applied fields they examined (up to $\sim$165 Oe (13.2 kA/m)).[20] The relationship between nanoparticle size, number of domains and SAR is shown in Fig. 2.

Andrä[45] compiled data from several studies and compared the efficacy of different particles. He noted that the SAR value appeared

Table 1. This table describes many of the nanoparticle hyperthermia studies which have been done in biological settings.

Group	Year	Particles used	Experimental setting	Effect seen
Jordan *et al.*[126]	1999	Dextran or aminosilane-coated magnetite. Superparamagnetic. 3–13 nm crystal diameters.	*In vitro*	Similar cytotoxic efficacy of water bath and mNP hyperthermia when used to heat cell cultures.
Hilger *et al.*[127]	2001	Magnetite nanoparticles of several different shapes, aspect ratios and hydrodynamic diameters.	*Ex vivo* (human breast tissue) and *in vivo* (tumors in mice)	Significant average temperature increases in both *ex vivo* and *in vivo* treated tissues. During experiments, there was little increase in mouse core body temperature.
Hilger *et al.*[47]	2002	Coated magnetite. Superparamagnetic. 10 nm and 200 nm hydrodynamic diameter.	*In vivo* (tumors in mice)	Heterogenous tumor heating. 12–73°C temperature increase seen within tumors.
Ito *et al.*[128]	2003	Magnetite nanoparticles coated with lipid membrane. Administered with Interleukin-2 (IL-2).	*In vivo* (tumors in mice)	Significant improvement in mouse survival and tumor regrowth delay.
Maier-Hauff *et al.*[48]	2007	Aminosilane-coated iron oxide. Superparamagnetic. 15 nm crystal diameter.	*In vivo* (human brain tumors)	Little toxicity seen in human patients after brain tumors heated to 42.4–49.5°C and treated with therapeutic radiation.

(*Continued*)

Table 1. (*Continued*)

Group	Year	Particles used	Experimental setting	Effect seen
DeNardo *et al.*[16]	2007	Dextran- and PEG-coated iron oxide, conjugated to Chimeric L6 antibody. Superparamagnetic. 20 nm hydrodynamic diameter.	*In vivo* (tumors in mice)	Significant tumor growth delay.
Kikumori *et al.*[129]	2009	Iron-based magnetic nanoparticles (10 nm crystals) loaded into liposomes. Liposomes conjugated to Trastuzumab antibody.	*In vivo* (tumors in mice)	Significant tumor necrosis and growth delay with some complete responses.
Dennis *et al.*[19]	2009	Ferromagnetic, dextran-coated nanoparticles. Average hydrodynamic diameter of approximately 100 nm.	*In vivo* (tumors in mice)	Significant tumor regrowth delay.
Hoopes *et al.*[130]	2009	Ferromagnetic, dextran-coated nanoparticles. Average hydrodynamic diameter of approximately 100 nm.	*In vitro* and *in vivo* (tumors in mice)	Significant tumor regrowth delay. Additive effects seen with chemotherapy and radiation.

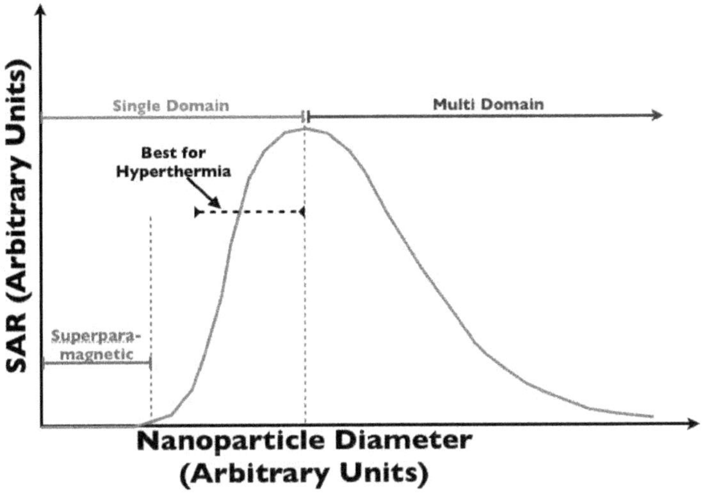

Fig. 2. This figure shows the dependence of SAR on nanoparticle diameter. Single-domain particles, whose size is close to the single-domain/multi-domain transition size, are desirable for their high SAR and smaller size.

to increase linearly with increasing frequency over the frequency range studied. The best heating occurred for iron oxide particles — mainly Fe_2O_3 — with sizes in the range 20–100 nm.[45]

Rand *et al.*[51,52] injected large, uncoated multi-domain ferrosilicone particles (100–1000 nm) into rabbits, and applied a low-frequency AMF of 2 kHz at a high field strength of 1000 Oe (80 kA/m). The rabbit's kidneys were determined to reach 55°C in 1–2 min. After the kidneys cooled, they performed further heat treatments, raising the kidney temperature to 43°C up to three times. They found extensive cancer cell necrosis. In later treatments, they raised the temperature to 50°C, but cooled the kidneys more slowly after treatment. This latter treatment killed all kidney tumor cells. All animals survived the treatments. They found that rabbits exposed to these magnetic fields for up to 30 min did not show ill effects even after three years with the presence of the nanoparticles in the lungs and kidneys.

Since this preliminary work has been completed, there have been few additional studies using multi-domain ferromagnetic nanoparticles *in vivo* for cancer therapy. This is due to a shift toward using superparamagnetic and single-domain ferromagnetic nanoparticles.

7. Challenges of mNPH

Recently, Keblinski *et al.*[53] used a diffusive heat equation to show that, because of the large thermal diffusivity in cells, which are essentially water, it is impossible for either a single-particle or many particles to produce significant localized heating. A large concentration of particles, however, are capable of producing significant global heating in a tissue. The results of these calculations are similar to those done by Rabin.[54]

An extension of the work by Keblinski and Rabin is the implication that the SAR of the nanoparticles determines the minimum size of treatable tumor. Hergt *et al.*[55] showed that if a tumor contains no more than 0.1 mg/mm^3 of nanoparticles, with SAR values of 50, 500 and 5000 W/g, the minimum size of tumor that can be heated to a temperature sufficient for hyperthermia treatment is 2, 0.6 and 0.1 mm. It is worth noting that 5000 W/g may be unachievable due to biological constraints on AMF strength and frequency and the properties of materials used to make nanoparticles.

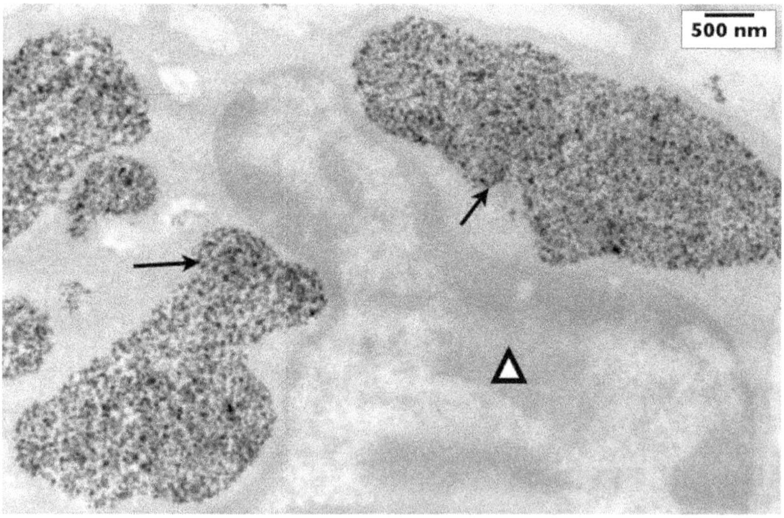

Fig. 3. This TEM image demonstrates ferromagnetic nanoparticles inside of vesicles within a murine adenocarcinoma cell (arrows). The cell's nucleus (triangle) is shown adjacent to the nanoparticle collections. Nanoparticles were injected into this mouse tumor five hours before the tumor was excised and fixed for TEM.

Clustering of nanoparticles is commonly observed in tumors.[56] Figure 3 shows the clustering of nanoparticles within a mouse tumor. This clustering has been shown to affect the SAR in gel–nanoparticle systems.[19,57] Thus, there is significant evidence that the arrangement of nanoparticles in cellular structures is critical to their role in AMF heating. Little has been done, however, to fully understand or exploit this behavior. Abraham *et al.*[58] have shown that magnetic fields on the order of 0.3–3 T (comparable to those experienced in MRI coils) are sufficient to drive the formation of chains of nanoparticles, and other linked structures.

8. Non-iron oxide magnetic nanoparticles

As noted, one of the most important characteristics of magnetic nanoparticles for anti-cancer hyperthermia is high SAR. High nanoparticle SAR allows for high CEM43°C in the tumor while minimizing the eddy current and diamagnetic heating in normal tissue. Iron-core, iron oxide-shell nanoparticles have been successfully developed to improving the SAR of iron oxide nanoparticles while simultaneously improve the utility of therapeutic nanoparticles as MRI contrast agents.[59] The ability to visualize the biodistribution of nanoparticles before heating them is projected to aid in treatment planning.

Nanoparticles with a Fe core and passivating epitaxial shell of MgO have been synthesized via chemical vapor condensation[60] for hyperthermia applications. Nanoparticles produced by Chatterjee *et al.* are encapsulated in polyethylene glycol and can include drugs which are released upon thermal activation.[61] Cobalt[62] and iron–cobalt alloys[63,64] have attractive SAR values but may have toxic properties.[41]

Another novel form of mNP have self-limited heating properties (tunable T_C). Their maximum temperature is typically set to that required for cytoxicity in tumors.[65–68] Unfortunately, as with the nanoparticles containing Co, Cu and Ni, this requires the use of elements such as Sr, La, Y, Mn, Ag or Al, whose toxicity effects as nanoparticles are unknown.

9. Nanoparticle selection

There does not appear to be an ideal particle for all magnetic heating applications. Iron oxide particles, often coated with dextran, are the most commonly used because they have excellent biocompatibility with almost no toxicity[15,69] and very high SAR/heating values.[10]

The optimum particle for heating depends on the AMF frequency and field strength, and nanoparticle size (ability to enter tumor) and shape. Hergt *et al.*[70] illustrated the importance of these points by examining the power loss per unit weight for three different average sizes of Fe_3O_4 particles, some of which were equi-axed, and some of which were lenticular (from 250–1500 nm). Each showed different hysteresis loops. They found a crossover in power loss behavior, where the particles that showed the largest power loss at low applied fields exhibited the least loss at high fields.

For power loss due to Néel relaxation, the optimum particle size decreased with increasing frequency.[70] A key feature of Néel relaxation power loss of a superparamagnetic nanoparticle is that sizes below the optimum lose power at significantly lower rates than particles that are the optimum size, indicating that a monodispersed particle size is the ultimate goal. Hergt *et al.*[70] showed that the power loss per unit weight for ferrofluid (single-domain) Fe_3O_4 nanoparticles increased with increasing particle size at 300 kHz and 82 Oe (6.56 kA/m). Later, Hergt *et al.*[55] showed that by changing the particle size distribution in a batch of ferrofluidic Fe_3O_4 nanoparticles with average initial particle size of 13 nm, such that the average particle size increased, while the distribution width decreased, the power loss at 410 kHz increased dramatically.

10. Synthesis of magnetic nanoparticles

10.1. *Standard precipitation*

The conventional method of producing magnetite nanoparticles utilizes the coprecipitation of a 2:1 mixture of Fe^{3+} and Fe^{2+}, in a nonoxidizing alkaline ($pH = 8-14$) environment. The overall reaction is:

$$Fe^{2+} + Fe^{3+} + 8OH^- \rightarrow Fe_3O_4 + 4H_2O. \quad (4)$$

An-oxygen-free environment is required to prevent the following reaction from producing Iron (III) hydroxide:

$$Fe_3O_4 + 0.25O_2 + 4.5H_2O \rightarrow 3Fe(OH)_2. \tag{5}$$

When carried out in bulk solution, the reaction kinetics must be carefully tailored to control the particle size distribution. Such control is obtained by separating the process into nucleation and growth steps. Supersaturating the salt solution ensures that nucleation occurs simultaneously. Ideally, after nucleation, only growth takes place, resulting in a narrow size distribution. A wide variety of reaction conditions can be varied to tailor the size, magnetic properties, and surface properties.[69]

10.2. *Nanoreactors*

To more easily control the size distribution during synthesis, various techniques have been employed to physically confine synthesis reactions. An archetypical example is the water in oil emulsion system which typically consists of water, reagents, a surfactant, a co-surfactant, and oil. In this case, iron salt reagents are present in a stable aqueous dispersion within an oil phase. Dispersion of water in the oil phase is made possible by surfactants and co-surfactants, which lower the water/oil interfacial tension. Varying system temperature along with the amount of surfactant/co-surfactant allows control over the size of the nanoreactor. Phospholipids can naturally form vesicles around magnetite particles[71] and are used in an analogous fashion to water in oil emulsion confinement.[72] Synthesis and stabilization of mNPs has been accomplished inside dendrimers,[73] and cyclodextrins.[74] Ferittin, a protein that stores iron in "cage" like fashion, is used as a nanoreactor as well.[75–77] Size distributions having standard deviations on the order of 1 nm have been achieved using ferritin proteins; and, through genetic modification, cancer-specific targeting peptides can be incorporated into ferrittin cages giving this technology innate targeting capabilities.[78]

10.3. *Sol–gel*

Additional wet chemical methods include sol–gel and polyol methods. In these methods, molecular iron oxide precursors (i.e., iron salts) are "polymerized" into nanoparticulate structures through OH group linkages in a solvent at room temperature; this creates the sol-phase of the process. Upon completion of the precursor sol-phase further heat treatments are applied to generate the final chemical and structural state.[69] For example, silica-encapsulated γ-Fe_2O_3 particles in the 6–15 nm range have been produced by 400°C heat treatment of Fe $(NO_3)_3 9H_2O$ sols in tetraethylorthosilicate.[79] By varying the solvents, salts, reagent concentrations, reaction temperature, pH, and agitation, particle size, composition and microstructure can be controlled. This method has the advantage of allowing the formation nanocomposite structures,[69] such as Fe_2O_3–SiO_2.[80] In a related process, polyols (polyaclohols) are used to solubilize metal-oxide precursor molecules. The polyol is then boiled, during which the metal precursors reduce and nucleate to form particles. Polyols are advantageous due to the higher reaction temperature allowing for better crystallinity and *in situ* coating of hydrophilic polyol groups which permits aqueous dispersion of the particles.[69] Nanoparticles were successfully produced in this manner using tri-ethylene glycol.[81]

Hydrothermal synthesis routes usually involve either hydrolysis or oxidation of iron salts or neutralization of mixed metal hydroxides.[69,82] Solvent type, reaction temperature, and presence of a surfactant are primarily used to control particle size by influencing the kinetics of growth and nucleation. For example, higher temperatures may favor nucleation over growth of existing nuclei, resulting in smaller particle size.[83] Other high temperature synthesis routes include thermal decomposition of iron precursors, such as iron pentacarbonyl. Park *et al.* produced monodispersed magnetite particle solutions with sizes ranging from 4 to 11 nm, depending on reaction temperature.[84]

Additional high temperature synthesis routes employing aerosol and vapor methods have been found. Maghemetite particles from 5 to 60 nm have been produced by the spray pyrolosis method. Iron precursors, typically in an organic solvent, are aerosolized and sprayed into reactors where the precursor nucleates as the solvent evaporates; particle morphology is dependent on the precursor solution.[69,85] Laser pyrolysis of iron pentacarbonyl vapors in a flowing ethylene/air gas stream has been used to produce magnetite nanoparticles with very narrow size distributions, and can be tuned by changing the ethylene/air gas composition, flow rate, or laser power.[86–89]

10.4. *Stabilization*

Bare magnetic nanoparticles do not form stable aqueous colloidal suspensions. Creation of a stable ferrofluid requires nanoparticles be coated with a surfactant that augments either stearic or electrostatic repulsive forces. The choice of surfactant is critical to the end-use of a given nanoparticle technology; many commonly used surfactants are not biocompatible, limiting medical applications of iron oxide nanoparticles. Generally, coatings are applied *in situ* during synthesis and thus play a role in the above synthesis. Citric acid, for example, has been used to stabilize magnetite particles produced via coprecipitation of iron salts; its concentration during synthesis has an effect on nanoparticle size.[90] The carboxyl groups on citric acid coordinate to the particle's surface adding hydrophilic and negatively charged properties.[69] It has been found, however, that excess carboxylates negatively impact the crystallinity of iron oxide nanoparticles.[91]

Inorganic materials have been used extensively to stabilize magnetic nanoparticles. Silica and other silicon-based coatings are useful because they can prevent agglomeration, improve chemical stability and be bio-inert.[92] These coatings are usually added via silanization with various organosilanes,[93–95] or from silicic acid solutions.[96] Gold is another appropriate inorganic colloidal stabilizer; by using iterative hydroxylamine seeding Au^{3+} ions have been deposited onto 9 nm magnetite nanoparticles to create hydrophilic particles 60 nm in diameter. Despite the thickness of this coating, magnetic properties of the particles remain unaffected.[97]

Some of the most widely used stabilizers of iron oxide nanoparticles are polymer-based. There are many different polymeric stabilizers; some of the most widely adopted are dextran and polyethylene glycol

(PEG). Dextran, a glucan, is widely adopted for its accepted biocompatibility. Adsorption of dextran is believed to be facilitated by hydrogen bonding of hydroxyl groups to the oxide surface.[98] It is most often applied *in situ* during co-precipitation of iron salts[99] but has also been applied to particles post-synthesis.[99] PEG is another favored surfactant; it is not only biocompatible but increases a nanoparticle's blood circulation time[100] and prevents nanoparticles from being phagocytosed by the macrophages in the liver and spleen (the reticuloendothelial system).[69] It should be noted that different nanoparticles coatings can affect the magnetic properties of nanoparticles.[101–104]

Heat-labile polymer-mNP constructs are a promising development as they introduce both highly focused chemotherapeutics and highly focused heating, which would reduce systemic toxicity. The TI would also be further improved if the chemotherapeutic were one with synergistic or additive properties when used in conjunction with hyperthermia. Polymers which are both thermally responsive and biodegradable have been created which undergo transformations at physiologically acceptable temperatures and can be used to carry chemotherapeutics. An example of this is dextran-g-poly(NIPAAm-co-DMAAm) which adapts an "expanded hydrophilic structure" at temperatures below its lower critical solution temperature (LCST).[105] This LCST can be "tuned" with the addition of co-monomer units. At temperatures above the LCST, the polymer adapts "compact hydrophobic structure" which exposes the chemotherapeutic conjugated to the iron oxide core.[106]

11. Enhanced Permeability and Retention (EPR) effect

For a tumor to grow beyond approximately two millimeters in diameter, tumor cells must excrete a variety of molecular signalers to initiate blood vessel growth and recruit nutrients.[107] The growth of new blood vessels is termed "neovascularization" or "angiogenesis". Tumoral angiogenesis typically is disorganized, occurring rapidly. This type of vascularization results in large (600–800 nm) fenestrations (gaps) between adjacent tumor endothelial cells.[108] These fenestrations permit substances injected into the blood — for instance, gadolinium contrast used to increase signal within tumor tissues during MRI imaging — to accumulate within tumors, even without any targeting moiety present.[109] By injecting nanoparticles systemically, it is hoped that a large percentage of the injected dose will accumulate within tumors due to the EPR effect.[110]

The EPR effect is demonstrated in Fig. 4.

For an intravenously-administered molecule to be able to reach the tumor, it must avoid clearance by (predominantly) four organs: kidneys, liver, spleen and bone marrow.[111] The degree and mode of clearance is significantly dependent upon nanoparticle size and surface chemistry. The kidneys will rapidly clear most molecules less than approximately 10^4 atoms (several nanometers) in size.[111] The reticuloendothelial system (RES) is composed of immune cells — predominantly macrophages — present in the liver and spleen which remove certain

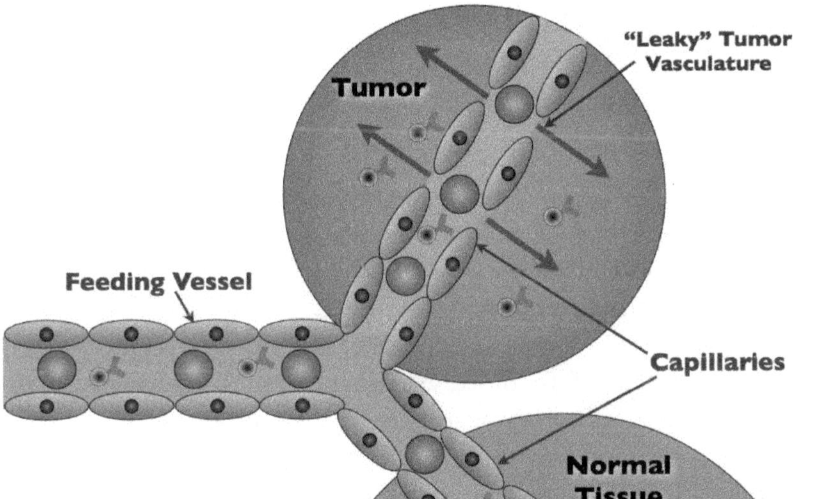

Fig. 4. The EPR (enhanced permeability and retention) effect allows for preferential diffusion of substances present in the blood into tumors (as shown with the schematic of targeted nanoparticles in this figure).

macromolecules from circulation, especially when they are hydrophobic, charged[112,113] and large (approximately 100–300 nm hydrodynamic diameter).[114]

Nanoparticle size and surface characteristics will affect their tumor localization and overall biodistribution *in vivo*. As noted, nanoparticles over 100 nm in diameter and particles with more hydrophobic coatings will be rapidly depleted from circulation through RES filtration.[100] Smaller particles are therefore more desirable from a distribution standpoint as well as for penetration and diffusion by the EPR effect. Nanoparticles of decreasing size, however, have higher surface area to volume ratios which favors plasma protein adherence. With significant protein agglomeration, the particles will again be recognized and cleared by reticuloendothelial macrophages.[115] Since surface coatings, along with targeting moiety attachment, to the nanoparticle will determine the final hydrodynamic diameter, the ability to decrease surface thickness while ensuring stability and maintaining sizeable crystal cores is invaluable.

12. Nanoparticle targeting

Specific epitopes and receptors associated with cancer cells may be targeted using functional groups. Due to their mutated genotype, tumor cells often produce unique or overexpressed markers (antigens) which distinguish them from normal cells. These markers may then be exploited for targeting purposes. For example, the breast cancer marker Her2 is frequently over-expressed as a surface receptor in breast tumors and is therefore of targeting interest.[116] Another strategy involves targeting tumor-associated antigens such as VEGF, which is a factor involved in angiogenesis.[117]

Various organic and inorganic polymer coatings can be chemically-modified to display functional groups, forming the basis for conjugation of other targeting ligands. Examples of synthetic polymer coatings include poly(vinyl alcohol), poly(lactic-co-glycolic acid) and PEG.[118–121] Natural polymers like dextran and chitosan are also commonly used.[119,122] Although some of these polymers are intrinsically cationic or anionic, they may all be modified with the addition of terminal groups such as amines, carboxylic acids and thiols to influence surface charge.

Upon the application of functionalized coatings, nanoparticles may have a variety targeting moieties added (demonstrated in Fig. 5), depending on the intended cancer target or associated function. Folic acid is one of the most frequently conjugated ligands, as it preferentially targets cancer cells and folate receptor binding results in particle endocytosis.[123,124] Other common targeting ligands include therapeutically relevant peptides and derivations of antibodies. Proven anti-cancer antibodies such as Herceptin (anti-Her2) have been conjugated in full IgG form successfully to nanoparticles. The decreased size and increased availability of engineered Fab (fragment,

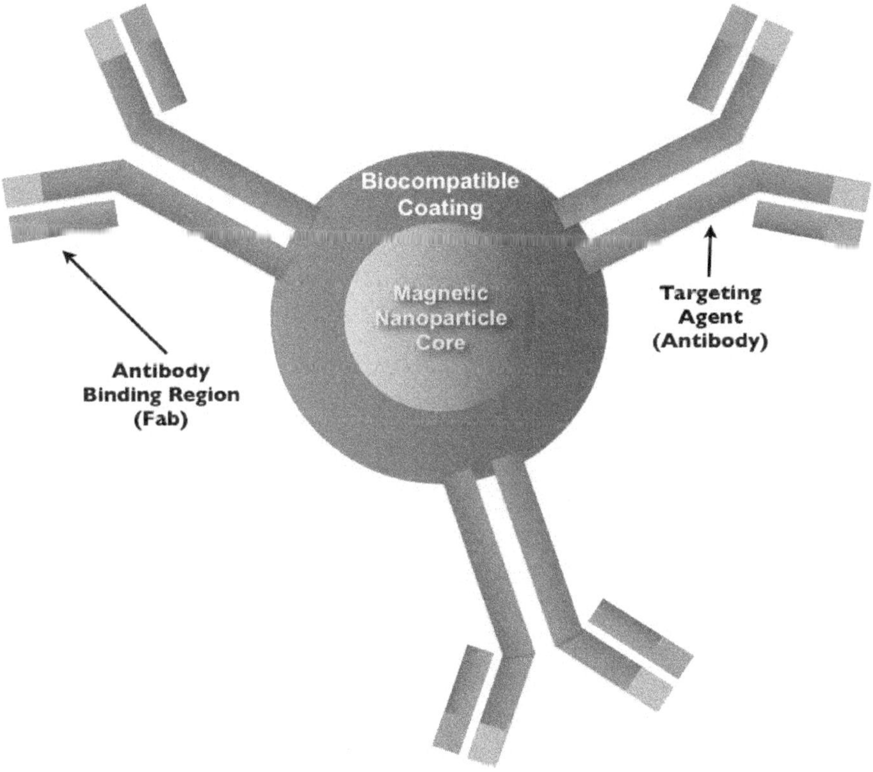

Fig. 5. A schematic of a nanoparticle conjugated to targeting agents. In this schematic, the nanoparticle is conjugate to several antibodies.

antigen binding) or scFv (single-chain variable fragment) fragments of these antibodies, however, can provide more flexibility in determining the final hydrodynamic diameter as well as available coupling chemistries.[125] The number of ligands which can be conjugated to a given nanoparticle depends on available particle surface binding sites, particle surface area and the stearics of the ligand. The latter condition may be mediated by using linker molecules (such as bi-functionalized PEG) as spacers between the ligand and the particle surface, but at the expense of increased size.

13. Conclusion: Requirements for magnetic nanoparticles used in cancer therapy

Producing localized hyperthermia of malignant lesions, using nanoparticles and AMF, has the potential to either directly kill the cancer cells or enhance susceptibility to radiation or chemotherapy. Several critical developments are needed to make nanoparticle-based hyperthermia clinically viable:

(i) The nanoparticles need to be coated for biocompatibility, low toxicity and evasion of the RES and kidney filtration.
(ii) Nanoparticles in tumors must be selectively heated via focused AMF, leaving nanoparticles that collect in potentially vulnerable regions (liver, kidney) unheated.
(iii) Nanoparticles must absorb enough power to achieve cytolytic tumor temperatures (CEM43°C of greater than 60), without significant heating of the surrounding tissue.
(iv) It is desirable that the nanoparticles be observable *in vivo* noninvasively — such as with MRI or fluorescence imaging — to ensure that they are localized in the tumor.
(v) The temperature rise in the tumor must be monitored in real time during the hyperthermia treatment to allow for high TI and to compensate for changes blood flow and physiological response to heating.
(vi) The treatment effectiveness needs to be accurately assessed so that the issues such as nanoparticle dose and administration

technique, temperature, treatment time and the number of treatments effect can be optimized.

(vii) For treatment of nonlocalized tumors (metastases), the nanoparticles must be targeted to improve selectivity of nanoparticles to tumors and supporting tissues.

(viii) Although there is potential for use of mNPH as a nontargeted monotherapy, the greatest potential for mNPH is likely due to its ability to act as an adjuvant or targeted therapy; these possibilities must be further explored.

Acknowledgments

The authors gratefully acknowledge the support of the Norris Cotton Cancer Center (Dartmouth Hitchcock Medical Center), NCI support grant: P30 CA023108-32.

References

1. M. S. Tallman *et al.*, *N. Engl. J. Med.* **337**, 1021 (1997).
2. C. H. Pui, L. L. Robison and A. T. Look, *Lancet* **371**, 1030 (2008).
3. A. Jemal *et al.*, *CA: A Cancer J. Clin.* **58**, 71 (2008).
4. L. Roizin-Towle and J. P. Pirro, *Int. J. Radiat. Oncol. Biol. Phys.* **20**, 751 (1991).
5. S. R. McWhinney, R. M. Goldberg and H. L. McLeo, *Mol. Cancer Ther.* **8**, 10 (2009).
6. S. Marchini, M. D'Incalci and M. Broggini, *Curr. Med. Chem. Anti-Cancer Agents* **4**, 247 (2004).
7. J. H. J. Hoeijmakers, *Nature* **411**, 366 (2001).
8. E. M. Rosen, S. Fan, S. Rockwell and I. D. Goldberg, *Cancer Invest* **17**, 56 (1999).
9. R. K. Gilchrist *et al.*, *Ann. Surg.* **146**, 596 (1957).
10. K. W. Chan and C. K. Chou, *Int. J. Hyperthermia* **9**, 831 (1993).
11. P. Wust *et al.*, *Lancet Oncol.* **3**, 487 (2002).
12. A. Jordan *et al.*, *Int. J. Hyperthermia* **9**, 51 (1993).
13. S. M. Moghimi, A. C. Hunter and J. C. Murray, *Pharmacol. Rev.* **53**, 283 (2001).
14. A. Ito *et al.*, *Cancer Lett.* **212**, 167 (2004).
15. S. J. DeNardo *et al.*, *Clin. Cancer Res.* **11**, 7087s (2005).
16. S. J. DeNardo *et al.*, *J. Nucl. Med.* **48**, 437 (2007).
17. M. E. Wieder *et al.*, *Photochem. Photobiol. Sci.* **5**, 727 (2006).
18. B. E. O'Neill and K. C. P. Li, *Int. J. Hyperthermia* **24**, 506 (2008).

19. C. L. Dennis *et al.*, *Nanotechnology* **20**, 395103 (2009).
20. A. Jordan *et al.*, Magnetic fluid hyperthermia, *Scientific and Clinical Applications of Magnetic Carriers*, eds. U. Häfeli, W. Schütt, J. Teller and M. Zborowski (Plenum Press, New York, 1997), pp. 569–595.
21. A. Ito, F. Matsuoka, H. Honda and T. Kobayashi, *Cancer Gene Therapy* **10**, 918 (2003).
22. J. R. Oleson *et al.*, *Amer. J. Clin. Oncology* **11**, 368 (1988).
23. M. R. Horsman and J. Overgaard, *Clin. Oncol.* **19**, 418 (2007).
24. K. S. Ryu *et al.*, *Gynecol Oncol.* **94**, 325 (2004).
25. D. Needham and M. W. Dewhirst, *Adv. Drug Deliv. Rev.* **53**, 285 (2001).
26. A. A. Petryk, A. J. Giustini, P. Ryan, R. A. Strawbridge and P. J. Hoopes, *Energy-Based Treatment of Tissue and Assessment V* **7181**, 71810N (2009).
27. T. K. Jain *et al.*, *Mol. Pharm.* **2**, 194 (2005).
28. J. Zhang and R. D. K. Misra, *Acta Biomater.* **3**, 838 (2007).
29. M. Takemoto *et al.*, *Int. J. Hyperthermia* **19**, 193 (2003).
30. P. L. Ausmus, A. V. Wilke and D. L. Frazier, *Cancer Res.* **52**, 4965 (1992).
31. M. Kim *et al.*, *IEEE Trans. Magnetics* **42**, 979 (2006).
32. K. R. Sekhar *et al.*, *Cancer Res.* **67**, 695 (2007).
33. H. H. Kampinga and E. Dikomey, *Int. J. Rad. Biol.* **77**, 399 (2001).
34. S. M. Cassim, A. J. Giustini, A. A. Petryk, R. A. Strawbridge and P. J. Hoopes, *Energy-Based Treatment of Tissue and Assessment V* **7181**, 71810O (2009).
35. Q. A. Pankhurst, J. Connolly, S. K. Jones and J. Dobson, *J. Appl. Phys. D* **36** R167 (2003).
36. S. A. Sapareto and W. C. Dewey, *Int. J. Radiat. Oncol. Biol. Phys.* **10**, 787 (1984).
37. M. Oudkerk *et al.*, *Radiology* **203**, 449 (1997).
38. R. Ivkov *et al.*, *Clin. Cancer. Res.* **11**, 7093s (2005).
39. D.-H. Kim *et al.*, *Nat. Mater.* **9**, 1 (2009).
40. S. Mornet *et al.*, *Prog. Solid State Chem.* **34**, 237 (2006).
41. R. Hergt, S. Dutz, R. Muller and M. Zeisberger, *J. Phys.: Condens. Matter* **18**, S2919 (2006).
42. D. J. Griffiths, *Introduction to Electrodynamics*, 3rd edn. (Prentice-Hall, Upper Saddle River, NJ, 1999), pp. 280–281.
43. I. Baker, Q. Zeng, W. Li and C. R. Sullivan, *J. Appl. Phys.* **99**, 08H106 (2006).
44. W. Andrä, C. G. d'Ambly, R. Hergt, I. Hilger and W. A. Kaiser, *J. Magn. Magn. Mater.* **194**, 197 (1999).
45. W. Andrä, Magnetic Hyperthermia, *Magnetism in Medicine*, eds. W. Andrä and H. Nowak (Wiley-VCH, Berlin, 1998), pp. 455–470.
46. F. Gazeau, M. Lévy and C. Wilhelm, *Nanomedicine* **3**, 831 (2008).
47. I. Hilger *et al.*, *Investigative Radiol.* **37**, 580 (2002).
48. K. Maier-Hauff *et al.*, *J. Neurooncol.* **81**, 53 (2007).
49. T. Fischer, *Materials Science for Engineering Students* (Elsevier, Burlington, MA, 2009), pp. 414–415.
50. R. F. Butler and S. K. Banerjee, *J. Geophys. Res.* **80**, 4049 (1975).
51. R. W. Rand, H. D. Snow, D. G. Elliott and M. Snyder, *Appl. Biochem. Biotech.* **6**, 265 (1981).

52. R. W. Rand, H. D. Snow and W. J. Brown, *J. Surg. Res.* **33**, 177 (1982).
53. P. Keblinski, D. G. Cahill, A. Bodapati, C. R. Sullivan and T. A. Taton, *J. Appl. Phys.* **100**, 54305-1 (2006).
54. Y. Rabin, *Int. J. Hyperthermia* **18**, 194 (2002).
55. R. Hergt *et al.*, *J. Magn. Magn. Mater.* **280**, 358 (2004a).
56. A. J. Giustini, R. Ivkov and P. J. Hoopes, *Energy-Based Treatment of Tissue and Assessment V* **7181**, 71810M (2009).
57. A. S. Eggeman, S. A. Majetich, D. Farrell and Q. A. Pankhurst, *IEEE Trans. Magnetics* **43**, 2451 (2007).
58. V. S. Abraham, S. S. Nair, S. Rajesh, U. S. Sajeev and M. R. Anantharaman, *Bull. Mater. Sci.* **27**, 155 (2004).
59. G. Zhang, Y. Liao and I. Baker, *Mater. Sci. Eng. C* **30**, 92 (2010).
60. C. Martinez-Boubeta *et al.*, *Nanomedicine: NBM* **6**, 362 (2010).
61. J. Chatterjee, M. Bettge, Y. Haik and C. J. Chen, *J. Magn. Magn. Mater.* **293**, 303 (2005).
62. H. Bonnemann *et al.*, *Inorg. Chim. Acta.* **350**, 617 (2003).
63. X. X. Zhang, G. H. Wen, G. Xiao and S. Sun, *J. Magn. Magn. Mater.* **261**, 21 (2003).
64. A. Hutten, D. Sudfeld, I. Ennen, G. Reiss, K. Wojczykowski and P. Jutzi, *J. Magn. Magn. Mater.* **293**, 93 (2005).
65. A. A. Kuznetsov, O. A. Shlyakhtin, N. A. Brusentsov and O. A. Kuznetsov, *Eur. Cells Mater.* **3**, 75 (2002).
66. J. Giri, A. Ray, S. Dasgupta, D. Datta and D. Bahadur, *Bio-Med. Mater. Eng.* **13**, 387 (2003).
67. O. V. Melnikov *et al.*, *J. Biomed. Mater. Res. Part A* **91**, 1048 (2009).
68. S. Vasseur *et al.*, *J. Magn. Magn. Mater.* **302**, 315 (2006).
69. S. Laurent *et al.*, *Chem. Rev.* **108**, 2064 (2008).
70. R. Hergt *et al.*, *IEEE Trans. Magnetics* **34**, 3745 (1998).
71. M. Decuyper and M. Joniau, *Langmuir* **7**, 647 (1991).
72. C. Sangregorio *et al.*, *J. Appl. Phys.* **85**, 5699 (1999).
73. E. Strable *et al.*, *Chem. Mater.* **13**, 2201 (2001).
74. D. Bonacchi *et al.*, *Chem. Mater.* **16**, 2016 (2004).
75. F. C. Meldrum *et al.*, *Science* **257**, 522 (1992).
76. D. P. E. Dickson *et al.*, *Nanostruct. Mater.* **9**, 595 (1997).
77. K. K. Wong *et al.*, *Chem. Mater.* **10**, 279 (1998).
78. M. Uchida *et al.*, *J. Amer. Chem. Soc.* **128**, 16626 (2006).
79. F. del Monte *et al.*, *Langmuir* **13**, 3627 (1997).
80. S. Solinas, G. Piccaluga, M. P. Morales and C. J. Serna, *Acta Mater.* **49**, 2805 (2001).
81. W. Cai and J. Q. Wan, *J. Coll. Interf. Sci.* **305**, 366 (2007).
82. M. A. Willard, L. K. Kurihara, E. E. Carpenter, S. Calvin and V. G. Harris, *Encyclopedia of Nanoscience and Nanotechnology*, ed. H. S. Nalwa (American Scientific Publishers Valencia, CA, 2004), p. 815.
83. D. Chen and R. Xu, *Mater. Res. Bull.* **33**, 1015 (1998).
84. J. Park *et al.*, *Ange. Chem.-Int. Edn.* **44**, 2872 (2005).
85. T. González-Carreño *et al.*, *Mater. Lett.* **18**, 151 (1993).

86. S. Veintemillas-Verdaguer *et al.*, *Mater. Lett.* **35**, 227 (1998).
87. S. Veintemillas-Verdaguer *et al.*, *J. Phys. D Appl. Phys.* **37**, 2054 (2004).
88. M. P. Morales *et al.*, *J. Magn. Magn. Mater.* **266**, 102 (2003).
89. R. Alexandrescu *et al.*, *Appl. Surf. Sci.* **248**, 138 (2005).
90. A. Bee *et al.*, *J. Magn. Magn. Mater.* **149**, 6 (1995).
91. C. Liu and P. M. Huang, *Soil Sci. Soc. Amer. J.* **63**, 65 (1999).
92. A. I. Lesnikovich *et al.*, *J. Magn. Magn. Mater.* **85**, 14 (1990).
93. S. Mornet *et al.*, *J. Magn. Magn. Mater.* **293**, 127 (2005).
94. A. del Campo *et al.*, *J. Magn. Magn. Mater.* **293**, 33 (2005).
95. M. Yamaura *et al.*, *J. Magn. Magn. Mater.* **279**, 210 (2004).
96. M. D. Butterworth, S. A. Bell, S. P. Armes and A. W. J. Simpson, *Coll. Interf. Sci.* **183**, 91 (1996).
97. J. L. Lyon *et al.*, *Nano Lett.* **4**, 719 (2004).
98. M. C. Bautista *et al.*, *J. Magn. Magn. Mater.* **293**, 20 (2005).
99. R. S. Molday and D. MacKenzie, *J. Immunol. Meth.* **52**, 353 (1982).
100. A. K. Gupta and M. Gupta, *Biomaterials* **26**, 3995 (2005).
101. D. F. Chan, D. B. Kirpotin and P. A. Bunn, Jr., Physical chemistry and *in vivo* tissue heating properties of colloidal magnetic iron oxides with increased power absorption rates, *Scientific and Clinical Applications of Magnetic Carriers*, eds. U. Häfeli, W. Schütt, J. Teller and M. Zborowski (Plenum Press, New York, 1997), pp. 607–618.
102. A. E. Berkowitz and J. A. Lahut, *AIP Conf. Proc.* **10**, 966 (1973).
103. A. E. Berkowitz, J. A. Lahut, I. S. Jacobs, L. M. Levinson and D. W. Forester, *Phys. Rev. Lett.* **34**, 594 (1975).
104. A. H. Morrish, Studies of magnetic properties of fine particles, *Surface Properties of Small Particles*, eds. J. L. Dormann and D. Fiorani (Elsevier, Rome, 1992), pp. 181–190.
105. J. Zhang and R. D. K. Misra, *Acta Biomater.* **3**, 838 (2007).
106. Q. Yuan, R. Venkatasubramanian, S. Hein and R. D. K. Misra, *Acta Biomater.* **4**, 1024 (2008).
107. S. B. Coffelt, R. Hughes and C. E. Lewis, *Biophys. Acta* **1796**, 11 (2009).
108. X. Wang, L. Yang, Z. Chen and D. M. Shin, *CA: A Cancer J. Clin.* **58**, 97 (2008).
109. K. Greish, *J. Drug Targeting* **15**, 457 (2007).
110. D. Sutton *et al.*, *Pharm. Res.* **24**, 1029 (2007).
111. H. Maeda, *Advances in Enzyme Regulation* **41**, 189 (2001).
112. X. Shan *et al.*, *Coll. Surf. B Biointerf.* **72**, 303 (2009).
113. C. Chouly, D. Pouliquen, I. Lucet, J. J. Jeune and P. Jallet, *J. Microencapsulation* **13**, 245 (1996).
114. M. Gaumet, R. Gurny and F. Delie, *Eur. J. Pharm. Sci.* **36**, 465 (2009).
115. V. P. Torchilin and V. S. Trubetskoy, *Adv. Drug Del. Rev.* **16**, 141 (1995).
116. D. J. Slamon, *Cancer Invest.* **8**, 253 (1990).
117. J. Chen, H. Wu, D. Han and C. Xie, *Cancer Lett.* **231**, 169 (2006).
118. A. Petri-Fink, M. Chastellain, L. Juillerat-Jeanneret, A. Ferrari and H. Hofmann, *Biomaterials* **26**, 2685 (2005).

119. H. Pardoe, W. Chua-anusorn, T. G. St. Pierre and J. Dobson, *J. Magn. Magn. Mater.* **225**, 41 (2001).
120. S. J. Lee *et al.*, *Coll. Surf. A: Physicochem. Eng. Asp.* **255**, 19 (2005).
121. Y. Zhang, N. Kohler and M. Zhang, *Biomaterials* **23**, 1553 (2002).
122. Y. C. Chang and D. H. Chen, *J. Coll. Interf. Sci.* **283**, 446 (2005).
123. H. Choi *et al.*, *Acad. Radiol.* **11**, 996 (2004).
124. F. Sonvico *et al.*, *Bioconjugate Chem.* **16**, 1181 (2005).
125. P. Holliger and P. J. Hudson, *Nat. Biotech.* **23**, 1126 (2005).
126. A. Jordan *et al.*, *J. Magn. Magn. Mater.* **194**, 185 (1999).
127. I. Hilger *et al.*, *Radiology* **218**, 570 (2001).
128. A. Ito *et al.*, *Cancer Sci.* **94**, 308 (2003).
129. T. Kikumori, T. Kobayashi, M. Sawaki and T. Imai, *Breast Cancer Res. Treat.* **113**, 435 (2009).
130. P. J. Hoopes *et al.*, *Energy-Based Treatment of Tissue and Assessment V* **7181**, 71810P (2009).

https://doi.org/10.1142/9789819809028_0009

Chapter 9

Sizes and Sufficient Quantities of MSC Microspheres for Intrathecal Injection to Modulate Inflammation in Spinal Cord Injury*

Suneel Kumar[†], Joanne Babiarz[‡] and Sayantani Basak[§]

Department of Cell Biology & Neuroscience
Rutgers University, 604 Allison Rd.
Piscataway, NJ 08854 USA
[†]sk1350@rci.rutgers.edu
[‡]jbabiarz@dls.rutgers.edu
[§]sbasak@rci.rutgers.edu

Jae Hwan Kim

Department of Cell Biology & Neuroscience
Rutgers University, 604 Allison Rd.
Piscataway, NJ 08854 USA
Department of Anatomy
Yonsei University College of Medicine
Seoul 120-752, Republic of Korea
jhchriskim@gmail.com

Jeffrey Barminko

Department of Biomedical Engineering
Rutgers University, Piscataway, NJ 0885 USA
The Mount Sinai Hospital
One Gustave L. Levy Place New York, NY 10029
jeffrey.barminko@mssm.edu

*To cite this article, please refer to its earlier version published in the *Nano LIFE*, Vol. 5, No. 4 (2015) 1550004 (14 pages), DOI: 10.1142/S179398441550004X

Andrea Gray

Department of Biomedical Engineering
Rutgers University, Piscataway, NJ 0885 USA
andrea.gray@rutgers.edu

Parry Mendapara

Department of Cell Biology & Neuroscience
Rutgers University, 604 Allison Rd.
Piscataway, NJ 08854 USA
parry.mendapara@rutgers.edu

Rene Schloss¶ and Martin L. Yarmush||

Department of Biomedical Engineering
Rutgers University, Piscataway, NJ 0885 USA
¶*schloss@soemail.rutgers.edu*
||*yarmush@rci.rutgers.edu*

Martin Grumet**

W. M. Keck Center for Collaborative Neuroscience
Rutgers Stem Cell Research Center
Department of Cell Biology & Neuroscience
Rutgers University, Piscataway, NJ, 08854 USA
mgrumet@rci.rutgers.edu

Microencapsulation of mesenchymal stem cells (MSC) in alginate facilitates cell delivery, localization and survival, and modulates inflammation *in vivo*. However, we found that delivery of the widely used ~0.5 mm diameter encapsulated MSC (eMSC) by intrathecal injection into spinal cord injury (SCI) rats was highly variable. Injections of smaller (~0.2 mm) diameter eMSC into the lumbar spine were much more reproducible and they increased the anti-inflammatory macrophage response around the SCI site. We now report that injection of small eMSC > 2 cm caudal from the rat SCI improved locomotion and myelin preservation 8 weeks after rat SCI versus control injections. Because preparation of sufficient quantities of small eMSC for larger studies was not feasible and injection of the large eMSC is problematic, we have developed a procedure to prepare medium-sized eMSC (~0.35 mm diameter) that can be delivered more reproducibly into the lumbar rat spine. The number of MSC incorporated/capsule in the medium sized capsules was ~5-fold greater than that in small capsules and the total yield of eMSC was ~20-fold higher than that for the small capsules. Assays with all three sizes of eMSC capsules showed that they

**Corresponding author.

inhibited TNF-α secretion from activated macrophages in co-cultures, suggesting no major difference in their anti-inflammatory activity *in vitro*. The *in vivo* activity of the medium-sized eMSC was tested after injecting them into the lumbar spine 1 day after SCI. Histological analyses 1 week later showed that eMSC reduced levels of activated macrophages measured by IB4 staining and increased white matter sparing in similar regions adjacent to the SCI site. The combined results indicate that ~0.35 mm diameter eMSC reduced macrophage inflammation in regions where white matter was preserved during critical early phases after SCI. These techniques enable preparation of eMSC in sufficient quantities to perform pre-clinical SCI studies with much larger numbers of subjects that will provide functional analyses of several critical parameters in rodent models for CNS inflammatory injury.

Keywords: Microcapsules; alginate; mesenchymal stem cells; intrathecal; inflammation.

1. Introduction

Polymerized alginate is biocompatible and has been approved for clinical treatments.[1,2] Alginate microspheres of various sizes have been prepared with encapsulated cells for several applications including to control cell differentiation within the capsules[3] and as a source for secretion of desired factors.[4–6] Encapsulation involves extrusion of a mixture of alginate with cells into microdroplets that become cross-linked into microspheres after they fall into a bath containing divalent cations. Capsule sizes typically range from as small as ~0.1 mm, containing only a few cells, up to ~0.5 mm to 1 mm, containing hundreds to thousands of cells, but perfusion of factors throughout larger capsules may be limited by diffusion.[4] Encapsulation promotes cell survival and protects cells from immune rejection *in vivo* while allowing secreted factors to be released from the capsules. The capsules are useful for delivering factors locally when they can be delivered to specific sites including in the brain, spinal cord, eye, cochlea, bone, kidney capsule, pancreas and heart.[4,5]

A major use of cells encapsulated in microspheres is to release growth factors, cytokines and small proteins into the surrounding milieu. Genetically engineered cell lines over-expressing neuroprotective factors including ciliary neurotrophic factor (CNTF), glial cell line-derived neurotrophic factor (GDNF) and fibroblast growth factor (FGF) have been encapsulated in alginate and implanted into the central nervous system (CNS) to yield improvement in several models of neurodegenerative disorders.[4,6,7] Different types of cells [(e.g., fibroblasts, Schwann cells and mesenchymal stem cells (MSC)] and cell lines [baby hamster kidney cells (BHK) and myoblasts] have been transfected to release various factors from capsules that are bioactive.[5] For example, eMSC transfected to release GLP-1 were found to be neuroprotective but protection was also reported for the eMSC alone.[8]

While only a few studies have used eMSC without transfection of exogenous proteins, many studies have demonstrated that migratory MSC improve recovery in wide range of injuries and disorders both in animal models and, in a few cases, in the clinic.[9–12] There is convincing evidence *in vitro* that MSC act to a great extent via their secreted anti-inflammatory and growth factors but other possible mechanisms of action cannot be ruled out when the cells are injected *in vivo*.[9,11,13] Effects using encapsulated cells *in vivo* can be attributed to their secreted factors because the cells are segregated from the host by the capsule.[5,8] Encapsulation of MSC in alginate has been found to upregulate the expression of many cytokines dramatically and many of the secreted factors are anti-inflammatory both *in vitro* and *in vivo*.[14]

Proinflammatory cytokines play a critical role in expanding damage after CNS trauma and treatment with MSC can control inflammation and improve survival of neural tissue and functional outcomes.[15,16] Spinal cord contusion in the rat is a widely used model to study molecular processes of secondary damage over time caused by inflammatory and other factors, and mediated by inflammatory cells including macrophages.[17] Beneficial effects of MSC in spinal cord injury (SCI) have resulted following various injection methods but the fate of the MSC is unclear making it difficult to study their mechanisms of action. Studies with eMSC are not complicated by direct interactions of the cells with the host and therefore reveal actions only of MSC secreted factors.

Functional improvement with encapsulated cells in the CNS has been observed when the capsules are injected into or adjacent to injury sites, which can accommodate large capsules but this requires invasive surgical procedures and exposes the capsules and cells to an inflammatory and cytotoxic environment.[5,7,18] This may be avoided by placing the capsules at a location distant from the site of inflammation as long as the factors secreted by the cells gain access to the site of inflammation. We have injected small ($\sim$0.2 mm) eMSC intrathecally into the rat lumbar spine ($>$2 cm from SCI site), which had anti-inflammatory effects after SCI.[14] A major limitation in the use of $\sim$0.2 mm alginate capsules is the small number of live MSC that could be encapsulated. To overcome this limitation and thereby facilitate more extensive quantitative studies, we report here a method that yields much higher numbers of cells in intermediate-sized microspheres, which when injected intrathecally, reduced pro-inflammatory macrophages and preserved white matter tissue after SCI.

2. Materials and methods

2.1. *MSC culture*

Human bone marrow-derived mesenchymal stem/stromal cells (MSC) were purchased from Texas A&M at passage 1 and cultured, as previously described,[14] in minimum essential medium (MEM)-α (Gibco Life Technologies, USA) medium containing no deoxy- or ribonucleosides, and supplemented with 10% fetal bovine serum (FBS, Atlanta Biologicals, USA), 1 ng/mL basic fibroblast growth factor (bFGF), 2 mM L-glutamine, 100 U/mL penicillin and 100 μg/mL streptomycin (Gibco). MSC were plated at 5000 cells/cm^2 and allowed to proliferate to $\sim$70% confluence. Only low passages (2–4) were used for experiments.

2.2. *Alginate microencapsulation*

Microencapsulation of MSC was performed as described.[14,19] Briefly, MSC were detached using trypsin–EDTA (Gibco), washed and mixed with 2.2% (w/v) alginate (Sigma Aldrich, USA) solution to obtain an initial cell density of 4–6$\times 10^6$ cells/mL. An electrostatic bead generator was used to form microdroplets, which were subsequently cross-linked in a $CaCl_2$ bath. Microcapsules were washed with phosphate buffered saline (PBS, Gibco) and briefly incubated with 0.05% (w/v) poly-L-Lysine (Sigma Aldrich, USA) in PBS. Encapsulated cells were re-suspended in cell culture medium and transferred to 25 cm^2 tissue culture flasks. MSC viability in the capsules was assessed using a calcein and ethidium homodimer assay (Molecular Probes, USA).[19] Capsules were imaged in an inverted fluorescent microscope (IX81, Olympus, Tokyo, Japan) and diameters were measured using SlideBook image analysis software version 5.0 (Intelligent Imaging Innovations, USA). Large- ($n = 5$) and medium- ($n = 4$) sized capsules were prepared using 0.17 mm inner bore extrusion needles, which yielded a total of $\sim 10^6$ live cells in a single preparation, and 0.12 mm inner bore needles were used for the small capsules ($n = 6$), which yielded ~50,000 cells/preparation (Table 1). Encapsulations were performed within 1 h to maximize cell viability, which decreased at longer times of exposure to unpolymerized alginate, and therefore the low flow rate (0.5 mL/h) with the narrower 0.12 mm needles yielded much fewer eMSC than with the larger 0.17 mm needles, which had a much higher flow rate of 20 mL/h. The percent encapsulated/input is the ratio of the total number of cells encapsulated divided by the total cell input in the alginate mixture. To reduce variability among preparations of small eMSC, three preparations were pooled, the average numbers of live cells/capsule were measured, and aliquots from the pool were used for 2–3 replicates. Individual preparations of large and medium sized capsules yielded sufficient quantities for many replicates. Ejection

Table 1. Analysis of MSC encapsulation parameters.

MSC capsules	Diameter (μm) +/− Std.	Viability (%)	Live cells/ capsule	Total live cells encapsulated	Encapsulated/ input (%)
Large	450 ± 65	88 ± 7	124 ± 43	$\sim 10^6$	~25
Medium	378 ± 29	83 ± 7	73 ± 15	$\sim 10^6$	~25
Small	214 ± 27	83 ± 13	14 ± 5	~50,000	~1.25

efficiency of eMSC through 23 gauge thin walled needles (0.52 mm inner diameter, NIPRO) was calculated as the number of ejected capsules recovered divided by (the average number of capsules/mL) × (the volume ejected in mL).

2.3. *Co-culture of macrophages with eMSC*

Macrophages were isolated and co-culture assays were performed as described[20] except with adaptations made for the use of capsules. Briefly, peripheral blood mononuclear cells were collected from blood of healthy donors (Blood Center of New Jersey) after centrifugation in Ficoll density gradients (GE Healthcare, USA). Monocytes were isolated by magnetic cell sorting using anti-CD14 coated beads (Miltenyi Biotec, USA), and $CD14^+$ monocytes were cultured in 175 cm^2 flasks (BD Biosciences, USA) at 10^7 cells/flask in Advanced RPMI 1640 medium (Gibco) supplemented with 10% FBS (Atlanta Biologicals, Lawrenceville, GA), 100 U/mL penicillin, 100 μg/mL streptomycin and 2 mM L-glutamine (Gibco). Macrophages were incubated with 5 ng/mL GM-CSF (R&D Systems, USA) for 7 days and replated at 1×10^4 cells/mL or 5×10^4 cells/mL in 96 or 24-well plates (Corning, USA), respectively, and allowed to attach overnight. To activate the macrophages, the medium was replaced with medium containing 1 μg/mL lipopolysaccharide (LPS) (Sigma-Aldrich). Transwell inserts containing small, medium or large eMSC in medium with 1 μg/mL LPS were then added to the wells in a 1:1 macrophage:MSC ratio. Wells containing only macrophages and medium with or without LPS were included as positive and negative controls, respectively. After 48 h, co-culture supernatants were collected, stored at −20°C and then analyzed for secreted tumor necrosis factor (TNF)-α by ELISA[14] (Biolegend, USA).

2.4. *SCI and transplantation*

Adult female Sprague-Dawley rats (77 ± 2 days old, Taconic, USA) were used for all experiments with protocols approved by the Animal Care and Use Committee of Rutgers, The State University of New Jersey. For SCI surgery, rats were anesthetized with 2% isoflurane

(IsoFlo; Abbott Laboratories, USA), the spinal cord was exposed by laminectomy at T9–T10, and then contused by dropping a 10-g rod on the exposed cord from a height of 12.5 mm using a MASCIS Impactor as described.[14,21] Following contusion, the muscles and skin were closed separately. Cefazolin (25 mg/kg) was administered daily for 7 days by subcutaneous injection after SCI to all rats. Food and water were provided *ad libitum*. One day after SCI, saline, capsules without MSC, 5×10^4 free MSC or 3×10^4 eMSC were injected intrathecally into the lumbar spine (L4–L5) over a period of 30 s using a thin-walled needle (23G X 1 inch, inner diameter = 0.52 mm, outer diameter = 0.64 mm, NIPRO) attached to 250 μL Hamilton syringe. The needle was left in place for another 60 s to prevent leakage. After the injection, the muscles and skin were sutured separately. Locomotor recovery was assessed weekly using the 21-point Basso, Beattie and Bresnahan (BBB) scoring method[22] by a team that was unaware of experimental treatments. Rats injected with 0.2 mm eMSC were allowed to survive for 8 weeks and those injected with 0.35 mm eMSC survived for 8 days (7 days after injection).

2.5. *Magnetic resonance imaging of intrathecal transplanted capsules*

Alginate capsules were prepared with 100 nm chitosan-coated magnetite nanoparticles (ChMNP, 6 mg/mL) and $\sim 4 \times 10^3$ ChMNP-containing 0.2 mm diameter capsules were prepared without or with MSC, and implanted intrathecally into the rat cauda equina. MRI was performed on rats under isoflurane anesthesia using a T1-weighted fast spin echo sequence with the M2™ Compact High-Performance MRI at the Rutgers Molecular Imaging Center. Imaging was performed at indicated times after ChMNP capsule implantation to track the capsules in the spinal cord over time. Noncontused rats were transferred to the Rutgers Molecular Imaging Center one day after ChMNP capsules injection and MRI was performed first on day 2 and at the indicated times up to 42 days. Contused rats remained in the Nelson Biological Labs animal facility for ~2–3 weeks until they gained bladder control and no longer required special care.

2.6. *Tissue processing for immunofluorescence and quantitation*

Animals were sacrificed, perfused with 4% paraformaldehyde either 8 days or 8 weeks after SCI. Spinal cords were dissected and post-fixed with 4% paraformaldehyde at 4°C overnight. For cryosections, spinal cords were equilibrated in graded sucrose (10–30%) for 72 h at 4°C, embedded in optimal cutting temperature compound (OCT) compound (Fisher Scientific, USA) and cut into 20 μm cross sections. For immunofluorescence, sections were blocked with 10% normal goat serum at room temperature for 2 h and incubated with Isolectin IB4 Alexa-488 conjugate (1:100, Invitrogen). Image analysis was performed using Zeiss 510 confocal laser scanning microscope and analyzed using LSM software. IB4 stained tile scans encompassing the entire cross section were taken from the 8-day rats at ~2.2 mm distal to the SCI epicenter. For quantitation in the dorsal midline of the SCI site, a circle (1900 μm circumference) was drawn between and below the dorsal horns using Zeiss LSM Image Browser tool. A constant threshold was applied to obtain superthreshold pixels of IB4 staining within the fixed circular areas and averages of the resulting percentages were calculated.

2.7. *White matter sparing*

For analysis of spared white matter, cryosections from 8-week rats ranging from −3 mm (rostral) to +3 mm (caudal) to injury epicenter at 1 mm intervals were stained with Eriochrome Cyanine-R (ECR) as described.[23] Sections were dehydrated at room temperature in a series of graded ethanol solutions for 5 min each and cleared in histoclear (National Diagnostics, USA) solution for 5 min. The sections were then rehydrated in a reverse-graded ethanol series. Sections were stained for 10 min with a solution of 0.16% ECR, 0.4% sulfuric acid, 0.4% iron chloride and 0.12% HCL. Sections were then rinsed with water for 10 min, mounted in Permount media (Fisher Scientific, USA) and scanned with Super Coolscan 8000 (Nikon, Japan). Images were analyzed using NIH ImageJ software to obtain super-threshold areas for each section using a constant threshold for all sections that were stained at the same time with ECR. Percent white matter is defined as the super-threshold area divided by the total area outlined in each section. Averages of spared white matter tissue were calculated. For analysis of spared white matter, rats were sacrificed after 8 days and sections at 2.2 mm caudal to the SCI epicenter were used.

2.8. *Statistical analysis*

BBB scoring and white matter sparing data were analyzed using repeated measure ANOVA followed by Tukey HSD test. Macrophage TNF-α secretion data were analyzed using ANOVA followed by Fisher's least significant difference (LSD) test. White matter sparing and IB4 staining data were analyzed using Student's t-test. Statistical significance was accepted for p values of <0.05 and the mean $\pm$ SD are indicated.

3. Results

3.1. *Localization of MSC capsules by MRI in the spinal cord*

In a previous SCI study we showed one week after intrathecal injection that fluorescent capsules were detected in the lumbar spine.[14] To determine their distribution over more extended times in the living rat, we injected capsules containing magnetic nanoparticles (ChMNP) intrathecally, and MRI localized them to the cauda equina for 6 weeks after injection (Fig. 1). Signals were detected at all time points, indicating that the capsules persisted for 6 weeks *in vivo* but no contrast enhancement was detected in an uninjected rat [Fig. 1(a)]. Cross-section images at day 2 and 42 indicated that the capsules were restricted to the spinal column [Figs. 1(b) and 1(c)] and horizontal imaging showed that they remained close to where they were injected in the cauda equina at 1–6 weeks after injection in a noncontused rat [Figs. 1(d) and 1(e)]. Optical sections through the spinal cord showed the distribution of ChMNP capsules at several levels from dorsal to

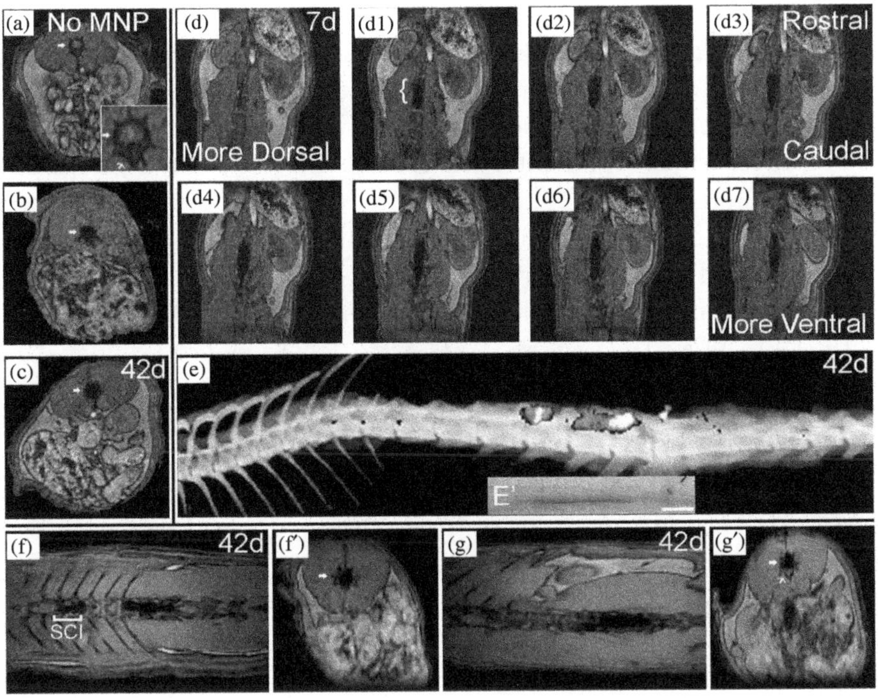

Fig. 1. MRI visualization of ChMNP capsules in rat spinal cords without and with contusion. Noncontused rats without (a) or with (b)–(e) intrathecal injection of ChMNP capsules were imaged at indicated times after injection. In the axial image, without ChMNP capsules note the gray region in panel A (arrow) corresponding to the spinal cord and the bony vertebral body, which is marked by a thin arrow (a) and at higher magnification in the insert. Signals (black) were detected with ChMNP capsules after 2 days (b) and they persisted for 42 days (c) in axial images. Horizontal images at 7 days (d1–d7) show localization of ChMNP capsules along the spinal axis (bracket in d1) localized in serial sections from dorsal to ventral encompassing ~2.2 mm. A 3D reconstruction of super-threshold MRI signals superimposed on an X-ray (e) shows a ventrolateral distribution, which is within the ventral distribution of ChMNP particles in brown (e′) in a bright field image of the same spinal cord after dissection from the spine. SCI Rats at 42 days after intrathecal injection of ChMNP capsules without (f, f′) or with (g, g′) eMSC were imaged ($n = 2$, 3, respectively). A bracket marks the SCI site at T9-10 in the horizontal image (f) with signals of ChMNP particles in dorsal regions of T13- L2; the signal extends more caudally to L3-4 (f′) but was primarily ventral (not shown). Horizontal image (g) with signals of ChMNP particles in eMSC in ventral regions of L3- L5; note the signal is in the spine above the vertebral body (g′).

ventral [Figs. 1(d)– 1(d7)]. The most intense mass of capsules was localized within ∼1 cm along the rostro-caudal axis of the spinal cord within ∼3 spinal segments after 1–6 weeks in the live rat [Fig. 1(e)]. Histological analysis after sacrifice confirmed that most capsules were found in this same region after the spinal cord was removed from the spinal column [Figs. 1(e) and 1(e′)].

To determine whether similar distributions of ChMNP capsules were obtained in SCI rats, we injected them intrathecally one day after contusion. Injections of ChMNP capsules without [Fig. 1(f)] and with MSC [Fig. 1(g)] in SCI rats were localized primarily in the lumbar spine after 42 days; the distributions in each rat were very similar to that observed ∼3 weeks after injection (data not shown), suggesting no gross movement of the capsules. ChMNP capsules extended rostrally as far as L13 [Fig. 1(f)] and caudally to L5 [Fig. 1(g)] and L6 [Fig. 1(e)]. Distributions of ChMNP capsules without and with MSC were typically located more ventrally in the spine [Figs. 1(e) and 1(g)] and less frequently in dorsal regions [Fig. 1(f)]. The combined results indicate that the ChMNP alginate capsules without or with eMSC remained in and around the cauda equina in the lumbar spine for 6 weeks without any gross movement in both control and contused rats.

3.2. *Injection of eMSC in SCI inhibits inflammation and promotes locomotor recovery*

We observed previously that one week after intrathecal injection of ∼0.2 mm eMSC at a location >2 cm caudal from the SCI site at T9-10, expression in the injury site was increased for CD206, a marker for anti-inflammatory/reparative M2 macrophages.[14] In a longer-term study with survival for 8 weeks following SCI and lumbar injection of small eMSC, we observed a temporal trend toward improved hindlimb locomotion that reached significance between eMSC and the saline control groups at 7 and 8 weeks [Fig. 2(a)]. The ∼2 point differences observed in this region of the nonlinear BBB scale (i.e., between 9–10 and 11–12) represents a difference between weight support and walking.[22] The BBB scores for a third group of SCI rats

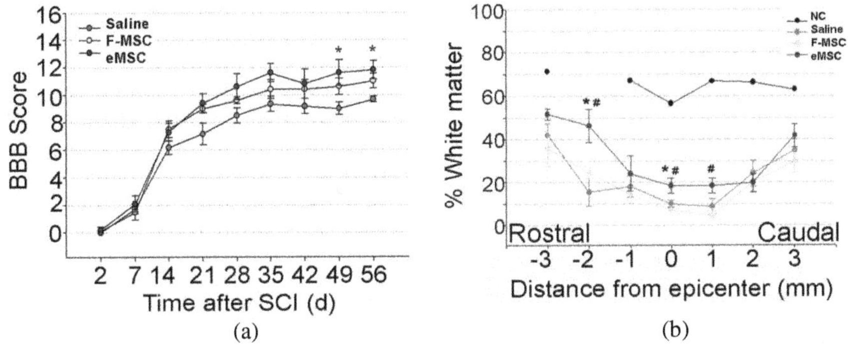

Fig. 2. Effects of small eMSC on recovery after SCI. (a) Post-injury locomotor function assessed using BBB scoring was done weekly for 8 weeks by trained observers in SCI rats injected with 5×10^4 free human MSC (F-MSC), small encapsulated MSC (3×10^4), or saline 1 day after SCI. Data is represented as mean ± SD. The eMSC ($n = 5$) showed consistently higher scores than F-MSC ($n = 5$) and saline group ($n = 6$) and attained significance at week 7 and 8 (*, $p < 0.05$ ANOVA repeated measures with Tukey HSD test). (b) Percent preserved white matter at 8 weeks after SCI was calculated by measuring ECR staining in cross sections from rats treated with saline ($n = 4$), F-MSC ($n = 5$) and eMSC ($n = 3$) at the indicated positions relative to the injury epicenter; (NC, normal control). Significant differences were detected in the percent of preserved white matter between eMSC versus saline groups (*, $p < 0.05$) or versus F-MSC (#, $p < 0.05$).

that were injected with free nonencapsulated MSC, fell in between the eMSC and saline controls but the differences were not statistically different by comparison to the other two groups [Fig. 2(a)]. This suggests that ~0.2 mm eMSC are more effective than free MSC in improving locomotion when injections were made 1 day after rat SCI. Histological analyses after sacrifice showed that levels of white matter were significantly higher in the eMSC group by comparison to the saline group but no significant differences were observed by comparison to the free MSC group [Fig. 2(b)]. The weaker improvements observed with the free MSC may be explained by their disappearance from the spinal cord within one week after injection while eMSC retrieved at the same time showed an average MSC survival of ~50% in the capsules by live/dead staining (data not shown).

3.3. *Optimization of MSC capsules for intrathecal injection in rats*

3.3.1. *Properties of small and large MSC capsules*

A major limitation in these experiments using the small ~0.2 mm alginate capsules was the low number of MSC that could be encapsulated due to the slow flow rates through the narrow bore extrusion needles used to generate them. The average number of live eMSC per 1-h encapsulation for the small microspheres was ~50,000, whereas the average for the large capsules with the larger inner diameter of 0.17 mm needle was ~10^6 (Table 1). Thus, we were able to generate on average >20 times more cells/encapsulation in large capsules than in the small capsules.

In control experiments, we analyzed the reproducibility of capsule ejection through 0.52 mm inner diameter thin-walled needles to model the intrathecal delivery by measuring the numbers of capsules that were ejected into a tube *in vitro*. An average of >90% of the expected numbers of capsules were ejected with the small capsules but <30% were ejected with the large capsules and the yield was highly variable (Fig. 3). For these ejections that modeled the intrathecal rat injection procedure, it was necessary to concentrate the eMSC into a small volume (~0.15 mL), which often caused the large capsules to aggregate and become trapped in the hub of the injection needles. This trapping resulted in highly variable numbers of large capsules ejected in repeated samples of equal volume. Capsule trapping in the syringe hub was not a problem with small eMSC (Fig. 3) or with the large capsules prepared without cells (data not shown). The variable yields that occurred with large eMSC made them unsuitable for quantitative studies *in vivo*.

Given the limited number of small capsules that could be prepared, we attempted to increase the number of cells/small capsule or to produce intermediate sized capsules. We varied multiple parameters using the small bore needle (inner diameter of 0.12 mm) for capsule generation including different flow rates and voltages, alginate densities and cell input (up to 8 million/preparation) but we could not get much higher yields and the properties of the capsules (i.e., shape and fragility) were often inferior (data not shown). We then varied these parameters

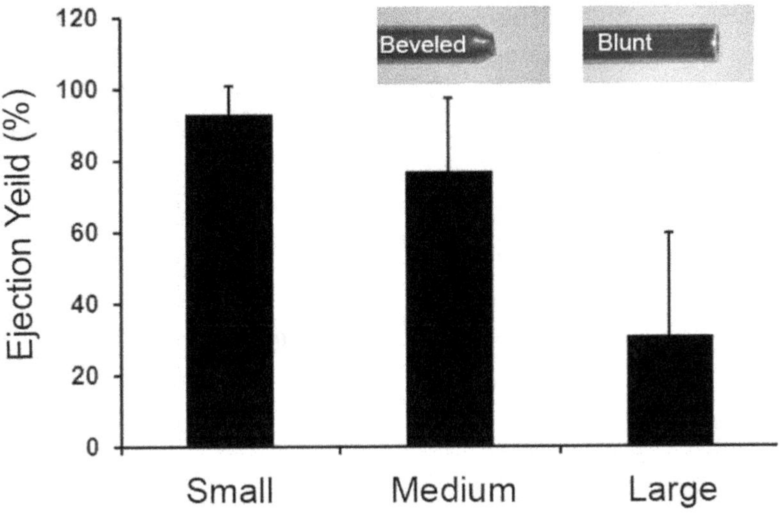

Fig. 3. Efficiency of eMSC ejection through narrow bore needles. Graph shows the effect of capsule size on eMSC ejection yield (%, mean $\pm$ SD) in 2–3 experiments for three different eMSC sizes (small $\sim$0.2 mm, medium $\sim$0.35 mm and large $\sim$0.5 mm). The ejection yield with larger capsules was much lower than the small and medium size capsules due to aggregation (see text). The inserts show tips of 0.17 inner diameter needles with blunt or beveled ends, which gave large- and medium-sized capsules, respectively.

using the larger needle with inner diameter of 0.17 mm in attempts to generate smaller capsules but we could not find conditions to produce eMSC that could pass reproducibly through the 0.52 mm injection needles (Fig. 3). However, we found that a needle with the same inner diameter of 0.17 mm with a beveled tip, instead of the blunt tip used previously (Fig. 3 inserts), yielded relatively uniform eMSC of $\sim$0.35 mm, which contained five times as many cells as in the small eMSC (Table 1). The beveled needle tip has a narrower outer diameter at the ejection orifice than the blunt needle (Fig. 3 inserts), which resulted in the formation of smaller diameter micro-drops before they fell from the needle tip into the $CaCl_2$ bath where they were cross-linked.

Then we analyzed the reproducibility of ejecting the $\sim$0.35 mm eMSC through 0.52 mm inner diameter thin-walled needles and compared the results with those for the larger eMSC described above.

An average of $\sim$80% of the expected numbers of $\sim$0.35 mm eMSC were ejected, which is much improved by comparison to the <30% ejected with the large capsules (Fig. 3). Unlike the larger $\sim$0.5 mm eMSC which tended to aggregate and clog the thin-walled needles used for intrathecal injections, these problems were not observed with $\sim$0.35 mm eMSC, which were collected with more reproducible yields than the larger $\sim$0.5 mm eMSC (Fig. 3).

3.3.2. *Properties of medium-sized $\sim$0.35 mm MSC capsules*

We characterized these medium-sized $\sim$0.35 mm eMSC by comparison to the small and large eMSC. While the number of live cells/capsule was much higher in the medium and large than in small capsules, the percent of live MSC was comparable among the three different sized capsules (Table 1). Comparable yields of incorporated cells were obtained for the large and the medium sized capsules generated using the inner diameter needle of 0.17 mm. However, the smaller capsules generated using the inner diameter needle of 0.12 mm required much slower flow rates such that during a 1-h encapsulation only $\sim$50 000 cells were obtained in capsules (Table 1). Encapsulations were limited to 1 h to avoid lower yields of live cells that resulted when MSC were exposed to unpolymerized alginate for longer durations (J. Barminko, unpublished observations). Thus, large numbers of cells were obtained in medium-sized capsules (Table 1), which could be ejected through narrow bore needles used for intrathecal delivery in SCI experiments (Fig. 3).

3.4. *MSC capsules inhibit secretion of TNF-α from activated macrophages in vitro*

To compare the immunomodulatory properties of the different sized eMSC, we tested their effects in co-cultures with LPS-activated human macrophages.[20] LPS induced secretion of TNF-α and these levels were decreased by co-culture with the different sized eMSC (Fig. 4). Decrease in TNF-α levels were obtained in all cases, with the medium eMSC showing the most robust affect (Fig. 4). Thus, the

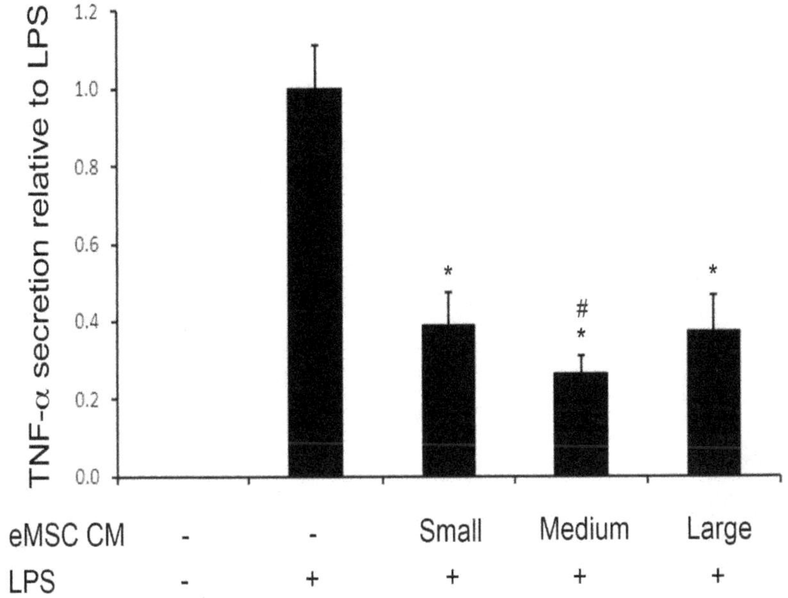

Fig. 4. Different sizes of eMSC reduce TNF-α secretion when cultured with activated macrophages. Culture supernatants collected from transwell co-cultures of LPS-activated macrophages with eMSC at 1:1 ratio were assayed for TNF-α by ELISA and normalized to levels in LPS activated macrophages supernatants without added eMSC. Differences between the LPS only control and each of the three different sized eMSC were significant (*, $p < 0.05$) and the difference between the medium-sized capsules and the large and small capsules was also significant (#, $p < 0.05$).

medium-sized eMSC were more effective than the large eMSC in reducing secretion of a key pro-inflammatory cytokine from activated human macrophages.[14]

3.5. *MSC capsules reduce levels of activated macrophages in SCI*

Given the immunomodulatory effects of the medium-sized eMSC *in vitro*, we injected them 1 day after SCI in rats to evaluate their effects on inflammation *in vivo*. To test the effects on pro-inflammatory microglia and macrophages we immunostained for the isolectin IB4 in sections from rat SCI one week after eMSC injection. IB4 binding is

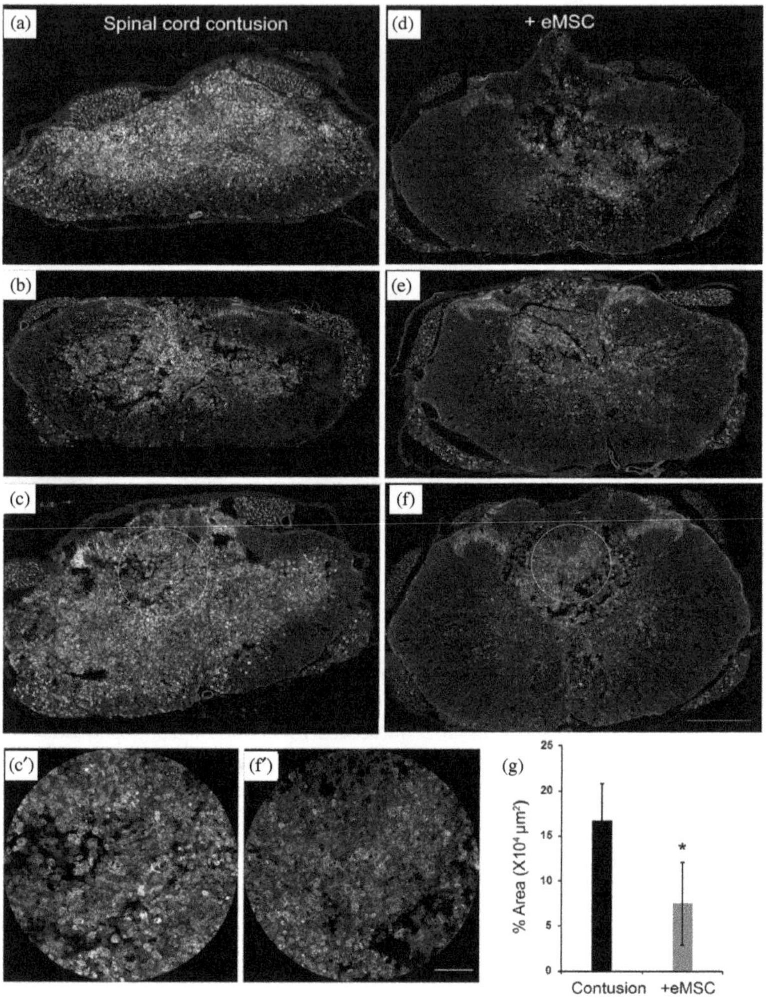

Fig. 5. Effect of medium-size eMSC transplantation on activated macrophages in SCI. Tissues from SCI rats one week after injection with ~0.35 mm eMSC (d)–(f) or saline as a control (a)–(c) were cryosectioned in cross sections and were incubated with Isolectin IB4 Alexa-488 conjugate. Confocal imaging showed more robust staining in control than eMSC treated sections in white matter and gray matter regions. Quantitation (g) of IB4 staining regions in equivalent dorsal midline circles drawn in spinal cord cross sections (for example, C′ and F′ are magnified images from C and F, respectively) were measured as super-threshold areas at ~2.2 mm caudal to the injury epicenter. IB4 levels decreased significantly (*, $p < 0.05$) in the eMSC group ($n = 3$) as compared to the control ($n = 4$) group. Scale bars are 500 μm in panels (a)–(f) and 100 μm in panels C′ and F′.

an early marker for activated macrophages[24] and microglia.[25] IB4+ staining in SCI cross sections indicated the presence of many robustly labeled pro-inflammatory macrophages one week after injection in SCI rats with control treatment [Figs. 5(a)–5(c)] but much less staining was observed after injection of eMSC [Figs. 5(d)–5(f)]. While the IB4 staining varied among different rats within each group, there appeared to be less staining in the eMSC group [Figs. 5(d)–5(f)] in white matter regions than in the controls [Figs. 5(a)–5(c)]. The IB4 staining was most intense in the dorsal central region of the SCI site, and quantitation in these regions (C′ versus F′) showed significantly lower average levels in the eMSC rats by comparison to controls [Fig. 5(g)].

3.6. *MSC capsules promote white matter sparing in SCI*

Pro-inflammatory macrophages and cytokines have been associated with CNS demyelination.[26] We found that ECR staining for myelin showed more white matter sparing with eMSC [Figs. 6(d)–6(f)] by comparison to controls [Figs. 6(a)–6(c)]. Quantitation of ECR staining confirmed larger superthreshold areas of white matter with eMSC treatment compared to controls [Fig. 6(g)]. The combined results indicate that intrathecal injection of medium-sized eMSC reduced levels of pro-inflammatory macrophages and increased white matter

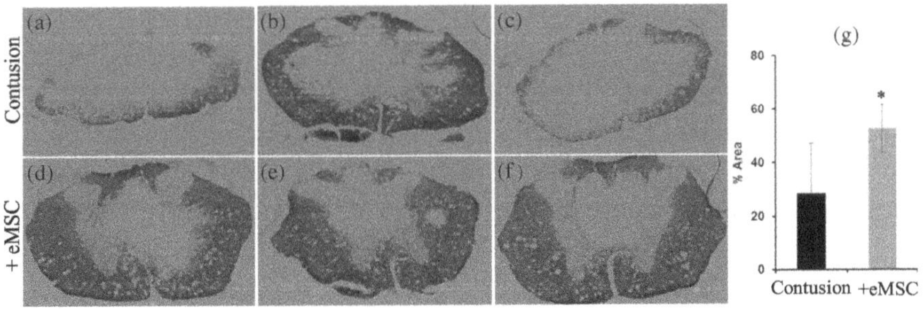

Fig. 6. Medium-size eMSC increased white matter sparing. Spinal cord cross sections in regions adjacent to those analyzed in Fig. 5 from spinal cord contusion control (a)–(c) and ∼0.35 mm eMSC (d)–(f) injected groups were stained for ECR. The percent of white matter (g) is significantly higher in eMSC group ($n = 7$) as compared to control group ($n = 3$) (*, $p < 0.05$).

sparing in the corresponding regions of the spinal cord [compare Figs. 5(a)–5(f) with 6(a)–6(f)] after a one-week treatment after SCI.

4. Discussion

Transplantation of encapsulated cells has shown success *in vivo*[4,27] but very few studies have demonstrated benefits in the CNS.[14] In this and a previous study,[14] we provide the first evidence that intrathecal eMSC injections are immunomodulatory and promote recovery after contusive SCI. We showed previously that small eMSC increased M2 anti-inflammatory macrophages 1 week after injection,[14] and we report here that after 8 weeks they improved locomotor recovery and white matter sparing. Medium-sized eMSC decreased M1 pro-inflammatory macrophages and promoted white matter sparing one week after acute injection in SCI. These improvements in white matter sparing [Fig. 2(b)] and locomotion [Fig. 2(a)] are consistent with previous studies demonstrating a positive relationship between white matter sparing and locomotion after SCI of different severities.[22] We also report methods for encapsulating ~20 times more human MSC in medium-sized capsules than was possible previously in the small capsules, which were used for minimally invasive intrathecal injection of eMSC into the rat spine after SCI. The results indicate that alginate capsules without or with MSC remain in the lumbar spine for at least 6 weeks and suggest that eMSC have immunomodulatory effects at a distance of >2 cm in more rostral thoracic SCI sites.

Relatively large (>0.5 mm diameter) capsules have been used for many applications where they can be delivered locally, although smaller capsules are preferred due to their excellent surface-volume ratio and oxygen permeability.[4] However, few studies have compared the properties of different sized capsules *in vivo*[28,29] and we are not aware of any comparison that has been reported for injection of different sized alginate capsules into the CNS. A comparison performed with various sizes of encapsulated islets concluded that capsules <0.35 mm were more biocompatible than larger capsules, which were more fibrotic.[28] We have compared three different sizes of capsules ($\sim$0.2 mm, 0.35 mm and 0.5 mm) and found that they have relatively similar activities to modulate inflammation *in vitro*. However, their use differed substantially *in vivo* for minimally invasive intrathecal delivery, which required small volumes and narrow bore needles to avoid excessive damage and leakage of cerebrospinal fluid (CSF). We found that for quantitative studies injections of concentrated suspensions of large alginate capsules were problematic because of high variability in the number of capsules that could be injected. Similar problems have not been reported with injection of much larger volumes through wider bore needles.[8,28] We have shown here and previously[14] that MSC capsules ranging from 0.2–0.35 mm can be injected intrathecally through narrow-walled needles and that they had significant anti-inflammatory effects in SCI. The $\sim$0.35 mm medium-sized capsules are advantageous because they allow encapsulation of many more cells than in the small capsules, thereby providing sufficient quantities for injection in large controlled physiological studies.

Encapsulation of MSC is also advantageous because the capsule protects cells from direct contact with the host while the MSC secrete immunomodulatory factors. MSC respond rapidly to pro-inflammatory cytokines by releasing anti-inflammatory cytokines and factors, making them particularly well suited to suppress inflammation.[30] Encapsulated MSC were comparable to free MSC *in vitro* in decreasing macrophage secretion of TNF-α, a major pro-inflammatory cytokine,[14] suggesting that prolonged survival of MSC in capsules may modulate inflammation in a host for longer times than free MSC, which disappear rapidly. Encapsulation of MSC also upregulates the expression of many cytokines for extended times even without activation, and eMSC are anti-inflammatory and neuroprotective both *in vitro* and *in vivo* as shown here and previously.[8,14]

A typical response to injury involves an early pro-inflammatory activation of M1 macrophages followed by a transition to a later phase with increased levels of M2 anti-inflammatory macrophages that promote resolution and repair, but in severe injuries the M1 phase persists and the M2 response is suppressed.[31] Pro-inflammatory stimuli (e.g., LPS) activate macrophages into a pro-inflammatory M1 phenotype[26] and this activation has been detected as an increase in the percent of IB4+ macrophages.[24] IB4 binds robustly to both microglia indigenous to CNS tissue and macrophages that migrate into the CNS after injury.[32] This suggests that the reduction in IB4+ staining in SCI with eMSC treatment represents a decrease in M1 macrophages that is mediated by factors secreted by the MSC. Human eMSC also increased M2 macrophages in rat SCI,[14] which is consistent with increased levels of anti-inflammatory cytokines such as IL-10 in M1 activated macrophages *in vitro*[14] and in rat SCI (unpublished observations).

Effects of MSC in a wide range of animal models have been attributed primarily to their anti-inflammatory properties mediated by secreted cytokines and growth factors but it has not been possible to evaluate direct interactions with host cells *in vivo* because MSC migrate widely, are difficult to locate and survive only transiently. Very small fractions of intravenously injected MSC migrate to sites of injury and disease while most get trapped in organs including the lungs and liver. Their transient survival makes it difficult to analyze their relative contributions *in vivo* via secretion versus cell–cell interactions.[33] A comparison of different MSC delivery methods in the CNS indicated that intrathecal lumbar injection was superior to intraspinal or intravenous delivery.[34] However, the transient fate of MSC *in vivo* may require very large or repeated cell doses to be maximally effective. Even when MSC have been localized with intrinsic markers *in vivo*, it is difficult to prove their mechanism of action.[35] Given that encapsulation of cells excludes direct interactions with host cells, the effects of eMSC must be due to their secretion of relatively small proteins and factors that can diffuse into the host.[30]

Encapsulation is also advantageous because it allows MSC to survive longer and perhaps be effective at lower doses, to be localized *in vivo*, and to be retrieved from the host.[8,36] In rat SCI for example, a comprehensive review of MSC transplantation indicated that improved locomotion was observed with intravenous doses of 10^6 MSC and intraspinal doses of at least 250,000 cells.[16] We showed locomotor improvement with 30,000 MSC when they were encapsulated, suggesting that encapsulation may allow reduced MSC dosing for efficacy. Delayed injections of MSC indicated their benefit even four weeks after SCI,[35] suggesting that multiple doses may be required for maximal activity but this may be avoided using the longer lasting eMSC. Because CSF circulates only within the CNS, delivery of eMSC may be particularly effective by injection into CSF in brain ventricles[8] and the cauda equina.[14] Imaging demonstrated that alginate capsules with or without MSC remain for as long as 6 weeks in the CNS near their injection sites in the cauda equina and they can be retrieved from the host for analysis[8] (JHK, SK and MG unpublished observations).

MSC have only been approved for clinical therapy in graft versus host disease (GvHD),[37] which probably differs from other applications because MSC normally reside in the bone marrow where they can survive for extended periods and integrate into that niche. Numerous studies indicate that MSC are safe but in many cases they have modest and variable immunomodulatory effects in the CNS for a variety of reasons including some suggested above but their mechanisms of action *in vivo* are not yet clear.[15,16,38,39] Studies with eMSC have shown that protective effects of MSC can be enhanced by genetically overexpressing bioactive proteins, demonstrating the efficacy of proteins secreted from eMSC.[8,36] However, the use of other cells as vehicles to deliver proteins may be problematic because they elicit much greater immune responses around capsules than with MSC, which are hypoimmunogenic.[36]

Safety for alginates has been demonstrated in the clinic for several applications[40] and in a clinical trial (NCT01298830) using eMSC expressing GLP-1.[18] These capsules were generated using a recently described proprietary method (USP 8790705) with concentric needles that yield high cell densities in an inner capsule core surrounded by a cell-free outer alginate shell.[29] Capsules containing immortalized human MSC without or with transfection to express GLP-1 yielded improved outcome but their delivery adjacent to injury sites may have contributed to enlarge brain ventricles.[8] It will be interesting to determine whether intrathecal delivery of similar capsules with large numbers of low passage human MSC at a distance from the target site avoids the deleterious consequences that may result when eMSC are delivered close to injury sites.

Alginate encapsulates MSC sufficiently well so that many of the human cells survive for at least 2 weeks[18] to 2 months in a rat host while only a minute fraction of the human cells are detectable in the rat within 1 week without encapsulation (JHK, SK, MG, unpublished observations). Xenogenic transplantation of human cells in animals usually requires immunosuppression or the use of immunocompromised animals, which may complicate interpretation of results in injuries and disease with major inflammatory components such as SCI. Alginate encapsulation provides protection in xenogenic transplantation of human cells in animals and will be useful for preclinical testing of cells that secrete bioactive factors.

Besides these studies, little data are available on the use and optimization of encapsulated cells in the CNS. Our results underscore advantages of intrathecal injections of medium-sized capsules for the widely used MASCIS model for rat SCI that may also be applicable to other CNS disorders by minimally invasive lumbar injection. Based on many reports of MSC efficacy,[9,11,15,30,33,41] early intrathecal injections of eMSC may be effective in treating other acute CNS injuries including traumatic brain injury and stroke, and extended eMSC survival may be beneficial in chronic inflammatory disorders such as multiple sclerosis.[10] Feasibility for these applications will require proof of concept with eMSC in preclinical models, which often involve delivery through small bore needles in rodent models as described here. While larger microcapsules are useful for various applications, the results described here highlight potential problems with injection of large eMSC and underscore advantages of delivering smaller capsules by minimally invasive procedures that use narrow bore needles.

Acknowledgments

These studies were supported by the New Jersey Commission for Spinal Cord Injury 10-2947-SCR-R-0 and the New Jersey Commission for Brain Injury Research CBIR12IRG019. JB and AG were supported in part by a DHHS-PHS-NIH Biotechnology Training Grant T32GM008339. We thank Derek Adler (Molecular Imaging Center), Dr. Noriko Kane-Goldsmith, Nabgha Farhat, Justyna

Michalik and Sean O'Leary for technical assistance. Suneel Kumar and Joanne Babiarz contributed equally to this paper.

References

1. A. Acarregui, A. Murua, J. L. Pedraz, G. Orive and R. M. Hernandez, *Biodrugs* **26**, 283 (2012).
2. T. Visted, R. Bjerkvig and P. O. Enger, *Neuro-Oncology* **3**, 201 (2001).
3. T. Maguire, E. Novik, R. Schloss and M. Yarmush, *Biotechnol. Bioeng.* **93**, 581 (2006).
4. G. Orive, E. Santos, J. L. Pedraz and R. M. Hernandez, *Adv. Drug Deliv. Rev.* **67–68**, 3 (2014).
5. M. P. Zanin, L. N. Pettingill, A. R. Harvey, D. F. Emerich, C. G. Thanos and R. K. Shepherd, *J. Control. Release* **160**, 3 (2012).
6. A. Gilert and M. Machluf, *J. Angiogenesis Res.* **2**, 20 (2010).
7. C. A. Tobias *et al.*, *J. Neurotrauma* **22**, 138 (2005).
8. A. M. Heile, C. Wallrapp, P. M. Klinge, A. Samii, M. Kassem, G. Silverberg and T. Brinker, *Neurosci. Lett.* **463**, 176 (2009).
9. A. I. Caplan, *J. Pathol.* **217**, 318 (2009).
10. F. E. Figueroa, F. Carrion, S. Villanueva and M. Khoury, *Biol. Res.* **45**, 269 (2012).
11. S. Ma, N. Xie, W. Li, B. Yuan, Y. Shi and Y. Wang, *Cell Death Differ.* **21**, 216 (2014).
12. V. Mundra, I. C. Gerling and R. I. Mahato, *Mol. Pharm.* **10**, 77 (2013).
13. D. J. Prockop, *Stem Cells (Dayton, Ohio)* **31**, 2042 (2013).
14. J. Barminko, J. H. Kim, S. Otsuka, A. Gray, P. Mendpara, R. Schloss, M. Grumet and M. L. Yarmush, *Biotechnol. Bioeng.* **108**, 2747 (2011).
15. A. M. Parr, C. H. Tator and A. Keating, *Bone Marrow Transplant.* **40**, 609 (2007).
16. W. Tetzlaff *et al.*, *J. Neurotrauma* **28**, 1611 (2011).
17. J. K. Alexander and P. G. Popovich, *Prog. Brain Res.* **175**, 125 (2009).
18. A. Heile and T. Brinker, *Dialogues Clin. Neurosci.* **13**, 279 (2011).
19. T. Maguire, A. E. Davidovich, E. J. Wallenstein, E. Novik, N. Sharma, H. Pedersen, I. P. Androulakis, R. Schloss and M. Yarmush, *Biotechnol. Bioeng.* **98**, 631 (2007).
20. J. A. Barminko, N. I. Nativ, R. Schloss and M. L. Yarmush, *Biotechnol. Bioeng.* **111**, 2239 (2014).
21. K. Hasegawa, Y.-W. Chang, H. Li, Y. Berlin, O. Ikeda, Kane-Goldsmith and M. Grumet, *Exp. Neurol.* **193**, 394 (2005).
22. D. M. Basso, M. S. Beattie and J. C. Bresnahan, *Exp. Neurol.* **139**, 244 (1996).
23. M. L. McEwen and J. E. Springer, *J. Histochem. Cytochem.* **53**, 809 (2005).
24. D. R. Tabor, C. H. Larry and R. F. Jacobs, *J. Leukoc. Biol.* **45**, 452 (1989).
25. C. H. Lee *et al.*, *Brain Res.* **1342**, 138 (2010).

26. A. D. Gaudet, P. G. Popovich and M. S. Ramer, *J. Neuroinflammation* **8**, 110 (2011).
27. R. Krishnan, M. Alexander, L. Robles, C. E. Foster, 3rd and J. R. Lakey, *J. Soc. Biomed. Diabet. Res.* **11**, 84 (2014).
28. R. Robitaille, J. F. Pariseau, F. A. Leblond, M. Lamoureux, Y. Lepage and J. P. Halle, *J. Biomed. Mater. Res.* **44**, 116 (1999).
29. C. Wallrapp, E. Thoenes, F. Thurmer, A. Jork, M. Kassem and P. Geigle, *J. Microencapsul.* **30**, 315 (2013).
30. D. J. Prockop and J. Y. Oh, *Mol. Ther.* **20**, 14 (2012).
31. M. L. Novak and T. J. Koh, *J. Leukoc. Biol.* **93**, 875 (2013).
32. F. Dehghani, A. Conrad, A. Kohl, H. W. Korf and N. P. Hailer, *Exp. Neurol.* **189**, 241 (2004).
33. H. Yagi, A. Soto-Gutierrez, B. Parekkadan, Y. Kitagawa, R. G. Tompkins, N. Kobayashi and M. L. Yarmush, *Cell Transplant.* **19**, 667 (2010).
34. C. Paul, A. F. Samdani, R. R. Betz, I. Fischer and B. Neuhuber, *Spine* **34**, 328 (2009).
35. M. Osaka, O. Honmou, T. Murakami, T. Nonaka, K. Houkin, H. Hamada and J. D. Kocsis, *Brain Res.* **1343**, 226 (2010).
36. A. Goren, N. Dahan, E. Goren, L. Baruch and M. Machluf, *FASEB J.* **24**, 22 (2010).
37. J. Kurtzberg *et al.*, *Biol Blood Marrow Transplant.* **20**, 229 (2014).
38. D. Drago, C. Cossetti, N. Iraci, E. Gaude, G. Musco, A. Bachi and S. Pluchino, *Biochimie* **95**, 2271 (2013).
39. J. Yoo, H. S. Kim and D. Y. Hwang, *J. Cell Biochem.* **114**, 743 (2013).
40. T. Andersen, B. Strand, K. Formo, E. Alsberg and B. Christensen, *Carbohydr. Chem.* **37**, 227 (2012).
41. R. S. Oliveri, S. Bello and F. Biering-Sorensen, *Neurobiol. Dis.* **62**, 338 (2014).

https://doi.org/10.1142/9789819809028_0010

Chapter 10

Effect of the Organic Functionality on the Synthesis and Antimicrobial Activity of Silver Nanoparticles*

P. C. Pandey[†,||], Atul Kumar Tiwari[†], Munesh Kumar Gupta[‡], Govind Pandey[§] and Roger J Narayan[¶,**]

[†]*Department of Chemistry*
Indian Institute of Technology
Varanasi, UP 221005, India
[‡]*Department of Microbiology*
Institute of Medical Sciences
Banaras Hindu University, Varanasi, India
[§]*Department of Pediatrics*
King George Medical University
Lucknow 226003, India
[¶]*Department of Biomedical Engineering*
University of North Carolina
and North Carolina State University
North Carolina, USA
[||]*pcpandey.apc@iitbhu.ac.in*
[**]*roger_narayan@unc.edu*

In this paper, the effects of the organic reducing agent and 3-aminopropyltrimethoxysilane on the synthesis and properties of mono-, bi-, and trimetallic noble metal nanoparticles were considered; the antimicrobial activity of these nanomaterials was also evaluated. It was shown that 3-aminoptopyltrimethoxysilane-treated noble metal cations undergo rapid conversion into nanoparticles in the presence of three organic reducing agents, namely, 3-glycidoxypropyltrimethoxysilane (3-GPTMS), cyclohexanone and formaldehyde; the nanoparticles were formed on the order of one minute under microwave incubation. Bimetallic nanoparticles were formed

*To cite this article, please refer to its earlier version published in the *Nano LIFE*, Vol. 10, No. 3 (2020) 2050002 (15 pages), DOI: 10.1142/S1793984420500026

by simultaneous or sequential reduction of metal cations; the formation of trimetallic nanoparticles containing gold, silver and palladium was demonstrated using a similar approach. The nanoparticles were characterized using UV-Visible light spectrophotometry, transmission electron microscopy and zeta potential measurements. All three nanoparticles exhibited a size $\leq$10 nm size. The nanoparticles showed antimicrobial activity against *Acinetobacter baumannii.* Scanning electron microscopy imaging showed an alteration in the size and shape of nanoparticle-treated bacterium, with bleb formation and cell wall disruption observed within 1 h of incubation at the MBC values of the nanoparticles. Fluorescence spectrophotometric imaging of silver nanoparticle-*Acinetobacter baumannii* interactions suggested selective binding of silver nanoparticles to surface proteins. Our results showed the preparation of the novel silver nanoparticles with potent Anti-*Acinetobacter baumannii* activity, which can serve as an alternative to conventional antimicrobial agents.

Keywords: 3-aminopropyltrimethoxysilane; 3-glycidoxypropyltrimethylsilane; antimicrobial agents; silver nanoparticles; minimum inhibitory concentration; minimum bactericidal concentration; dose-dependent kill kinetics.

1. Introduction

The use of functional alkoxysilanes such as 3-aminopropyltrimethoxysilane (3-APTMS) and 3-glycidoxypropyltrimethoxysilane (3-GPTMS) as potential stabilizing and reducing reagents for the synthesis of noble metal nanoparticles, including gold, silver and palladium nanoparticles as well as multi-metallic nanoparticles, has been described.[1–4] 3-APTMS is a hydrophilic compound with micellar activity; 3-GPTMS is a hydrophobic compound that provides control over the dispersibility of as made noble metal nanoparticles. All the noble metal cations, including gold, silver and palladium cations, can be precisely converted into monometallic, bimetallic or trimetallic nanoparticles through the active role of these functional alkoxysilanes[2] under ambient conditions within 5–14 h. The process of nanoparticle synthesis may be facilitated through the use of an organic reducing agent such as cyclohexanone[1–3] or formaldehyde,[2] which enables the formation of nanoparticles within 30 minutes to 6 h. This approach provides control over the dispersibility of the noble metal nanoparticles in a variety of solvents. Since the alkoxysilanes and the organic reducing agent are active under microwave processing, the rate of nanoparticle synthesis may be accelerated by microwave processing of a reaction mixture containing noble metal cations or a mixture of noble metal cations. Noble metal nanoparticles and their bi-or tri-metallic analogs can be made within 15–40 s when the 3-APTMS capped noble metal cations undergo microwave processing in the presence of small organic reducing agents (e.g., cyclohexanone, formaldehyde and 3-GPTMS).

Over the past few decades, the use of nanotechnology-based solutions to counter antimicrobial resistance has been considered; for example, silver nanoparticles (Ag-NPs)[5,6] offer a viable alternative to treat infections caused by multidrug-resistant (MDR) microorganisms[7,8] due to their broad-spectrum and potent antimicrobial properties.[9] Silver is considered[10] to be a Lewis acid, which has a tendency to react with a Lewis base, including phosphorous- and sulfur-containing biomolecules that belong to the cell membrane, proteins and DNA bases.[11–13] Ag-NPs initially accumulate on the cell wall and/or cell membrane, resulting in morphological changes such as shrinkage of the cytoplasm, membrane detachment, numerous electron-dense pits, and final disruption of the membrane.[13] In this study, the activity of three types of Ag-NPs, which were made using 3-GPTMS, cyclohexanone and formaldehyde, against multi-drug resistant *Acinetobacter baumannii* was investigated. Protein–nanoparticle interactions were evaluated using fluorescence imaging.[14–16] The antimicrobial activity of theAG-NPs against multi-drug resistant *Acinetobacter baumannii* was evaluated using 2D and 3D fluorescence spectroscopy.

2. Materials and methods

2.1. *Materials*

3-aminopropyltrimethoxysilane (3-APTMS), 3-glycidoxypropyltrimethoxysilane (3-GPTMS) chloroauric acid ($HAuCl_4$), bovine serum albumin (BSA) and silver nitrate ($AgNO_3$) were obtained from Aldrich Chemical Co. (Bengaluru, India). Bacterial culture media such as Muller–Hinton Broth (MHB), Muller–Hinton Agar (MHA), Nutrient Agar (NA) and Nutrient Broth (NB) were purchased from Hi-Media Laboratories Ltd. (Mumbai, India). Plastic wares were purchased from Tarsons Product Pvt. Ltd. (Kolkata, India). The antibiotics and other routine chemicals were purchased from Sigma Aldrich Inc. (St. Louis, MO, USA). The organic solvents used were obtained from Merck Millipore (Merck Life Science Private Limited, India). All of the reagents were of analytical grade.

2.2. *Bacterial strain*

We isolated one strain of *Acinetobacter baumannii* from the endotracheal tube secretions of one intensive care unit (ICU)-admitted male patient who had developed ventilator-associated pneumonia. This strain was identified based on the culture characteristics on MacConkey agar and blood agar, Gram staining, as well as biochemical tests such as catalase, oxidase, sugar fermentation and citrate utilization test. On antibiotic susceptibility testing, this strain was only sensitive to polymyxin B; it showed resistance to the other tested antibiotics, including amoxicillin–clavulanic acid, ceftazidime, gentamycin, amikacin, ciprofloxacin, levofloxacin, ampicillin–sulbactam, piperacillin–tazobactam and the carbapenem group of antibiotics.

2.3. *Synthesis of alkoxysilane functionalized noble metal (mono-, bi- and tri-metallic) nanoparticles*

The noble metal mono-, bi- and tri-metallic nanoparticles were made from 3-APTMS capped silver, gold and palladium cations in the presence of three different organic reducing agents, specifically (i) cyclohexanone, (ii) 3-GPTMS and (iii) formaldehyde.

2.4. *3-APTMS and cyclohexanone-mediated synthesis of Ag-NP-1 nanoparticles*

Ethylene glycol di-acetate (120 μL) and a methanolic solution of 1-vinyl 2-pyrrolidone (540 mM, 100 μL) were placed in a 2 mL glass vial, followed by the addition of a methanolic solution of $AgNO_3$ (10 mM, 10 μL), 3-APTMS (150 μL) of the desired concentration

(0.5–5 M) and cyclohexanone (20 μL). The reaction mixture was thoroughly mixed on a vertex mixture for 30 s and processed in a microwave for 15 s. The microwave processing cycle was repeated 3–5 times, resulting in the appearance of a deep yellow color that indicated the formation Ag-NP-1.

2.5. *3-APTMS and 3-GPTMS-mediated synthesis of Ag-NP-2 nanoparticles*

Ethylene glycol di-acetate (120 μL) and a methanolic solution of 1-vinyl 2-pyrrolidone (540 mM, 100 μL) were placed in 2 mL glass vial, followed by the addition of a methanolic solution of $AgNO_3$ (10 mM, 10 μL), 3-APTMS (150 μL) and 3-GPTMS (2 M, 350 μL). The reaction mixture was thoroughly mixed on a vertex mixture for 30 s and processed in a microwave for 15 s. The microwave processing cycle was repeated 5–8 times, resulting in the appearance of a deep yellow color that indicated the formation of Ag-NP-2.

2.6. *3-APTMS and formaldehyde-mediated synthesis of Ag-NP-3 nanoparticles*

Ethylene glycol di-acetate (120 μL) and a methanolic solution of 1-vinyl 2-pyrrolidone (540 mM, 100 μL) were placed in 2 mL glass vial, followed by the addition of a methanolic solution of $AgNO_3$ (10 mM, 10 μL), 3-APTMS (150 μL), and formaldehyde (12 μL). The reaction mixture was thoroughly mixed on a vertex mixture for 30 s and processed in a microwave for 15 s. The microwave processing cycle was repeated 2–3 times, resulting in the appearance of a deep brown color that indicated the formation of Ag-NP-3.

2.7. *3-APTMS and cyclohexanone-mediated synthesis of Au-NP-1 nanoparticles*

Ethylene glycol di-acetate (100 μL) and a methanolic solution of $HAuCl_4$ (25 mM; 100 μL) were placed in 2 mL glass vial, followed by the addition of a methanolic solution of 3-APTMS (150 μL) and cyclohexanone (200 μL). The reaction mixture was thoroughly mixed on a vertex mixture for 30 s and processed in the microwave for 15 s.

The cycle was repeated 2–3 times in a microwave, resulting in the appearance of a deep pink color that indicated the formation of Au-NP-1.

2.8. *3-APTMS and 3-GPTMS-mediated synthesis of Au-NP-2 nanoparticles*

Ethylene glycol di-acetate (120 μL) and methanolic solution of $HAuCl_4$ (25 mM, 100 μL) were placed in 2 mL glass vial. A methanolic solution of 3-APTMS (150 μL) and 3-GPTMS (100 μL) were added to this mixture. The reaction mixture was thoroughly mixed on a vertex mixture for 30 s, and processed in a microwave for 15 s. The cycle was repeated 3–5 times in the microwave. The mixture showed a deep pink color, indicating the formation of Au-NP-2.

2.9. *3-APTMS and cyclohexanone-mediated sequential synthesis of Ag–Au–NP1 bimetallic nanoparticles*

Silver nanoparticles were synthesized as described above and diluted eight-folds in methanol. 100 μl of diluted Ag-NPs were mixed with a methanolic suspension of $HAuCl_4$ (100 μl, 25 mM), followed by the addition of cyclohexanone (200 μL), vortex mixing for 30 s, and processed in a microwave for 15 s. The microwave processing cycle was repeated 3–4 times.

2.10. *3-APTMS and 3-GPTMS-mediated simultaneous synthesis of Ag–Au–NP2 bimetallic nanoparticles*

Ethylene glycol di-acetate (120 μL) and a methanolic solution of 1-vinyl 2-pyrrolidone (540 mM, 100 μL) were placed in 2 mL glass vial, followed by the addition of a methanolic solution of $AgNO_3$ (10 mM, 10 μl) and $HAuCl_4$ (25 mM, 100 μl), 3-APTMS (150 μl) and 3-GPTMS (2 M, 350 μl). The reaction mixture was thoroughly mixed on a vertex mixture for 30 s and placed in a microwave for 15 s. The microwave processing cycle was repeated 5–8 times, resulting in the appearance of a deep reddish color that indicated the formation of Ag–Au bimetallic nanoparticles.

2.11. 3-APTMS and cyclohexanone sequential synthesis of Pd–NP and Pd–Ag bimetallic nanoparticles

120 μl of ethylene glycol di-acetate was placed in a vial. A methanolic solution of $PdCl_2$ (50 μl, 10 mM) was added; the mixture was mixed in a cyclomixer for 30 s. 3-APTMS (100 μl) was added to the mixture and mixed, followed by the addition of formaldehyde (50 μl). The reaction mixture was processed in a microwave for 60 s (4 cycles of 15 s). The appearance of a black color was associated with the formation of Pd nanoparticles. A five-folds dilution of Pd nanoparticles (200 μL) was placed in a vial, followed by the addition of $AgNO_3$ (10 mM, 10 μL); the mixture was mixed in a cyclomixer for 30 s. 20 μL of cyclohexanone was added to the mixture and vortexed. The reaction mixture was processed in a microwave, which was operated for 3–4 cycles of 15 s.

2.12. Sequential synthesis of Pd–Ag–Au trimetallic nanoparticles

Pre-synthesized Pd–Ag bi-metallic NPs were diluted 10-fold in methanol. After dilution, 100 μL of diluted NPs were dispensed in a vial, followed by the addition of a methanolic solution of $HAuCl_4$ (25 mM, 100 μL). Cyclohexanone was then added (200 μL); the reaction mixture was subsequently processed in a microwave for 15 s (4–5 cycles).

2.13. Characterization of functionalized Ag-NPs

The mono, bi- and tri-metallic nanoparticles were characterized using a U-2900 UV-vis spectrometer (Hitachi, Tokyo, Japan) over the scan range from 250 to 800 nm. Transmission electron microscopy analysis and selected area electron diffraction (SAED) were performed using a Techni G2 20 Twin instrument (FEI, Hillsboro, Oregon) at the IIT (BHU) Central Instrumentation Facility (CIF). Samples were made by diluting the nanoparticles in methanol and drop-casting the solution on a carbon-coated copper grid of 300 mesh. Zeta potential analysis was performed in a Zetasizer instrument (Malvern Panalytical, Malvern, United Kingdom). Scanning electron microscopy imaging was performed using an EVO instrument (Carl Zeiss Microscopy GmbH, Jena, Germany) in the CIF.

2.14. *Assessment of antibacterial activity*

The activity of the nanoparticles against *A. baumannii* was assessed using the agar well diffusion method. The MIC and MBC values of the nanoparticles were assessed using a two-fold serial dilution method. The MIC value was determined as the minimum concentration at which no turbidity was observed. The MBC value was determined as the minimum concentration at which no bacterial growth was observed on an MHA plate.

2.15. *Assessment by agar well diffusion method*

Ag-NP-1, Ag-NP-2 and Ag-NP-3 were assessed for antibacterial activity as described previously.[17,18] An overnight grown culture of *A. baumannii* in Muller–Hinton broth (MHB) medium was centrifuged; the pellet was inoculated in freshly prepared sterilized MHB medium and incubated for 4 h at 37°C. After incubation, a 0.5 MacFarland standard[19] of the bacterial strain containing 0.5×10^8 cfu/mL was prepared. A sterilized cotton swab was used for spreading these cells on freshly prepared MHA plates; the plates were kept undisturbed for 10 min under laminar flow. The wide mouth of sterilized 200 μl micropipette tips were used to make wells on the swabbed plates. All three synthesized nanoparticles were diluted two-fold in 1% DMSO; 20 μl of each nanoparticle was poured in the preformed wells. The same volume of respective test controls (without Ag-NP-1, Ag-NP-2 or Ag-NP-3) was poured in predetermined wells; polymyxin B sulphate and 4% DMSO were also poured in corresponding wells as positive and negative controls, respectively. After pouring of Ag-NP-1, Ag-NP-2, Ag-NP-3, and control samples, plates were kept undisturbed for 15 min under aseptic conditions under laminar flow for uniform spherical diffusion of the Ag-NPs and controls. The assay plates were incubated at 37 °C in an incubator for 24 h and observed for any zone of inhibition. All of the experiments were optimized and executed in triplicate; the mean zone of inhibition was recorded.

2.16. *Minimum inhibitory concentration and minimum bactericidal concentration*

The minimum inhibitory concentration (MIC) and minimum bactericidal concentration (MBC) of the nanoparticles against *A. baumannii* were determined by using the broth microdilution method in a flat bottom, sterile, 96 well microtiter plate as described previously.[20–22] In short, an overnight grown culture of *A. baumannii* in MHB medium was centrifuged; the pellet was resuspended in fresh MHB medium for 4 h to achieve log phase growth at 37°C. A 0.5 MacFarland bacterial suspension containing 0.5×10^8 cells/mL was then prepared. A working suspension of 112 μg/mL of Ag-NP-1, Ag-NP-2 and Ag-NP-3 was prepared in 4% DMSO; 100 μl of the suspension was placed in each well in a double dilution concentration ranging from 0.43 to 112 μg/ml. 100 μL of 0.5 MacFarland bacterial suspension was then added in each well. Test control (without Ag-NP), one bacterial control (without treatment), positive control with polymyxin B, and negative control with only media solution were evaluated. The microtiter plate was incubated at 37°C for 24 h and observed visually for complete inhibition (a visually clear well), which was taken as the minimum inhibitory concentration (MIC). Subsequently, a 5 μl of suspension from each well was inoculated on the MHA plates and observed for the growth. The minimum bactericidal concentration (MBC) was determined as the concentration at which no growth was observed after 24 h of incubation.

2.17. *Time kill assay*

The time kill assay was performed as described previously[23–25]; an overnight grown culture of *A. baumannii* in MHB was centrifuged. The pellet was suspended in MHB medium for 4 h at 37 °C to achieve log phase of growth. 100 μl of Ag-NP-1, Ag-NP-2 and Ag-NP-3 at the

MBC level and control were dispensed in a 96 well, flat bottom, sterile, polystyrene microtiter plate. Subsequently, 100 μl of 0.5 MacFarland standard of the *A. baumannii* suspension was poured into each nanoparticle solution and incubated at 37°C in a shaker incubator. 5 μl of culture from each test well were spread on MHA plates at different time intervals (0, 1, 2, 4, 6, 8, 12 and 24 h) and incubated overnight at 37°C to determine the surviving bacterial count values.

2.18. *Dose-dependent kill kinetic analysis*

A time kill assay, which involved understanding the effects of Ag-NP-1, Ag-NP-2 and Ag-NP-3 from 1.75 to 56 μg/mL on *A. baumannii*, was conducted. Data was collected 6 h after exposure of *A. baumannii* to Ag-NP-1, Ag-NP-2 and Ag-NP-3. 5 μl of the suspension was spread over the MHA plate, and the surviving cells were counted; the killing percentage was calculated using the following formula [26]:

$$\text{Percent cell reduction} = \frac{(A - B) \times 100}{A}$$

In this equation, A is the number of viable cells before treatment, and B is the number of viable cells after treatment. The dose-dependent kill curve graph was plotted using GraphPad Prism version 8.2.1 software.

2.19. *Scanning electron microscopy*

An overnight grown culture was reinoculated in fresh MHB medium for 4 h to achieve log phase of culture; the log phase culture was adjusted to 10^8 cfu/mL in fresh MHB medium and treated with each nanoparticle type for 1 h at 37°C in a shaker incubator. The cells were then harvested using centrifugation at 3500 rpm for 8 min; the pellet was resuspended in 0.1 M phosphate buffer (pH = 7), followed by centrifugation. The pellet was suspended in 2.5% glutaraldehyde solution for 30 min and again centrifuged; the pellet was washed with phosphate buffer followed by centrifugation. The washed pellet was resuspended in 1% OsO_4 in phosphate buffer for 45 min and washed with phosphate buffer; the cells were dehydrated with 35%, 50%, 75%, 95%, 99% ethanol each for 15 min. The dehydrated cells were dried in vacuum desiccator overnight and coated with gold prior to scanning electron microscopy imaging.

2.20. *Fluorescence imaging*

2D fluorescence spectra and 3D fluorescence imaging of log phase *A. baumannii* cells (10^4 cfu/mL) grown in nutrient broth and treated with nanoparticles were studied in ultra-pure sterilized water under at 37°C for 15 min in a 7000 fluorescence spectrophotometer (Hitachi, Tokyo, Japan) with excitation and emission matrix at 280 nm and 300 nm, respectively; a scan range of 300–500 nm was used in this study. Bovine serum albumin was chosen as standard protein to understand the process of nanoparticle-protein interaction; 2D and 3D fluorescence spectra of bovine serum albumin in the absence and in the presence of Ag–NP-1 nanoparticles were recorded.[16]

3. Results and discussion

3.1. *3-APTMS-mediated rapid synthesis of noble metal mono-metallic, bimetallic and trimetallic nanoparticles*

3-aminopropyltrimethoxysilane acts as a Lewis acid to facilitate interactions with metal cations and serves as potential stabilizer for many metal nanoparticles. 3-aminopropyltrimethoxysilane-treated metal cations initiate opening of the epoxide ring of 3-GPTMS, forming a covalent linkage with the nitrogen of the organoamine linked to trialkoxysilane; this approach results in reduction and stabilization of the noble metal cations and enables the synthesis of noble metal nanoparticles. This reaction scheme not only allows control over the reduction process of noble metal cations, but also enables various combinations of bimetallic and trimetallic noble metal nanoparticles to be produced. In addition, the ratio of organoamine-trialkoxysilane- and glycidyl-linked trialkoxysilane controls the dispersibility in desired polar and nonpolar solvents. The process of nanoparticles synthesis may also be controlled in the presence of organic aldehydes and ketones. We previously demonstrated that 3-APTMS treated noble metal cations can be converted into monometallic, bimetallic and trimetallic nanoparticles;[1–4,27,28] however, the time course for the formation of the nanoparticles is on the order of 1–8 h as a function of the type of organic reducing agent (e.g., 3-GPTMS, cyclohexanone or formaldehyde). Since the alkoxysilanes and the organic reducing agent are active under microwave processing, we sought to understand the role of microwave processing for functional alkoxysilane-assisted synthesis of nanoparticles. Interestingly, the time required for the conversion of noble metal cations into nanoparticles was reduced to the order of 15–45 s under microwave processing in the presence of an organic reducing agent (e.g., 3-GPTMS, cyclohexanone, or formaldehyde). The formation of monometallic gold nanoparticles, palladium nanoparticles, Ag–Au, Au–Pd bimetallic nanoparticles, and Ag–Au–Pd trimetallic nanoparticles was demonstrated. Figure 1 shows the formation of monometallic gold nanoparticles within less than 1 min in the presence of 3-APTMS with cyclohexanone [Fig. 1(A) (i)–(iii)] and 3-APTMS with 3-GPTMS [Fig. 1(B) (i)–(iii)]. The maximum absorbance between 519–530 nm indicate the formation of gold nanoparticles within less than 1 min was demonstrated [Fig. 1(i)]. The average size of gold nanoparticles was found to be < 10 nm in each case. It is noteworthy that an optimum concentration of 3-APTMS with an organic reagent like cyclohexanone and 3-GPTMS allowed the maximum conversion of metal cations into respective nanoparticles.

This process also enables the formation of silver-gold bimetallic nanoparticles under similar conditions. Figure 2(A) (i)–(iii) shows the characterization data from Ag-Au-NP1 bimetallic nanoparticles made by reduction of 3-APTMS treated noble metal cations in a sequential mode. Figure 2(B) (i)–(iii) shows characterization data from Ag-Au-NP2 bimetallic nanoparticles made 3-APTMS and 3-GPTMS-mediated simultaneous synthesis. The formation of bimetallic nanoparticles was also recorded within less than one minute. In addition, this process enables the formation of Pd-Ag-AuNP trimetallic nanoparticles under similar conditions. Initially, Pd-NPs were made from 3-APTMS treated palladium cations in the presence of

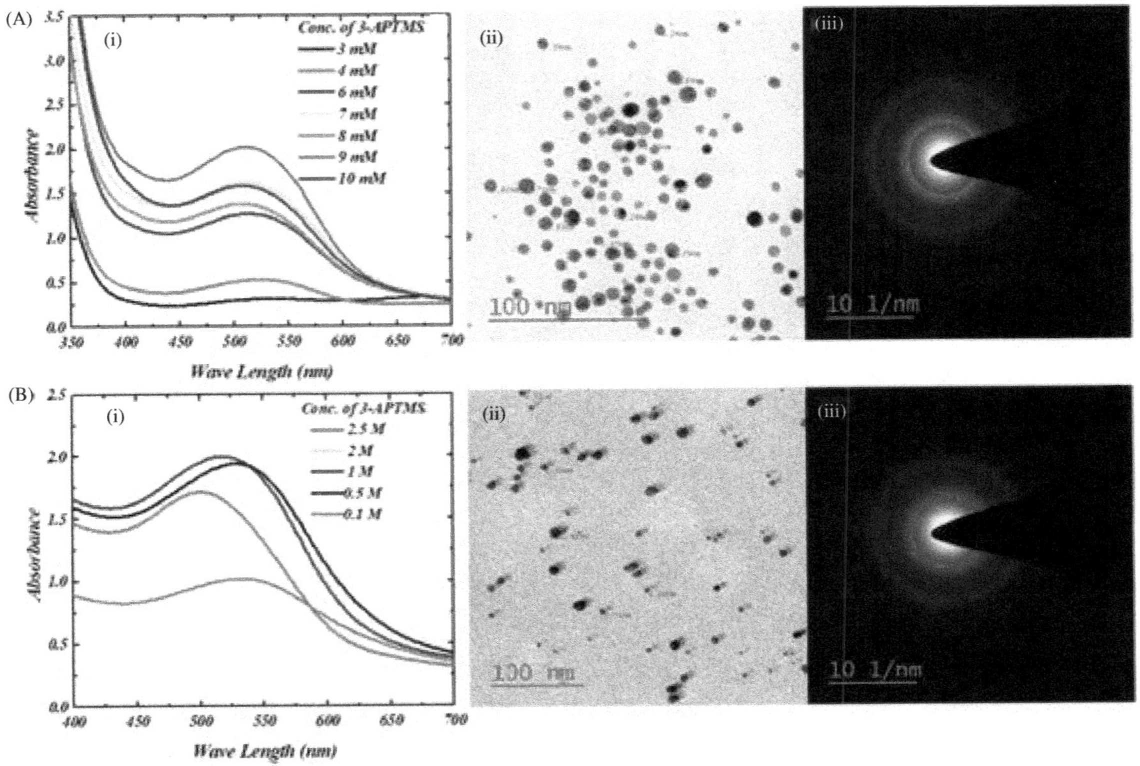

Fig. 1. (A) Characterization of Au-NP-1 nanoparticles by UV-Visible light spectrophotometry (i) transmission electron microscopy imaging (ii) and selected area electron diffraction pattern (iii). (B) Characterization of synthesized Au-NP-2 nanoparticles by UV-Visible light spectrophotometry (i) TEM imaging (ii) and selected area electron diffraction pattern (iii).

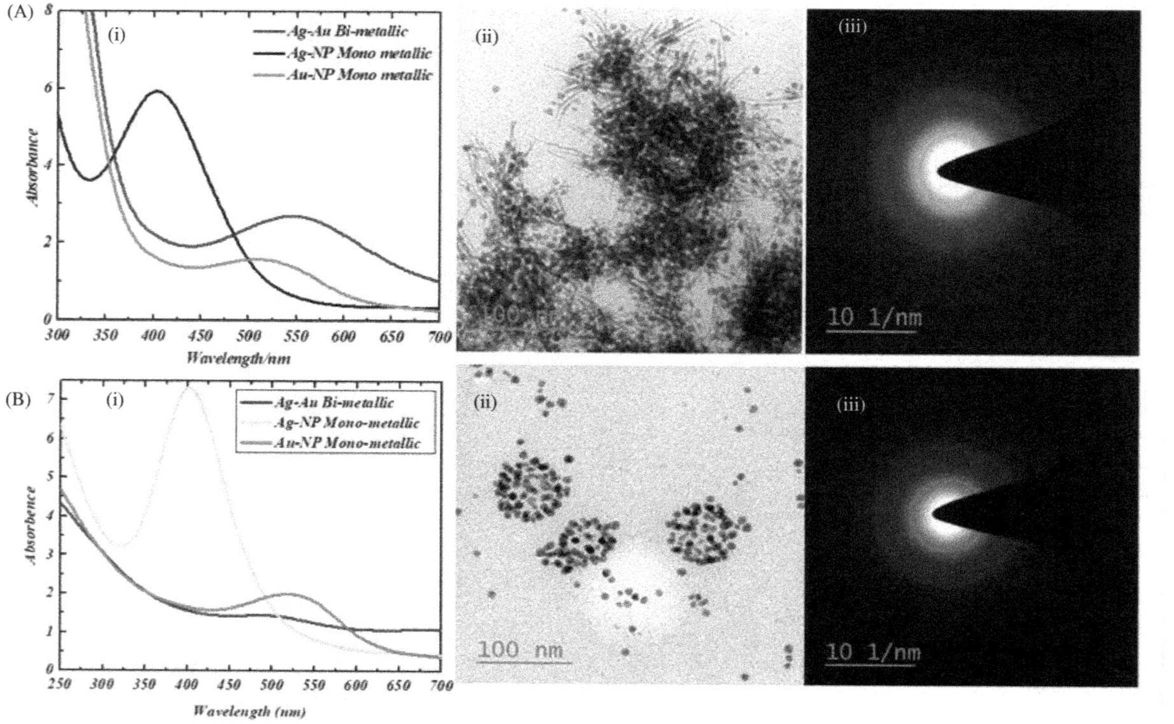

Fig. 2. (A) Characterization of Ag-Au-NP1 nanoparticles by UV-Visible light spectrophotometry (i) transmission electron microscopy imaging (ii) and selected area electron diffraction pattern (iii). (B) Characterization of synthesized Ag-Au-NP2 nanoparticles by UV-visible light spectrophotometry (i) TEM imaging (ii) and selected area electron diffraction pattern (iii).

formaldehyde under microwave processing for 1 minute. The Pd-Ag bimetallic nanoparticles as shown in Fig. 3 were made via a sequential mode of silver cation reduction in the presence of as made Pd-NPs (Fig. 3(A) (i)–(iii)) within less than 1 minute under microwave processing. As made bimetallic Pd-Ag nanoparticles were allowed to form Pd-Ag-Au nanoparticles by adding gold cations in the presence of cyclohexanone under similar conditions that were used for the formation of bimetallic nanoparticles. The results as shown in Fig. 3(B) (i)–(iii) justify the rapid formation of trimetallic nanoparticles and reveal the potential advantage of functional alkoxysilanes in the synthesis of noble metal nanoparticles and their multi-metallic analogs.

3.2. *Antimicrobial activity of noble metal nanoparticles and their multi-metallic analogs*

We attempted to understand the antimicrobial activity of the as made nanoparticles against *A. baumannii*. The results are shown in Fig. 4 for Au-NPs [Fig. 4(i)], Pd-Ag-NPs [Fig. 4(ii)], Ag-Au-NPs [Fig. 4(iii)] and Pd-Ag-Au-NPs [Fig. 4(iv)]. The zone of inhibition data under similar conditions for the nanoparticles is shown in Fig. 4(v). The results indicate that the AuNPs, bimetallic nanoparticles, and trimetallic nanoparticles do not possess significant antibacterial activity; on the other hand, the Pd-NP and Ag-NPs showed antimicrobial activity [Fig. 4(v)]. Since the Ag-NPs showed potent antimicrobial activity, a detailed investigation of the antimicrobial activity of these particles was performed.

3.3. *3-APTMS-mediated synthesis of silver nanoparticles as a function of organic reducing agents*

Figure 5(A) (i) shows the UV-visible light spectra recorded from Ag-NP-1, Fig. 5(A) (ii) shows the UV-visible light spectra recorded from Ag-NP-2 and Ag-NP-3 shows the UV-visible light spectra recorded from Ag-NP-3. An absorption maximum around 405 nm has been recorded for all these threeAg-NPs. The TEM and SAED pattern analysis as shown in Fig. 5(B) of Ag-NP-1 [(i) and (iv)], Ag–NP-2 [(ii)

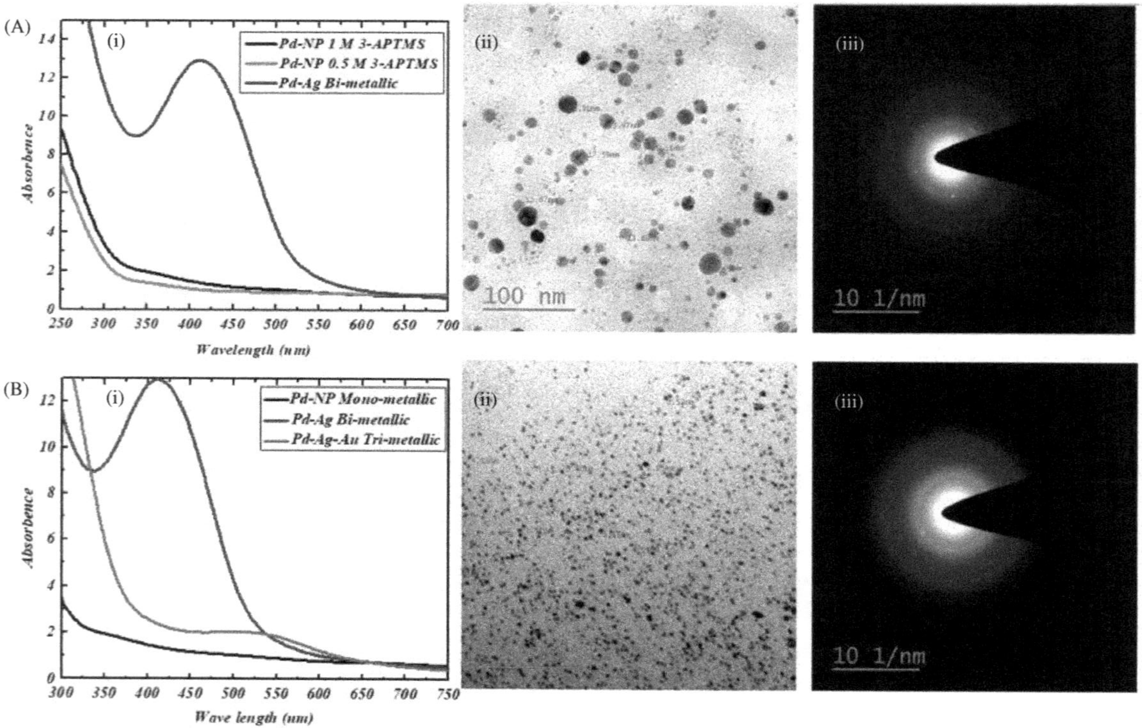

Fig. 3. (A) Characterization of Pd–Ag bimetallic nanoparticles by UV-visible light spectrophotometry (i), transmission electron microscopy imaging (ii), and selected area electron diffraction pattern (iii). (B) Characterization of synthesized Pd-Ag-Au trimetallic nanoparticles by UV-visible light spectrophotometry (i) TEM imaging (ii) and selected area electron diffraction pattern (iii).

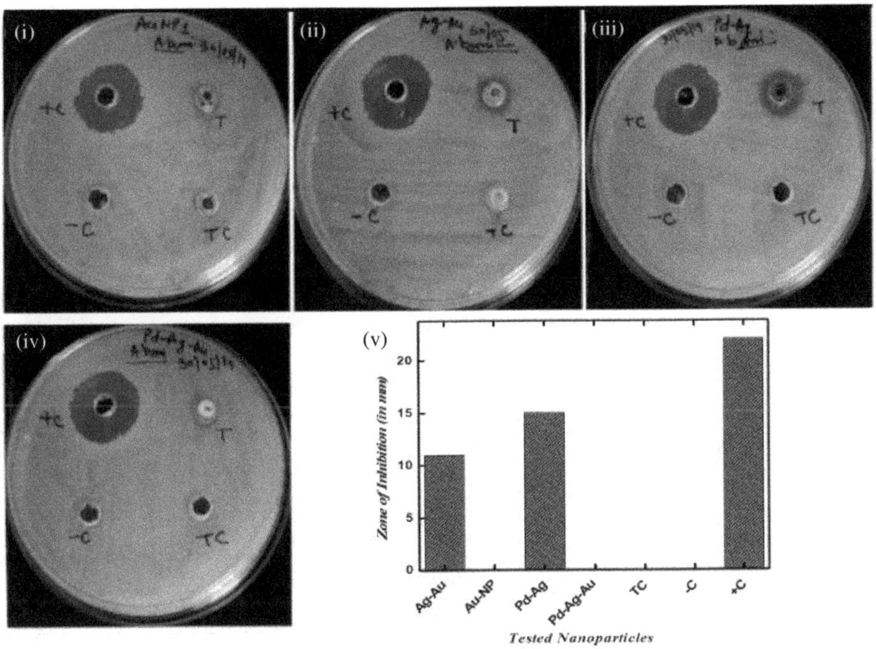

Fig. 4. Antibacterial assessment plates of mono-, bi- and tri-metallic nanoparticles against *A. baumannii* by the agar well diffusion method.

and (v)] and Ag–NP-3 [(iii) and (vi)]; the average size of the Ag-NP-1, Ag-NP-2 and AgNP-3 were 9.42, 8.77 and 7.42 nm, respectively. Zeta potential data [Fig. 5(C)] showed values around 25 mV for Ag-NP-3 [Fig. 5(C) (iii)], indicating higher stability than Ag-NP-1 and Ag-NP-2 [Fig. 5(C) (i) and (ii)].

3.4. *Antimicrobial activity of Ag-NP-1, Ag-NP-2 and Ag-NP-3 against A. baumannii*

3.4.1. *Agar well diffusion assay*

24 h incubated assay plates were visually examined for the zone of inhibition (ZOI) (Fig. 7). The assay was performed in triplicate; each ZOI was measured using the zone measurement scale (HiMedia, Mumbai, India). All threeAg-NPs showed a zone of inhibition; the test control (without silver cation) and negative

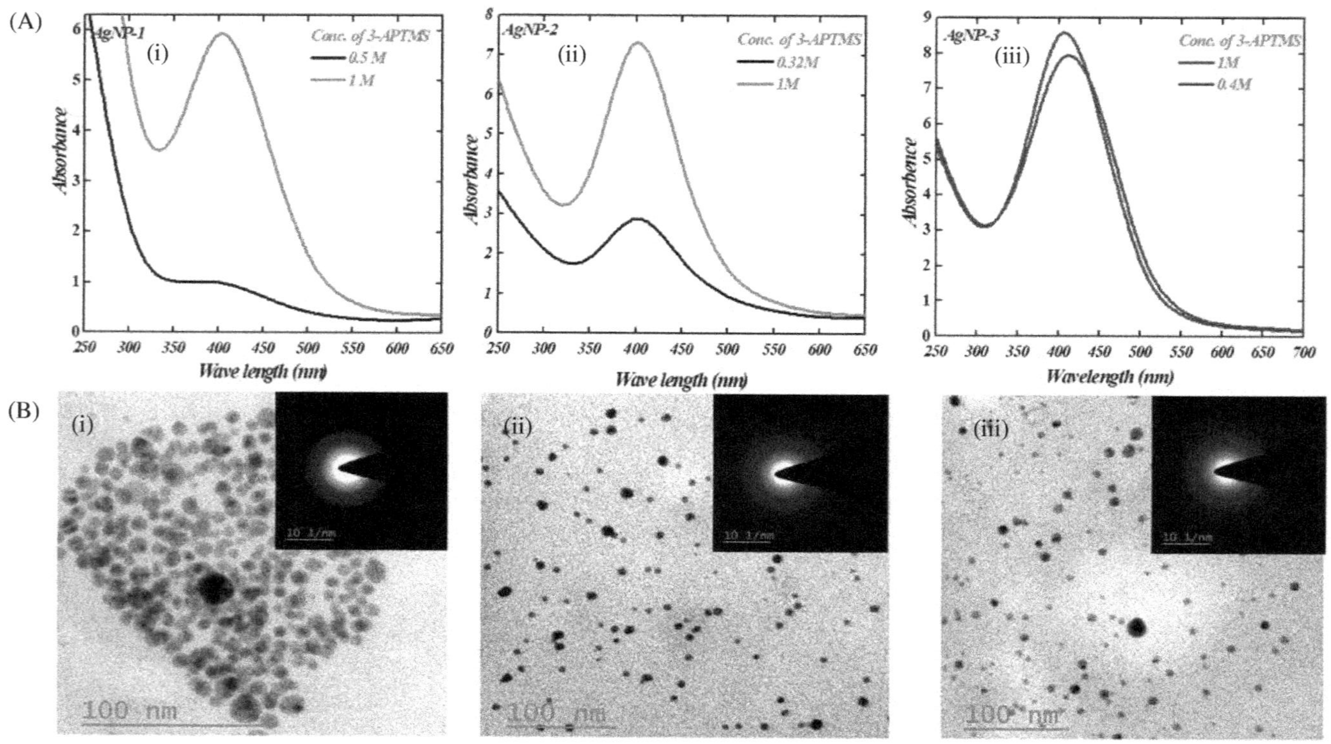

Fig. 5. (A) UV-Visible light spectrophotometry of Ag-NP-1 (i), Ag-NP-2 (ii) and Ag-NP-3 (iii). (B) Transmission electron microscopy images, selected area diffraction pattern (inset), and size distribution plots of Ag-NP-1 (i and iv), Ag-NP-2 (ii and v), and Ag-NP-3 (iii and vi). (C) Zeta potential analysis of Ag-NP-1 (i), Ag-NP-2 (ii), and Ag-NP-3 (iii).

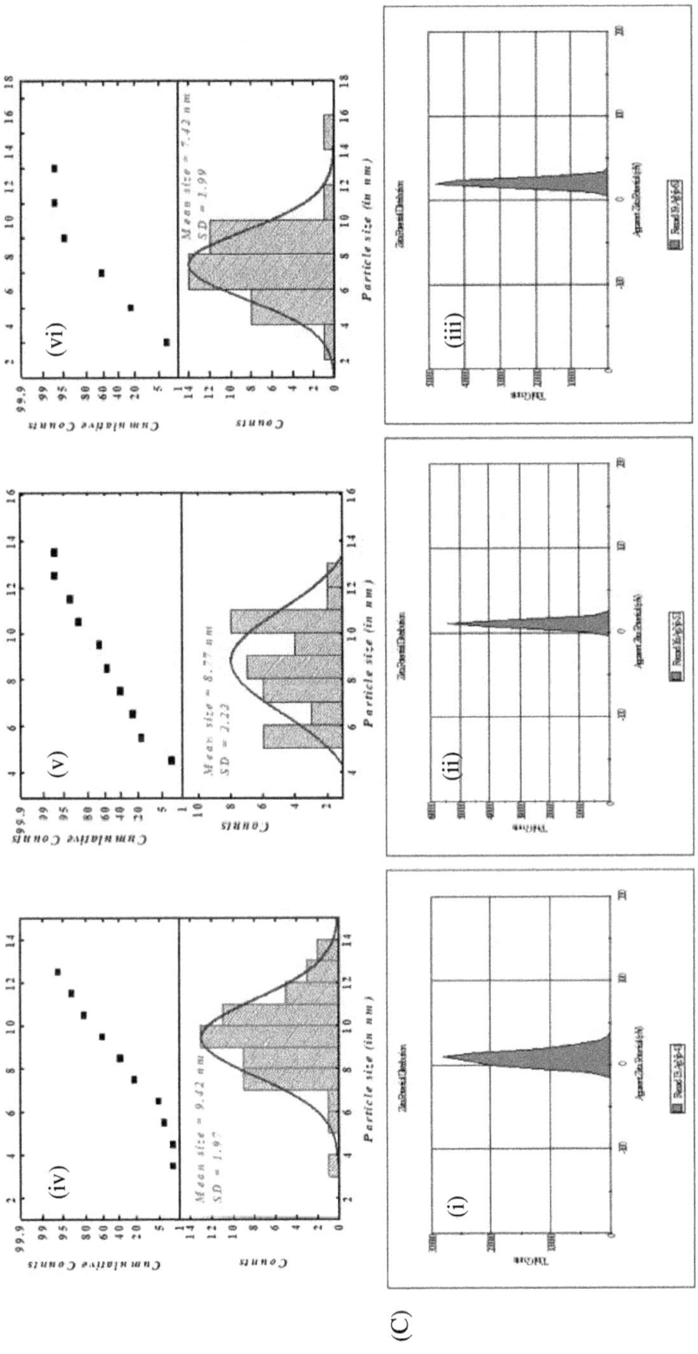

Fig. 5. (*Continued*)

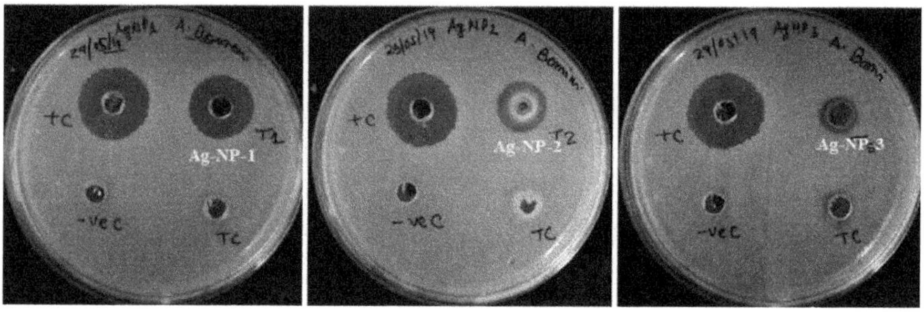

Fig. 6. Antibacterial assessment plates of Ag-NP-1, Ag-NP-2, and Ag-NP-3 nanoparticles against *A. baumannii* by the agar well diffusion method.

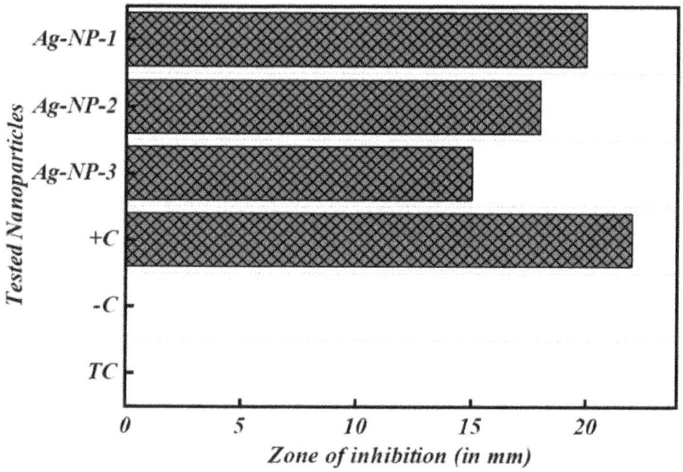

Fig. 7. Mean zone of inhibition diameter of each type of nanoparticle against *A. baumannii* planktonic cells. +C represents positive control, −C represents negative control, and TC represents test control.

control (4% DMSO) did not show any ZOI (Fig. 6). Among the three types ofAg-NPs, Ag-NP-1 and Ag-NP-2 showed more potent antibacterial activity than Ag-NP-3.

3.4.2. *MIC and MBC determination*

The MIC and MBC of each silver nanoparticle was determined by the broth microdilution method in a flat bottom, sterile microtiter

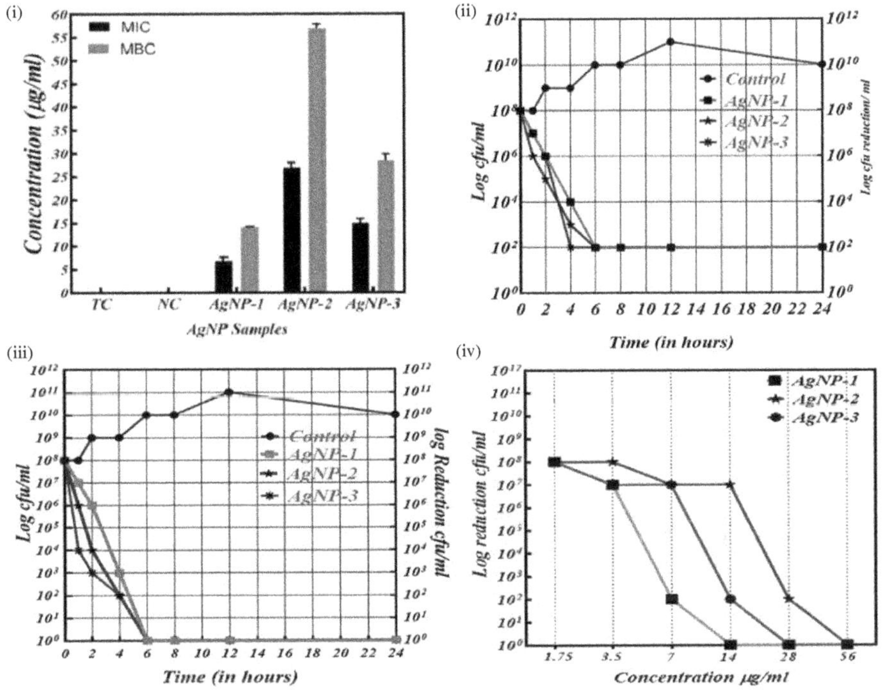

Fig. 8. (i) MIC (μg/mL) and MBC (μg/mL) values of Ag-NP-1, Ag-NP-2, and Ag-NP-3 against A. *baumannii* planktonic cells. TC represents Test control and NC represents negative control. (ii) Time kill curve of *A. baumannii* with 1x MIC concentration of each nanoparticle type at 37°C under aerobic conditions. Control is represented as untreated cells. (iii) Time kill curve of *A. baumannii*with 1x MBC concentration of each nanoparticle type at 37°C in under aerobic conditions. Control is represented as untreated cells. (iv) The dose-dependent kill curve at different concentration of Ag-NP-1, Ag-NP-2, and Ag-NP-3 against *A. baumannii* after six hours of treatment at 37°C under aerobic conditions; log reduction cfu/mL represents the log value of cfu/mL killed at their corresponding concentration (iv).

plates. The MIC of Ag-NP-1, Ag-NP-2 and Ag-NP-3 against *A. baumannii* were 7, 28 and 14 μg/mL, respectively. The MBC of Ag-NP-1, Ag-NP-2 and Ag-NP-3 against *A. baumannii* were 14, 56 and 28 μg/mL, respectively [Fig. 8(i)]. As shown in Fig 6, the agar well diffusion assay indicated that Ag-NP-3 had the lowest ZOI diameter among all of the assessed nanoparticles; however, MIC and MBC of Ag-NP-3 were lower than those of Ag-NP-2.

3.4.3. *Time kill assay*

A time kill assay for Ag-NP-1, Ag-NP-2 and Ag-NP-3 was performed at the MIC and MBC levels for these nanoparticles against *A. baumannii*. 5 μL of a Sbacterial suspension containing the MBC value of each type of silver nanoparticle (14 μg/mL of Ag-NP-1, 56 μg/mL of Ag-NP-2, or 28 μg/mL of Ag-NP-3) were sub-cultured on MHA plates over a duration of 0, 1, 2, 4, 6, 8, 12 and 24 h; no bacterial growth was observed after 6 h of incubation. A four-log reduction was observed [Fig. 8 (iii)] earlier with Ag-NP-3, followed by Ag-NP-2 and Ag-NP-1. Similarly, a time kill assay at the MIC value of each type of silver nanoparticles performed [Fig. 8 (ii)]. A two-log reduction was observed earlier with Ag-NP-3 than with the two other nanoparticles; a final two-log cells remained viable in the suspension at 4 h with Ag-NP-3, 6 h with Ag-NP-2 and 8 h with Ag-NP-1, which persisted even after 24 h.

3.4.4. *Dose-dependent kill kinetics*

Dose-dependent kill kinetics was evaluated by counting the surviving bacterial cells after six hours of exposure to double dilution concentration of each type of Ag-NP. It was shown that 10^2 cfu/mL remained survived in the medium after exposure to the MIC value of Ag-NP-1, Ag-NP-2, or Ag-NP-3 after six hours of incubation at 37°C. None of the cells survived in the medium after exposure to the MBC value of Ag-NP-1, Ag-NP-2, or Ag-NP-3 after six hours of incubation at 37°C. At lower concentrations (3.5 μg/mL), a one-log reduction was observed for Ag-NP-1 and Ag-NP-3; Ag-NP-2 did not show any inhibitory effect [Fig. 8(iv)].

3.4.5. *Scanning electron microscopy analysis*

Scanning electron microscopy examination of the silver nanoparticle-treated cells revealed that the silver nanoparticles caused a series of changes in *A. baumannii*, including size and shape alteration as well as bleb formation on the surface (Fig. 9) within one hour of treatment. Ag-NP-1 treated cells [Fig. 9(b)] showed a reduction in size with cell

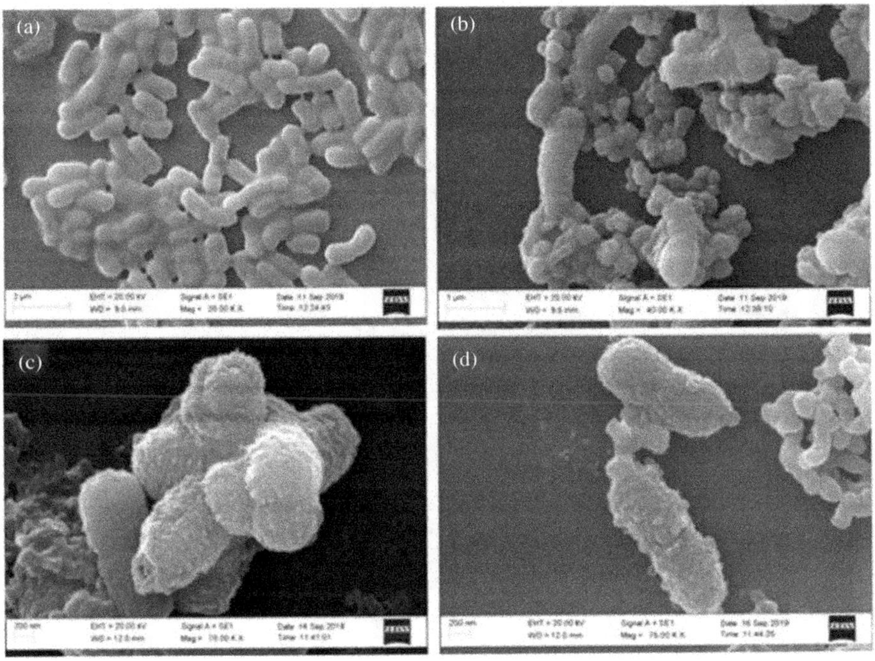

Fig. 9. Scanning electron microscopy images of control (a), Ag-NP-1 treated cells (b), Ag-NP-2 treated cells (c), and Ag-NP-3 treated cells (d) for 1 h at the appropriate MBC values in MHB medium at 37°C.

fragmentation and bleb formation. Ag-NP-2 treated cells [Fig. 9(c)] showed cell swelling with cell membrane breakage. Ag-NP-3 treated cells showed bleb formation, inducing the leakage of intracellular materials [Fig. 9(d)].

3.4.6. *Fluorescence imaging of silver nanoparticles with A. baumannii cell surface protein interaction*

Protein–nanoparticle interactions may be evaluated through fluorescence imaging.[15] Accordingly, we attempted to investigate the interaction of Ag-NP-1 with bovine serum albumin using 2D and 3D fluorescence imaging. Figure 10(a) shows the 2D fluorescence spectra in the absence (1) and the presence (2) of Ag-NP-1. The finding clearly predicts that after Ag-NP-1 interaction, the fluorescence intensity is

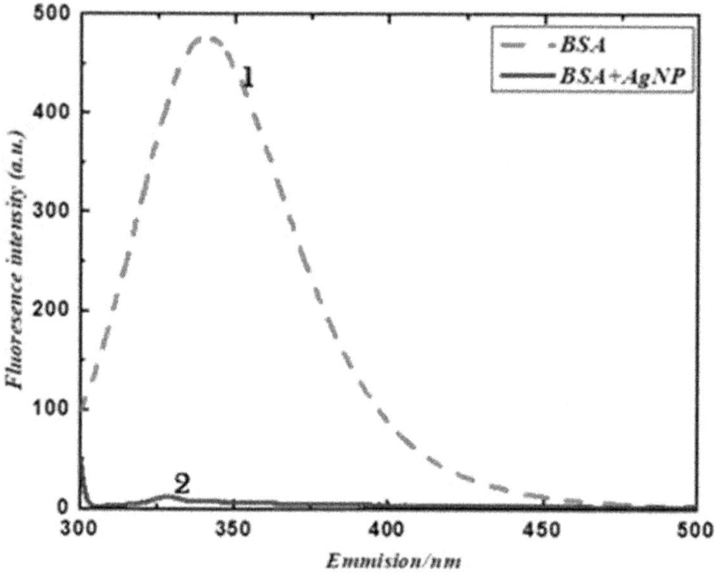

(a)

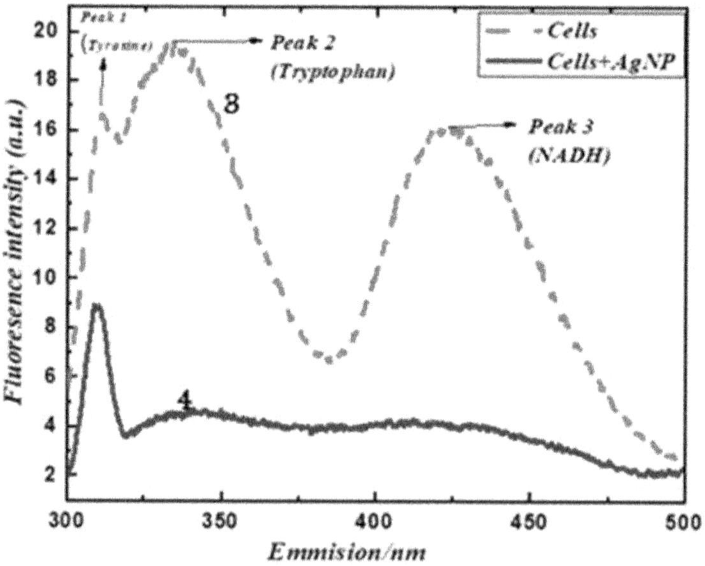

(b)

Fig. 10. (a) Fluorescence spectra of bovine serum albumin in the absence (1) and the presence of Ag-NP-1 (2). (b) Fluorescence spectra of *A. baumannii* in the absence (3) and the presence of Ag-NP-1 (4).

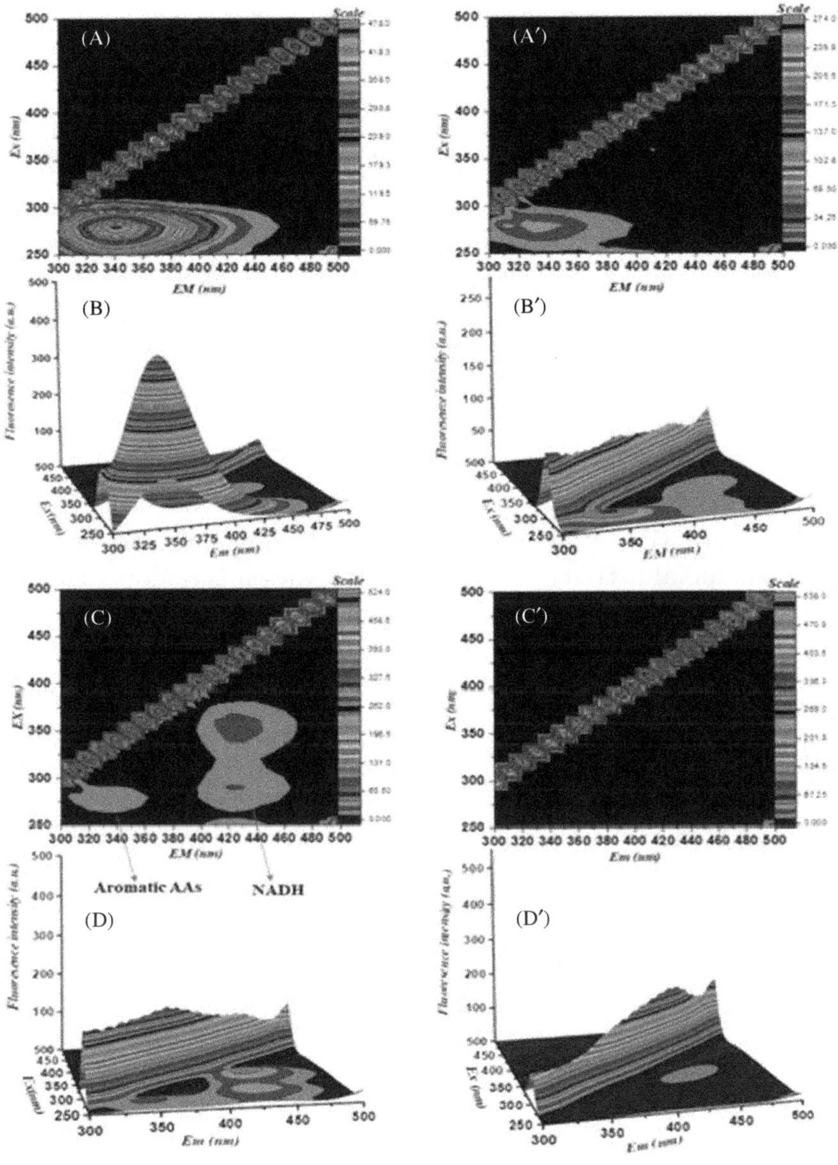

Fig. 11. 3D fluorescence images of bovine serum albumin in the absence (A, B) and the presence (A', B') of Ag-NP-1. A and A' show the contour images; B, B' show the surface images. 3D fluorescence images of *A. baumannii* in the absence (C and D) and the presence (C' D') of Ag-NP-1. C and D show the contour images; C' and D' show the surface images.

reduced close to zero, indicating selective binding of the silver nanoparticles to the protein. Similar observations were recorded for the interactions between Ag-NP-1 and *A. baumannii* (Fig. 10(b)). In order to understand the mechanism of surface protein binding to Ag-NP-1, 3D fluorescence imaging of the similar interactions is recorded as shown in Fig. 11. Figure 11 contains 3D fluorescence images of bovine serum albumin in the absence (A, B) and the presence (A', B') of Ag-NP-1. Images A and A' show the contour images; images B and B' show the surface images. 3D fluorescence images of *A. baumannii* in the absence (C and D) and the presence (C' D') of Ag-NP-1 were also obtained. Images C and D show the contour images; images C' and D' show the surface images.

The fluorescence of *A. baumannii* surface proteins diminished significantly in each case, indicating rapid interaction with silver nanoparticles; the surface and contour plots thus indicate selectivity in antimicrobial activity. A detailed observation is underway, which involves 3D spectrophotometric imaging of cell surface protein–nanoparticle interaction.

4. Conclusions

This study demonstrates the organic moiety-dependent rapid synthesis of noble metal mono-, bi- and trimetallic nanoparticles. Au, Ag–Au, Pd–Ag, and Pd–Ag–Au nanoparticles did not show significant antimicrobial activity; on the other hand, Pd-NPs and Ag-NPs were shown to be potent antimicrobial agents. Cyclohexanone, 3-GPTMS and formaldehyde allowed the formation of three different types of silver nanoparticles with $\leq$10 nm size, which showed antibacterial properties against a multi-drug resistant *A. baumannii* strain. The MIC and MBC of the Ag-NP-1 were the lowest among the tested silver nanoparticles. 2D and 3D fluorescence imaging showed selective cell surface protein–nanoparticle interactions. The above-presented work on the antibacterial activity of silver nanoparticles may enable the development of new therapies against deadly nosocomial infections.

References

1. P. C. Pandey and D. S. Chauhan, *Analyst*, **137**, 376 (2012).
2. P. C. Pandey, A. K. Pandey and G. Pandey, *J. Nanosci. Nanotechnol.* **14**, 6606 (2014).
3. P. C. Pandey and G. Pandey, *J. Mater. Chem. B.* **2**, 3383 (2014).
4. P. C. Pandey and G. Pandey, *Catalysis Sci. Technol.* **6**, 3911 (2016).
5. C. Burda, X. Chen, R. Narayanan and M. A. El-Sayed, *Chem. Rev.* **105**, 1025 (2005).
6. J. R. Morones, J. L. Elechiguerra, A. Camacho, K. Holt, J. B. Kouri, J. T. Ramírez and M. J. Yacaman, *Nanotechnol.* **16**, 2346 (2005).
7. G. Franci, A. Falanga, S. Galdiero, L. Palomba, M. Rai, G. Morelli and M. Galdiero, *Molecules* **20**, 8856 (2015).
8. M. Rai, A. Yadav and A. Gade, *Biotechnol. Adv.* **27**, 76 (2009).
9. M. A. Radzig, V. A. Nadtochenko, O. A. Koksharova, J. Kiwi, V. A. Lipasova and I. A. Khmel, *Colloids Surf. B.* **102**, 300 (2013).
10. B. Wiley, Y. Sun, B. Mayers and Y. Xia, *Chem. A Eur. J.* **11**, 454 (2005).
11. T. C. Dakal, A. Kumar, R. S. Majumdar and V. Yadav, *Front. Microbiol.* **7**, 1831 (2016).
12. M. A. Ansari, H. M. Khan, A. A. Khan, M. K. Ahmad, A. A. Mahdi, R. Pal and S. S. Cameotra, *J. Basic Microbiol.* **54**, 905 (2014).
13. I. Sondi and B. Salopek-Sondi, *J. Colloid Interf. Sci.* **275**, 177 (2004).
14. I. Lynch and K. A. Dawson, *Nano Today* **3**, 40 (2008).
15. L. R. Dartnell, T. A. Roberts, G. Moore, J. M. Ward and J. P. Muller, *PLoS One* **8**, e75270 (2013).
16. J. Mariam, P. M. Dongre and D. C. Kothari, *J. Fluorescence.* **21**, 2193 (2011).
17. A. W. Bauer, *Am. J. Clin. Pathol.* **45**, 149 (1966)
18. K. Q. Poletto and C. Reis, *Revista da Sociedade Brasileira de Medicina Tropical.* **38**, 416 (2005).
19. J. McFarland, *J. Am. Med. Assoc.* **49**, 1176 (1907).
20. J. M. Andrews, *J. Antimicrobial Chemotherapy.* **48**, 5 (2001).
21. I. D. Rankin, MIC Testing, *Manual de Pruebas de Susceptibilidad Antimicrobiano*, M. B. Coyle (ed.), Vol. 53 (American Society for Microbiology, 2005).
22. Z. Liu, Y. Wang, Y. Zu, Y. Fu, N. Li, N. Guo, R. Liu and Y. Zhang, *Mater. Sci. Eng. C.* **42**, 31 (2014).
23. J. J. Wade and M. A. Graver, *FEMS Microbiol. Lett.* **273**, 35 (2007).
24. N. S. Zainin, K. Y. Lau, M. Zakaria, R. Son, A. A. Razis and Y. Rukayadi, *Int. Food Res. J.* **20**, 3319 (2013).
25. K. Y. Lau, N. S. Zainin, F. Abas and Y. Rukayadi, *Int. J. Current Microbiol. Appl. Sci.* **3**, 499 (2014).
26. C. Y. Chen, G. W. Nace and P. L. Irwin, *J. Microbiol. Meth.* **55**, 475 (2003).
27. P. C. Pandey and R. Singh, *J. Nanosci. Nanotechnol.* **15**, 5749 (2015).
28. P. C. Pandey, R. Singh and A. K. Pandey, *Electrochim. Acta.* **138**, 163 (2014).

https://doi.org/10.1142/9789819809028_0011

Chapter 11

Quantification of Magnetic Nanoparticles in *ex vivo* Colorectal Lymph Nodes*

Lennert Molenaar[†], Melissa M. Horstman – van de Loosdrecht[†], Lejla Alic[†], Joop van Baarlen[‡], Jeroen J. H. J. Meijerink[§], Bennie ten Haken[†], Ivo A. M. J. Broeders[¶,‖,††] and Daan J. Lips[**]

[†]*Magnetic Detection & Imaging Group, Technical Medical Centre University of Twente, Enschede, The Netherlands*
[‡]*Department of Pathology, LabPON Hengelo, The Netherlands*
[§]*Department of Operating Rooms and MITeC Technology Center Radboud University Medical Center, Nijmegen, The Netherlands*
[¶]*Department of Surgery, Meander Medical Center Amersfoort, The Netherlands*
[‖]*Robotics and Mechatronics Group, University of Twente Enschede, The Netherlands*
[**]*Department of Surgery, Medisch Spectrum Twente Enschede, The Netherlands*
[††]*IAMJ.Broeders@meandermc.nl*

En-bloc tumor resection is the standard treatment for locally advanced colorectal cancer (CRC). An extensive histopathological assessment is necessary to evaluate the metastatic spread and adjuvant therapy. Sentinel lymph node biopsy decreases the histopathological burden when only sentinel lymph nodes (SLNs) are examined. This study aims to evaluate the spread of a magnetic tracer throughout the lymphatic system after *ex vivo* injection in en-bloc resected specimens of patients with CRC. To achieve this, lymph nodes (LNs) were quantified using a new magnetic detection method. Fifteen patients with CRC diagnosed with clinically negative LNs were included in this study and received 2–4 *ex vivo* magnetic tracer

---

*To cite this article, please refer to its earlier version published in the *Nano LIFE*, Vol. 12, No. 3 (2022) 2250006 (8 pages), DOI: 10.1142/S1793984422500064
[††]Corresponding author.

injections (total volume of 2 mL). Magnetic sample series were acquired to create a look-up table for magnetic tracer quantification. In 80% of the patients, at least one magnetic LN was detected. A total of 33 LNs were marked as magnetic, containing an average of 8.1 μg iron. In 71% of the patients, metastases were found in nonmagnetic LNs. *Ex vivo* injection leads to sub-optimal tracer spread and therefore inaccurate diagnosis. This study presents a novel magnetic detection method to quantify magnetic tracer in lymph nodes. Detecting the SLNs in en-bloc resected specimens and involving only these LNs in histopathological investigation enable a decrease in healthcare costs or an increased diagnostic potential.

Keywords: Colorectal cancer; DiffMag; sentinel lymph node; superparamagnetic iron oxide nanoparticles; superparamagnetic quantifier.

1. Introduction

Worldwide incidence of colorectal cancer (CRC) in 2018 was 1.8 million, causing 861,000 associated deaths.[1] This number would have been larger if not for screening, where premalignant lesions are detected and treated, preventing CRC.[2] Standard care for patients with CRC is radical en-bloc tumor resection that includes regional lymph nodes (LNs).[3] Patients with confirmed metastatic LNs are consecutively treated with adjuvant radiotherapy. Although this method is effective, it involves substantial time, effort and finances required by histopathological examination of a large number of LNs.[4]

Sentinel lymph node biopsy (SLNB) limits the excision of LNs to solely sentinel lymph nodes (SLNs) using perioperative SLN mapping. SLNs directly drain from the tumor and have the highest probability of containing metastases.[5] Even with apparent advantages of perioperative SLN mapping, more evidence is necessary before the procedure could become standard practice. During the current routine en-bloc resection, a section of colon and mesocolon is removed including fatty tissue with (S)LNs.[6] *In vivo* tracer injection or *ex vivo* tracer injection can potentially facilitate the identification of SLNs. Although tracer spread of *in vivo* injections is expected to be superior, added patient burden is also anticipated. *In vivo* injections can be given prior to surgery with an extra colonoscopy or at the start of the surgery. For optimal tracer spread, it is necessary to apply at least 20 min for the tracer to spread, which extends the total surgery time.

Therefore, investigating *ex vivo* injections as an alternative option could be beneficial, potentially enabling SLN identification without added patient burden and without extending surgery duration.

Under comparable diagnostic accuracy, the identification of SLNs potentially reduces health costs since fewer LNs need to be histopathologically processed. Additional benefit involves a strategy for SLN ultrastaging, instead of single sectioning of all LNs.[7] This potentially increases the diagnostic value by an increased identification rate of metastases, micro metastases and isolated tumor cells. However, isolated tumor cells have limited predictive value, therefore having no influence on the adjuvant treatment. Considering micro metastases are associated with an increased recurrence rate and an inferior prognosis,[8] adjuvant treatment is advised. With this strategy, the total histopathological workload is expected to remain similar. It is unknown which strategy would be more beneficial and cost-effective; decreasing histopathological investigation by investigating fewer LNs or performing extensive histopathological investigation on only the SLNs. Regardless the strategy of preference, it is beneficial to identify SLNs for a more refined histopathological process.

A variety of SLNB tracers are currently clinically available: Radioactive, fluorescent and magnetic tracers.[9] Radioactive tracers have proven to be effective.[10] However, they suffer from serious drawbacks under strict regulations, a short decay and shelf life, varying availability per clinical site/country and a radiation dose, although minimal, for users and patients. Fluorescent tracers do not suffer from these drawbacks, but detection time is limited and they have a low penetration depth of 5–10 mm,[11] which is in many clinical cases insufficient. Magnetic tracers (also referred to as magnetic nanoparticles and, in this case, specifically superparamagnetic iron-oxide nanoparticles [SPIONs]) have been suggested to alleviate a variety of the issues constituted by radioactive or fluorescence tracers, such as being widely available, having a long shelf life, logistically easy to use and no half-life, can be detected with MRI and are radiation-free.[12] With a great potential, SPIONs need assessment of clinical relevance in terms of relation between the amount of injected tracer and amount of trapped tracer in the (S)LNs.[13,14]

The SuperParamagnetic Quantifier (SPaQ)[15] is used to accurately quantify the amount of magnetic tracer trapped inside LNs. A unique feature of the SPaQ is its relatively large sample holder for static samples (diameter 20 mm) compared to other magnetometers, such as vibrating sample magnetometry (VSM) and magnetic particle spectroscopy (MPS).[16] This enables measurements on entire LNs. Due to the homogeneous magnetic field, precise orientation of the LN is irrelevant.

The aim of this study is the assessment of the clinical relevance for SPION-enhanced (S)LNs, which involves three research goals:

- Evaluation of tracer spread after an *ex vivo* peritumoral injection (with and without tissue massage).
- Quantification of the amount of tracer trapped inside the resected LNs.
- Evaluation of the performance of the SPaQ in a clinically relevant setting.

2. Methods

2.1. *The SuperParamagnetic quantifier*

The SPaQ is a relatively inexpensive in-house developed magnetometer with a sample holder placed in a homogeneous magnetic field (Fig. 1). The SPaQ uses an in-house developed control unit and laptop controlled acquisition software. The SPaQ is a mobile device that enables the use of the device in multiple clinical situations. In previous research, the SPaQ (in particle characterization mode) was used extensively for characterization of magnetic tracers.[15,17] Additionally, SPaQ functionality was extended to include a quantification mode, based on the patented differential magnetometry (DiffMag) detection principle.[18] This DiffMag principle (Fig. 2) is a nonlinear magnetic detection method specifically assessing magnetic tracer without influence of its surrounding. In case of a handheld device,[19] the height of the DiffMag signal reflects a combination of the amount of SPIONs and the distance between the detector and sample. Due to the homogeneous magnetic field in the SPaQ, the DiffMag

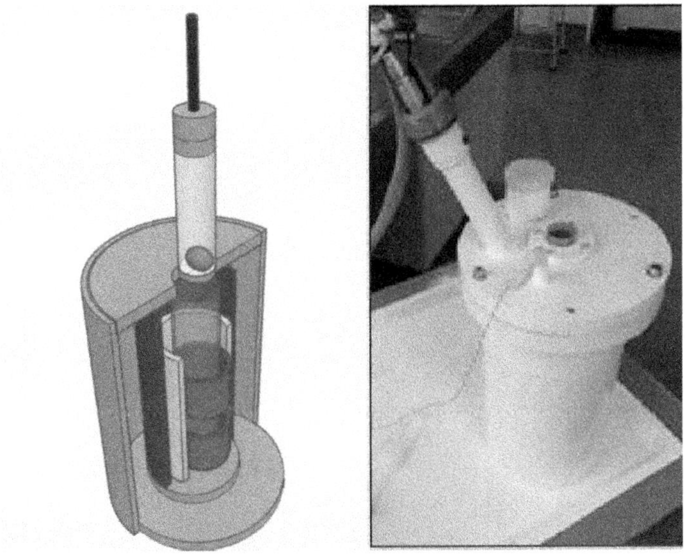

Fig. 1. (Color online) A simplified schematic cross-section and outer appearance of the SPaQ. The SPaQ has a height of 50 cm and width of 18 cm. The sample container has a diameter of 2 cm and a height of 2.5 cm. A vial with a LN (in blue) is lowered into the green shaft. An excitation coil (yellow) creates the homogenous magnetic field, and detection coils (red) measure the magnetic signal. The outer field coil (purple) serves as a shielding coil and improves the field homogeneity.

signal (expressed in μV) is directly proportional to the amount of SPIONs, resulting in an accurate assessment uninfluenced by sample orientation. A DiffMag signal below three standard deviations of the average background noise, assessed prior to each acquisition, is labeled as noise. The following SPaQ settings are used for characterizing the applied magnetic field: AC amplitude of 0.83 mT, AC frequency of 2.5 kHz and DC field strength of 4.99 mT. The DiffMag signal is refreshed every 0.5 s.

2.2. *Clinical trial*

Fifteen adult patients diagnosed with primary CRC (cT1–4) and clinically negative LNs were included in this study if scheduled for a hemicolectomy (left/right), a transverse colon resection or a sigmoid resection. Written informed consent was obtained prior to inclusion.

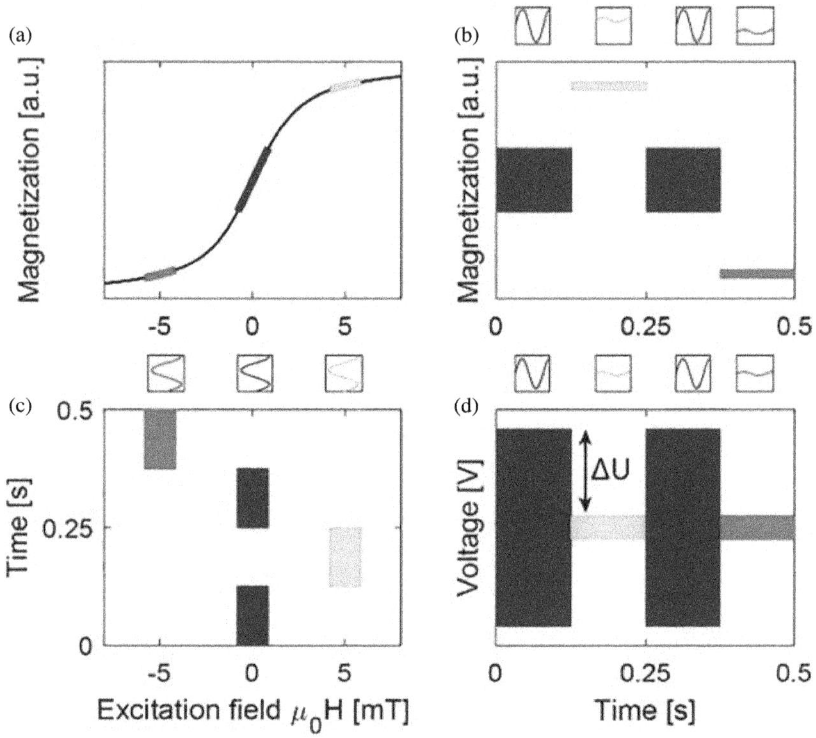

Fig. 2. (Color online) The DiffMag principle applied in the SPaQ. (a) Magnetization curve of magnetic particles. (b) AC field (blue) with DC offsets (red and green). (c) Magnetization of magnetic particles. (d) Measurement of nonlinear magnetic signal (ΔU).

Ethics committee approval was given by the Medical Ethical Committee Twente (Enschede, the Netherlands), under study number K19-13. The first 10 patients received two to four *ex vivo* peritumoral injections with a total of 2 mL Sienna+® (28 mg (Fe)/mL, Endomag, UK, Ltd.) diluted with Na Cl to a total volume of 4 mL and no tissue massage after injection (group 1). The next five patients received 3–4 *ex vivo* peritumoral injections with a total of 2 mL Magtrace® (28 mg (Fe)/mL, Endomag, UK, Ltd.) diluted with NaCl to a total volume of 4 mL and 1–2 min of tissue massage after injection (group 2). Figure 3(a) shows the resection specimen with the tracer injected after resection. For both groups, after a waiting period of at least 20 min (to promote tracer

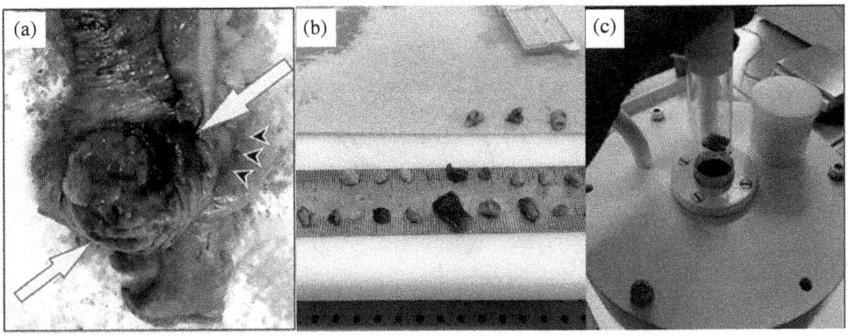

Fig. 3. (a) *Ex vivo* magnetic tracer injection in the primary tumor (white arrows) with visible tracer spread to lymph nodes (black arrows). (b) Resected lymph nodes during pathological research and (c) measurement of an individual lymph node.

distribution), the specimen was fixated in formalin and sent to the pathology department.

All LNs were harvested from the resection specimen (Fig. 3(b)) 24–72 h after the *ex vivo* tracer injection. Subsequently, the spread of magnetic tracer was assessed for all LNs by using the SPaQ (Fig. 3(c)). The total acquisition time for one LN (putting a LN in the sample holder, SPaQ measurement and removing the sample) was under 30 s. After the SPaQ measurements, all nodes were processed in accordance with the following histopathology protocol: For every found LN, two adjacent central slices were sectioned and stained with H&E for a general overview and with Prussian blue to identify SPIONs (Figs. 4(a) and 4(b)). This provided data for each LN whether it contains metastatic cells and/or magnetic tracer.

2.3. *Look-up table acquisition*

Assessing the amount of iron trapped inside the resected LNs is facilitated by a predefined SPaQ look-up table (LUT) for both Sienna+® and Magtrace®.

A relation between amount of iron and corresponding DiffMag signal (μV) was experimentally established and modeled as a first order polynomial by in-house developed software (Matlab environment, R2020a, Mathworks, Inc., Natick, MA). The DiffMag signal

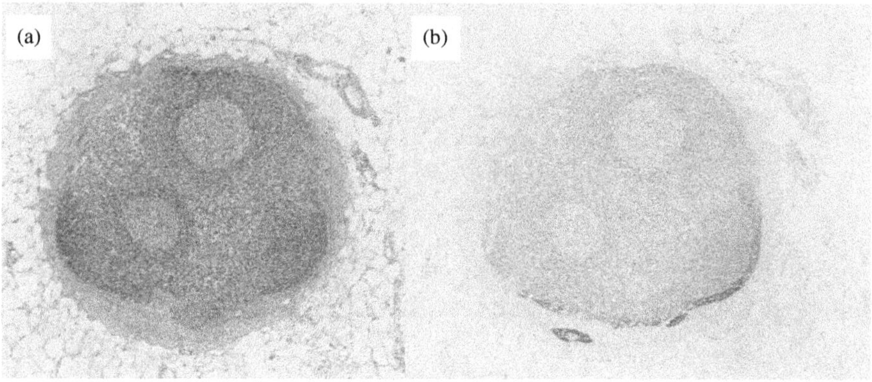

Fig. 4. (Color online) (a) Lymph node coupe with H&E staining and (b) Lymph node coupe with Fe staining (in blue the magnetic tracer).

corresponding to eight samples for both tracers were acquired 10 times using the SPaQ. The created LUT is available through a 4 TU repository for both Sienna+® and Magtrace®.[20]

2.4. *Correction factor*

It is necessary to apply a correction to the μg Fe found, since the LUT is created with measurements on liquid samples. Riahi *et al.* previously investigated the effect of environmental factors on the differential magnetic susceptibility.[17] Increasing the viscosity or completely blocking the rotation of magnetic nanoparticles by freeze-drying reduced the magnetic signal from 7% to 74%. In the colorectal LN measurements, the tracer is trapped in the LNs. Therefore, the estimated amount of tracer is increased with the correction factor.

3. Results

3.1. *Clinical results*

The clinical results of colorectal LNs using the SPaQ are summarized in Table 1 and further detailed in the Appendix A (Tables A.1 & A.2). The average number of magnetic LNs per patient was 1.9 (0–4) for

Table 1. An overview of the obtained clinical results based on the SPaQ measurements.

	Group 1	Group 2
Patients (N)	10	5
Tracer type	Sienna+®	Magtrace®
Average number of LNs (range)	21.3 (5–36)	27.6 (10–44)
Average number of magnetic LNs (range)	1.9 (0–4)	2.4 (0–4)
SPION detection rate	8/10 (80%)	4/5 (80%)
Number of patients with metastases in LNs	3	4
Number of patients with metastases in SLNs	1	1

group 1 and 2.4 (0–4) for group 2. Both patient groups showed an 80% SPION detection rate (i.e., in 80% of the patients at least one LN containing SPIONs was detected). During histopathological examination, LN metastases were found in a total of seven patients. In two of those patients, metastases were found in the LNs containing magnetic tracer, which we defined as SLNs (29%).

3.2. *Magnetic look-up table*

Figure 5 shows the DiffMag signals for both tracers (Sienna+® and Magtrace®) with the first-order polynomial fit.

3.3. *Amount of tracer trapped in LNs*

For the Sienna+® group, a total of 21 LNs were identified, with an average DiffMag signal of 249 μ V (range: 100–530) resulting in an average of 11.0 μg Fe (range: 2.0–29.2). For the Magtrace® group, a total of 12 LNs were identified, with an average DiffMag signal of 136 μV (range: 90–360) resulting in an average of 2.9 μg Fe (range: 0.8–12.8). After applying the correction factor, the average amount of Sienna+® was 11.8–19.1 μg Fe and 3.1–5.0 μg Fe for Magtrace®. When all 33 LNs were combined, the average μg Fe was 8.3 (8.9–14.4) μg Fe after correction. Further details can be seen in Table 2.

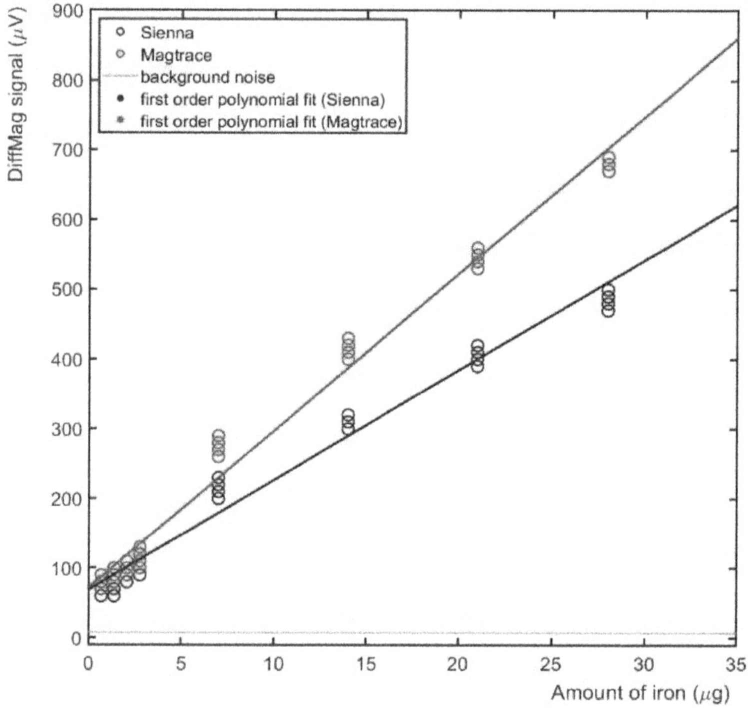

Fig. 5. (Color online) An overview of the two sample series with their corresponding first order polynomial line. The blue line represents the DiffMag signal for Sienna+® and the red line represents the DiffMag signal for Magtrace®. The green line represents the mean background noise.

Table 2. The clinically measured colorectal nodes with the corresponding calculated first polynomial based on the measured sample series.

	Sienna+®			Magtrace®	
LN #	DiffMag signal (μV)	First polynomial (μg Fe)	LN #	DiffMag signal (μV)	First polynomial (μg Fe)
1	420	22.2	22	360	12.8
2	520	28.6	23	240	7.5
3	200	8.3	24	120	2.1
4	410	21.6	25	120	2.1

Table 2. (*Continued*)

Sienna+®			Magtrace®		
LN #	DiffMag signal (μV)	First polynomial (μg Fe)	LN #	DiffMag signal (μV)	First polynomial (μg Fe)
5	440	23.5	26	90	0.8
6	160	5.8	27	90	0.8
7	190	7.7	28	90	0.8
8	100	2.0	29	90	0.8
9	170	6.4	30	110	1.7
10	200	8.3	31	90	0.8
11	440	23.5	32	110	1.7
12	160	5.8	33	120	2.1
13	100	2.0			
14	130	3.9			
15	200	8.3			
16	160	5.8			
17	280	13.4			
18	120	3.2			
19	200	8.3			
20	530	29.2			
21	100	2.0			
Average	249	11.0		136	2.9
After correction		11.8–19.1			3.1–5.0

4. Discussion

The spread of magnetic tracer throughout the lymphatic system after *ex vivo* injection was seen in 80% of the patients, despite the absence of natural lymph flow. No difference was observed in the SPION detection rate between the groups with and without tissue massage. In 29% of the patients with LN metastases, the metastases were detected in SLNs (magnetic LNs). Consequently, histopathological investigation of only these SLNs would result in inadequate medical treatment for 71% of patients. To enable successful clinical implementation of *ex vivo* SLN dissection, improved tracer spread is necessary.

An average amount of 8.9–14.4 μg of tracer was found trapped in LNs, after correction. When analyzing the standard deviation of both sample series with the SPaQ, good repeatability is suggested. When converted to μg Fe with the presented LUT, we can conclude that measurement deviations with the SPaQ are practically negligible. To our knowledge, there is only one previous study (breast cancer) reporting the amount of magnetic tracer (Resovist) trapped in the dissected LNs as assessed by a handheld magnetometer.[21] This study reported a mean of $140 \pm 40\,\mu$g Fe, which is significantly higher than that in our study (33 LNs with an average of 8.1 [8.7–14.1] μg Fe). Besides the differences (different tracer and cancer type), the main difference is the *ex vivo* injection, which presumably resulted in a much lower tracer spread throughout the tissue.

We established five unique aspects on valorization of the SPaQ as a clinical device. First, it is a relatively large sample holder, evaluating a complete LN instead of single plaques. Second, the SPaQ is relatively small and low in cost. Third, the device can easily be transported to a desired location, such as a pathology department. Fourth, the acquisition takes less than a second, making it possible to incorporate in current workflows without significant time investment. Last, LUT data were very concise, despite the high number of repeated acquisitions, proving the high reproducibility of the SPaQ.

To utilize the SPaQ to its full potential in a clinical setting, we envision an additional study using *in vivo* injections and a larger patient group. As illustrated earlier during SLN mapping by a fluorescent tracer,[22] changing the injection from *ex vivo* to *in vivo* is expected to lead to increased tracer spread. Until recently, *in vivo* tracer injections for patients with CRC were only considered feasible prior to the surgery during an additional colonoscopy or at the start of the surgery (extending surgery time). Currently, extended intended use allows the magnetic tracer to be injected up to 30 days prior to surgery. This leads to the opportunity to inject the tracer during the standard diagnostic colonoscopy. Comparing a time window of 30 days versus 12 h when using a radioactive tracer, the magnetic tracer provides great flexibility and has a major advantage regarding surgical planning.

5. Conclusion

This study presents a novel magnetic detection method to quantify magnetic tracer and assess magnetic tracer spread in colorectal LNs. With the expectation that *in vivo* tracer injection would greatly improve the tracer spread, the principle of *ex vivo* SLN dissection still has a great diagnostic potential. In regards to quantitative assessment of iron amount trapped in LNs, identification of the SLN(s) from a large number of resected LNs enables two options viable in histopathological investigation: Decrease of the ever increasing healthcare costs or increased diagnostic value.

Acknowledgments

This research has been sponsored by the Netherlands Organization for Scientific Research (NWO), under the research program Magnetic Sensing for Laparoscopy (MagLap), with project number 14322.

The authors declare no conflicts of interest related to this paper. Written informed consent was obtained prior to inclusion. Ethics committee approval was given by Medical Ethical Committee Twente (Enschede, the Netherlands), under study number K19-13.

The authors would like to thank Mike Liem, Pascal Steenvoorde, Eino van Duijn, Anneriet Dassen, Erik Krooshoop, Mariska Stellaard, Clemens Kormelink, Mark Selles and Quinten Eyck for their contribution to this research.

Appendix A

Table A.1. Sample series used to acquire the look-up table.

Sienna+®				
μg Fe	0.7	1.4	2.1	2.8
Volume (μL)	2.5	5	7.5	10
Concentration (μg/μL)	0.28	0.28	0.28	0.28
μg Fe	7	14	21	28
Volume (μL)	2.5	5	7.5	10
Concentration (μg/μL)	2.8	2.8	2.8	2.8

(*Continued*)

Table A.1. (*Continued*)

Magtrace®				
μg Fe	0.7	1.4	2.1	2.8
Volume (μL)	2.5	5	7.5	10
Concentration (μg/μL)	0.28	0.28	0.28	0.28
μg Fe	7	14	21	28
Volume (μL)	2.5	5	7.5	10
Concentration (μg/μL)	2.8	2.8	2.8	2.8

Table A.2. Overview of the demographic data of all included patients.

	Group 1	Group 2
Patients (N)	10	5
Number of males/females	7/3	3/2
Mean age	61.9	63
Mean BMI	27.6	25.1
Number of left/right hemicolectomies	1/6	0/2
Number of sigmoid resections	2	3
Number of transversum resections	1	0
Tumor stage (radiologists) cTx	4	2
Tumor stage (radiologists) cT1	1	0
Tumor stage (radiologists) cT1/2	1	0
Tumor stage (radiologists) cT2	1	1
Tumor stage (radiologists) cT2/3	2	1
Tumor stage (radiologists) cT3	1	1
Tumor location - coecum	4	2
Tumor location - colon ascendens	2	0
Tumor location - colon transversum	2	0
Tumor location - sigmoid	2	3

References

1. M. Arnold, M. S. Sierra, M. Laversanne, I. Soerjomataram, A. Jernal and F. Bray, *Gut* **66**, 683 (2017).
2. E. M. Montminy, A. Jang, M. Conner and J. J. Karlitz, *Med. Clin. North Am.* **104**, 1023 (2020).
3. S. Karki, S. Umar and A. Kasi, *Curr. Colorectal Cancer Rep.* **16**, 107 (2020).
4. Q. Alefan, R. Malhees and N. Mhaidat, *Curr. Probl. Cancer* **41**, 371 (2017).

5. A. Cousins, S. K. Thompson, A. B. Wedding and B. Thierry, *Biotechnol. Adv.* **32**, 269 (2014).
6. A. C. Currie, *Eur. Surg. Res.* **60**, 45 (2019).
7. S. Saha *et al.*, *Clin. Exp. Metastasis.* **35**, 463 (2018).
8. D. A. M. Sloothaak, S. Sahami, H. J. van der Zaag-Loonen, E. S. van der Zaag, P. J. Tanis, W. A. Bemelman and C. J. Buskens, *Eur. J. Surg. Oncol.* **40**, 263 (2014).
9. E. S. van der Zaag, W. H. Bouma, P. J. Tanis, D. T. Ubbink, W. A. Bemelman and C. J. Buskens, *Ann. Surg. Oncol.* **19**, 3449 (2012).
10. M. H. G. M. van der Pas, S. Meijer, O. S. Hoekstra, I. I. Riphagen, H. C. W. de Vet, D. L. Knol, N. C. T. van Grieken and W. J. H. J. Meijerink, *Lancet Oncol.* **12**, 540 (2011).
11. M. N. van Oosterom *et al.*, *IEEE Trans. Med. Imag.* **39**, 226 (2019).
12. Y. X. J. Wáng and J.-M. Idée, *Quantitative Imag. Med. Surg.* **7**, 88 (2017).
13. A. Kuwahata, M. Kaneko, S. Chikaki, M. Kusakabe and M. Sekino, *AIP Adv.* **8**, 056713 (2018).
14. E. R. Nieuwenhuis, B. Kolenaar, J. J. van Hof, J. van Baarlen, A. J. M. van Bemmel, A. Christenhusz, T. W. J. Scheenen, B. ten Haken, R. de Bree and L. Alic, *Cancers* **14**, 678 (2022).
15. M. M. van de Loosdrecht, S. Draack, S. Waanders, J. G. L. Schlief, H. J. G. Krooshoop, T. Viereck, F. Ludwig and B. ten Haken, *Rev. Sci. Instrum.* **90**, 024101 (2019).
16. S. Draack, T. Viereck, C. Kuhlmann, M. Schilling and F. Ludwig, *Int. J. Magn. Particle Imag.* **3**, 1703018 (2017).
17. K. Riahi, M. M. van de Loosdrecht, L. Alic and B. Ten Haken, *J. Magn. Magn. Mater.* **514**, 167238 (2020).
18. S. Waanders, M. Visscher, T. O. B. Oderkerk, H. J. G. Krooshoop and B. ten Haken, Method and apparatus for measuring an amount of superparamagnetic material in an object, *Espacenet.* The Netherlands, 2015, https://nl.espacenet.com/publicationDetails/biblio?II=17&ND=3&adjacent=true&locale=nLNL&FT=D&date=20151126&CC=US&NR=2015338376A1& KC=A1#.
19. S. Waanders, M. Visscher, R. R. Wildeboer, T. O. B. Oderkerk, H. J. G. Krooshoop and B. ten Haken, *Phys. Med. Biol.* **61**, 8120 (2016).
20. L. Molenaar, *Look-up table based on SPaQ measurements to quantify amount of iron in small samples* 2021, 4TU.ResearchData, https://doi.org/10.4121/15034902.
21. M. Sekino *et al.*, *Sci. Rep.* **8**, 1195 (2018).
22. M. Ankersmit, H. J. Bonjer, G. Hannink, L. J. Schoonmade, M. H. G. M. van der pas and W. J. H. J. Meijerink, *Tech. Coloproctol.* **23**, 1113 (2019).

https://doi.org/10.1142/9789819809028_0012

Chapter 12

Intratumoral Photosensitizer Delivery and Photodynamic Therapy*

Chen-Hua Ma[†], Jeffrey Yang[†], Jenna L. Mueller[†,‡] and Huang-Chiao Huang[†,‡,§]

[†]*Fischell Department of Bioengineering*
University of Maryland
College Park, MD 20742, USA
[‡]*Marlene and Stewart Greenebaum Cancer Center*
University of Maryland School of Medicine
Baltimore, MD 21201, USA
[§]*hchuang@umd.edu*

Photodynamic therapy (PDT) is a two-step procedure that involves the administration of special drugs, commonly called photosensitizers, followed by the application of certain wavelengths of light. The light activates these photosensitizers to produce reactive molecular species that induce cell death in tissues. There are numerous factors to consider when selecting the appropriate photosensitizer administration route, such as which part of the body is being targeted, the pharmacokinetics of photosensitizers, and the formulation of photosensitizers. While intravenous, topical, and oral administration of photosensitizers are widely used in preclinical and clinical applications of PDT, other administration routes, such as intraperitoneal, intra-arterial, and intratumoral injections, are gaining traction for their potential in treating advanced diseases and reducing off-target toxicities. With recent advances in targeted nanotechnology, biomaterials, and light delivery systems, the exciting possibilities of targeted photosensitizer delivery can be fully realized for preclinical and clinical applications. Further, in light of the growing burden of cancer mortality in low- and middle-income countries and development of low-cost light sources and photosensitizers, PDT could be used to treat cancer patients in low-income

*To cite this article, please refer to its earlier version published in the *Nano LIFE*, Vol. 11, No. 2 (2021) 2130003 (7 pages), DOI: 10.1142/S179398442130003X
[§]Corresponding author.

settings. This short article introduces aspects of interfaces of intratumoral photosensitizer injections and nano-biomaterials for PDT applications in both high-income and low-income settings but does not present a comprehensive review due to space limitations.

Keywords: Intratumoral injection; photosensitizer; photodynamic therapy; nanobiomaterials; cancer.

1. Administration routes for oncologic photosensitizers

Photodynamic therapy (PDT) is a photochemistry-based approach in which a photosensitizer is energized by red or near-infrared light to generate reactive oxygen species that kill or modulate target cells or tissues.[1,2] A photosensitizer is defined as a chemical entity that absorbs incident light and imparts a physical and chemical change on another chemical entity. There are two main types of photosensitized reactions to produce reactive oxygen species. In the Type I reaction, a photosensitizer at an excited state reacts with the substrate to produce radical ions or radicals via electron transfer or hydrogen atom abstraction. In the presence of oxygen, the photosensitizer radical ion can transfer the electron to oxygen to produce superoxide radical anion ($O_2^{\cdot-}$) or the radicals can further react to generate oxygenated species. In a Type II reaction, the excited photosensitizer directly transfers energy to the ground-state molecular oxygen without a radical ion intermediate to form singlet molecular oxygen ($^1O_2$). Common photosensitizers used in the practice of photodynamic therapy (PDT) include porphyrins, chlorins and dyes. These photosensitizers may be synthesized or induced endogenously in the heme biosynthetic pathway, such as 5-aminolevulinic acid (5-ALA)-induced protoporphyrin IX (PpIX). There are several reviews summarizing the history, development, and types of photosensitizers for PDT.[3,4]

Since Dougherty first reported successful PDT in a large cohort of cancer patients in 1978,[5] over 250 PDT clinical trials have been conducted to treat different types of cancer.[6,7] Photosensitizers are typically given to cancer patients or animals *via* intravenous injection, topical application, and oral administration. Out of the 17 completed cancer PDT clinical trials that were recently supported by NIH or other U.S. Federal agencies, 10 involved intravenous injections of photosensitizers, 5 delivered photosensitizers topically, and 2 administered photosensitizers orally (ClinicalTrials.gov). While intravenous injection remains the mainstream route of photosensitizer administration for cancer (i.e., accounts for 12 out of 24 of the ongoing trials), alternative photosensitizer injection routes, such as intratumoral (NCT04552990) and intravesical (NCT03945162) injections, are also starting to gain traction in clinical practices (Fig. 1). The most common intravenous photosensitizers include porfimer sodium (Photofrin®), WST-11 (TOOKAD® Soluble), verteporfin (Visudyne®, HS-201), temoporfin (tetra[m-hydroxyphenyl]chlorin, m-THPC, or Foscan®), and 2-(1-hexyloxyethyl)-2-devinyl pyropheophorbide-a (HPPH or Photochlor®) (Fig. 2). While topical and oral administration

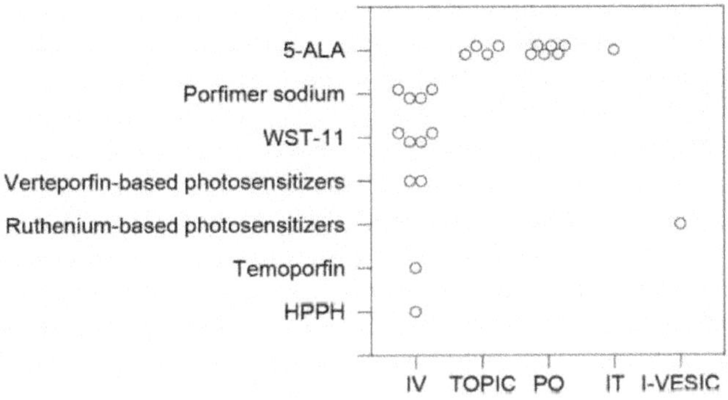

Fig. 1. Summary of photosensitizer administration routes for photodynamic therapy of cancer in clinical trials that are published by the U.S. National Library of Medicine.

Data collected from the clinicaltrials.gov website show different photosensitizers (y-axis) and their respective administration routes (x-axis). Each dot in the plot represents a clinical trial that is Active (not recruiting), Enrolling by invitation, Recruiting, or Not yet recruiting. Our summary indicates a majority of photosensitizers are currently administered intravenously in the clinic, with the exception of 5-ALA. In the plot, clinical trials that are Suspended, Terminated, Completed, Withdrawn, or have Unknown status were not included. Photosensitizers include 5-aminolevulinic acid (5-ALA or Gliolan®), porfimer sodium (Photofrin®), WST-11 (TOOKAD® Soluble), verteporfin-based PS (e.g., Visudyne®, HS-201), ruthenium-based PS (TLD1433), temoporfin (tetra[m-hydroxyphenyl]chlorin, m-THPC, or Foscan®), and 2-(1-hexyloxyethyl)-2-devinyl pyropheophorbide-a (HPPH or Photochlor®). Routes of administration include intravenous (IV, administration within or into a vein or veins), topical (TOPIC, administration to a particular spot on the outer surface of the body), oral (PO, administration to or by way of the mouth), intratumoral (IT, administration within a tumor), and intravesical (I-VESIC, administration within the bladder).

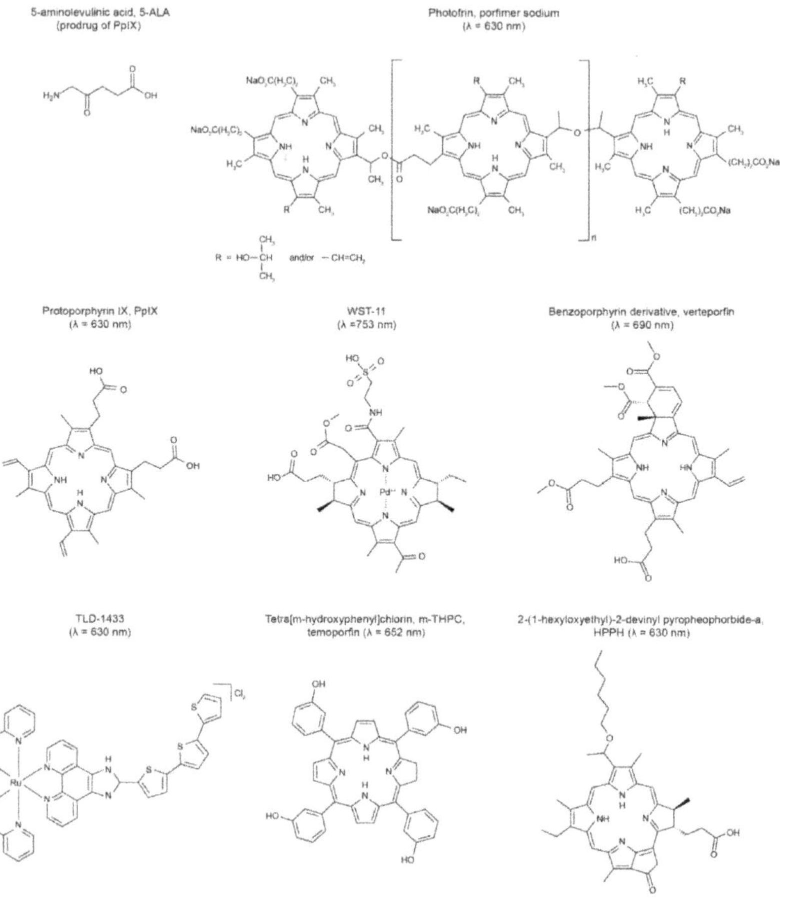

Fig. 2. Chemical structures of clinically used photosensitizers described in Figure 1.

All the listed photosensitizers, besides the ruthenium-based photosensitizer TLD-1422, contain the tetrapyrrole macrocycle structure. The porphyrin-based photosensitizers (e.g., Photofrin®, protoporphyrin IX) typically have a ring structure with 22 π-electrons, while the chlorin-type photosensitizer (i.e., tetra[m-hydroxyphenyl]chlorin) has one reduced double bond. These photosensitizers absorb light at red and near-infrared wavelengths, allowing for maximum penetration of light through tissues.

of 5-aminolevulinic acid (5-ALA or Gliolan®) are broadly accepted due to their simplicity, safety, convenience, and cost effectiveness, other groups have also demonstrated the feasibility and benefits (e.g., reduced skin phototoxicity) of intravenous[8] and intravesical[9] 5-ALA injections *in vivo*.

Advances in photosensitizer formulation, surgical device design, and light applicators[10] are creating tremendous opportunities to broaden photosensitizer injection routes to include intraperitoneal, intra-arterial, and intratumoral administrations. Intraperitoneal (or intracavitary) injection method has been reported to increase intratumoral photosensitizer concentrations compared to intravenous injection.[11–14] With significant progress being made towards antibody-photosensitizer conjugates (also known as photo-immunoconjugates),[15–18] we[19,20] and others[21,22] have shown that photo-immunoconjugates improve the selectivity and safety of photosensitizers, achieving a tumor-to-normal tissue ratio (T/N) of around 9–13 in ovarian cancer mouse models[19,21] and reducing bowel phototoxicity.[21] Additionally, there have been key innovations in the development of photosensitizing biomolecules,[18,23] light scattering agents, and intracavitary balloon catheter light applicators[24–28] that, together with advances in photo-immunoconjugates, make intraperitoneal photosensitizer delivery a more promising route of administration in clinical practice.[29]

Intra-arterial administration is another potential strategy to selectively deliver photosensitizers to diseased sites and reduce the drug-light interval (i.e., waiting time of light illumination after photosensitizer injection). The feasibility of intra-arterial photosensitizer injection has been demonstrated in veterinary medicine using canine[30,31] and swine models.[32] For example, Moore *et al.* showed that intra-arterial infusion selectively delivers lipid-formulated QLT0074 photosensitizers to the prostate with photosensitizer concentrations up to 18 times higher than that in the surrounding bladder, rectum and urethral tissues.[33] In a canine case study with adenocarcinoma of the left paranasal sinus, the combination of PDT with oral administration of 5-aminolevulinic acid and intra-arterial injection of chemotherapy (carboplatin and doxorubicin) achieved complete remission and long-term survival ($\sim$2 years) after initial disease presentation.[34] In view of these results, further clinical studies are warranted to evaluate the intra-arterial injection of photosensitizers and chemotherapy for PDT-based combination treatments.

2. Benefits and challenges of intratumoral photosensitizer injection

Intratumoral injection is particularly appealing for PDT of locally advanced, unresectable solid tumors.[35] First, directly injecting photosensitizers into a tumor can shorten the drug-light interval from a day to an hour[36] and reduce phototoxicity to normal tissues (e.g., skin), which are current drawbacks of intravenous photosensitizer injection.[1] Second, with growing clinical interest in interstitial PDT[37] and endoscopic ultrasound-guided PDT,[38,39] where one or more laser fibers are inserted into the tumor and/or margins, photosensitizers could potentially be delivered intratumorally immediately prior to optical fibers insertion through the same puncture or endoscopic approach. Finally, the use of nano-biomaterials[40,41] could further improve the distribution and retention of intratumorally injected photosensitizer, enhancing the safety, reliability, and efficacy of PDT. While direct intratumoral injections have significant advantages in photosensitizer delivery, several challenges remain to be addressed: (1) backflow (or retrograde flow) of photosensitizers along the catheter, (2) poor distribution, low retention, and quenching of photosensitizers within the tumor, (3) reabsorption of photosensitizers into the bloodstream, (4) lack of methods to quantitatively image photosensitizer distribution and concentrations, and (5) limited treatment efficacy with monotherapy. The following sections will provide examples of how novel formulations of photosensitizers, innovative light delivery systems, and PDT-based combination therapies could mitigate some of these challenges.

Intratumoral administration of photosensitizer-loaded nanoparticles to improve distribution and retention has been studied *in vivo* for many years. Liposomal photosensitizer is one of the most studied nanoformulations for PDT.[42–45] D'Hallewin *et al.* showed that intratumoral injection of liposomal formulation of meta-tetra(hydroxyphenyl)chlorin (Foslip®, 25 μL of 0.15 mg/mL) resulted in minimum reabsorption of meta-tetra(hydroxyphenyl)chlorin into the bloodstream (maxed at 1.5 ng/mg).[44] Using intratumorally injected Foslip® and a drug-light interval of 24 hours, around 70% of the tumor was necrotic after PDT. While light activation of

Foslip® did not result in a total cure likely due to the heterogeneous photosensitizer distribution, the authors suggested that repeated PDT sessions might be beneficial. Other organic and inorganic nanoparticles, such as polymeric nanoparticles,[46,47] upconversion nanoconstructs,[48,49] silica nanoparticles,[50,51] and gold nanoparticles[52,53] are also promising for intratumoral administration of photosensitizers and PDT. For example, Hu *et al.* showed that zeolite nanocarriers co-packaged with catalase and methylene blue photosensitizer improve intratumoral photosensitizer delivery and singlet oxygen yield for enhanced PDT outcomes.[54] Specifically, adding 0.05 mg/mL of catalase into methylene blue-loaded zeolite nanocarriers improved the singlet oxygen yield by approximately 3.7-fold upon light activation (635 nm, 50 mW/cm^2, 5 min). Using a xenograft mouse model of human SW1990 pancreatic cancer, the authors also showed that zeolite nanocarriers decrease the diffusion rate and increase the retention time of methylene blue in tumors by nearly 3-fold. Light activation of zeolite nanocarriers loaded with catalase and methylene blue completely inhibited tumor growth for 18 days and achieved 100% morbidity-free survival. Pluronic (F127) nanocomposite hydrogels have also been used to prolong the retention of micellar pyropheophorbide a (PPa) and imidazole derivative in 4T1 murine breast tumors. The pluronic composite gel increased the retention of PPa for up to 14 days and improved PDT-induced tumor growth inhibition by 54% compared to intratumorally injected PPa, which was cleared after 4 days with PDT-induced tumor growth inhibition of only ~28%.[55]

3. Implantable light sources and combination approaches for intratumoral photosensitizer injection

In addition to novel photosensitizer formulations that improve distribution and retention in target tissues, there have been recent developments in implantable light delivery systems that can perform repeated PDT. Clinically, light has been successfully delivered through chronically implantable balloon catheter systems to activate the photosensitizers for PDT.[24–28] Preclinically, Bansal *et al.* showed that a wireless light-emitting diode (LED) could be implanted near the MB49 bladder tumors to activate intratumorally injected chlorin e6 photosensitizers in mice.[56] Using wireless light delivery, two cycles of PDT suppressed MB49 tumor growth *in vivo* for 15 days. Multi-cycle PDT could be used to manage tumor burden post-surgery, particularly for residual or recurrent tumors.

It is increasingly evident that the most effective cancer treatments will likely involve a combination approach targeting multiple non-overlapping tumor growth and survival pathways. Photodynamic therapy and priming have been repeatedly shown to potentiate the efficacy of chemotherapy,[57–60] immunotherapy,[61–64] and biological agents.[11,65,66] We believe that intratumoral injection is an ideal method to deliver PDT-based combination regimen because the appropriate dosage can be optimized and easily controlled within a tumor for prolonged exposure. For example, Gupta *et al.* showed that nanoassemblies of anti-carcinoembryonic antigen (anti-CAE) monoclonal antibody and technetium-labeled hematoporphyrin derivative (PS-3) could be directly injected into murine Ehrlich ascites tumors for enhanced dye retention.[67] Tumor-selective accumulation of anti-CEA-PS-3 conjugates can be seen up to 2 hours after intratumoral administration. Non-specific diffusion of anti-CEA-PS-3 to the liver was observed at 6 hours after intratumoral injection and cleared from the system by 26 hours. No anti-CEA-PS-3 accumulation in muscle tissues was observed. Although PDT was not carried out in this study, these results suggest that cancer-targeted PDT can potentially be achieved soon after intratumoral administration of antibody-photosensitizer conjugates.

4. Future perspective: Is intratumoral photosensitizer injection an effective approach for global health PDT applications?

In low and middle-income countries (LMICs), where access to surgery, radiotherapy, and immunotherapy remains extremely limited, low-cost targeted therapies are desperately needed to reduce the global burden of cancer.[68] Currently, low-cost targeted therapies include cryoablation,[69–72] thermocoagulation,[71,73] and ethanol ablation,[74–77] which have been used to treat a variety of cancers, including cervical dysplasia,[69,71,73] breast tumors,[72] hepatocellular carcinoma,[74–76] thyroid tumors,[77] and renal tumors,[70] among others. However, these therapies are currently only used to treat superficial dysplasia or small tumors (< 3–5 cm in diameter) due to limited thermal diffusion[69,71] or poor retention of ethanol within tumors.[78,79] Recently, Morhard *et al.* demonstrated increased intratumoral retention of ethanol through: (1) slowing the infusion rate, which reduced backflow, and (2) adding the polymer ethyl cellulose to the injectate, which formed a gel in tissue, further improving retention of ethanol in a hamster cheek pouch model of oral squamous cell carcinoma.[80,81] These approaches could also enhance intratumoral delivery of low-cost photosensitizers for implementation of PDT in LMICs. Additionally, Mallidi *et al.* developed an inexpensive, portable, battery-powered LED light source for use in LMICs and found there was no significant differences in necrotic volume in a xenograft murine model of human squamous cell carcinoma when compared with a standard, high-cost laser source.[82]

In summary, intratumoral administration of photosensitizers could be achieved through minimally invasive techniques to significantly improve the T/N ratio, shorten the drug-light interval, and reduce any associated adverse events, compared to intravenous injection. Emerging intratumoral delivery platforms, such as nanoparticles and hydrogels, hold promise to further improve the retention and sustained delivery of photosensitizers, thereby enhancing the overall efficacy of PDT. With the development of low-cost light sources and intratumoral delivery of photosensitizers, PDT may provide an increasingly effective, yet affordable, method to treat cancer patients in both high-income countries and in LMICs.

Acknowledgments

This work is supported by the National Institutes of Health (NIH) R21EB028508 and R01CA260340 grants (H.H.) and the University of Maryland startup funds (H.H., J.M.).

References

1. J. P. Celli *et al.*, *Chem. Rev.* **110**, 2795 (2010).
2. M. S. Baptista *et al.*, *Photochem. Photobiol.* **93**, 912 (2017).
3. H. Abrahamse and M. R. Hamblin, *Biochem. J.* **473**, 347 (2016).
4. M. Lan *et al.*, *Adv. Healthc. Mater.* **8**, e1900132 (2019).
5. T. J. Dougherty *et al.*, *Cancer Res.* **38**, 2628 (1978).
6. D. Kessel, *J. Clin. Med.* **8**, 1581 (2019).
7. H. O. Alsaab *et al.*, *Cancers (Basel)* **12**, 2793 (2020).
8. C. S. Loh *et al.*, *Br. J. Cancer* **68**, 41 (1993).
9. S. C. Chang *et al.*, *Lasers Surg. Med.* **20**, 254 (1997).
10. S. H. Yun and S. J. J. Kwok, *Nat. Biomed. Eng.* **1**, 0008 (2017).
11. G. Cramer *et al.*, *Photochem. Photobiol.* **96**, 684 (2020).
12. R. R. Perry *et al.*, *Photochem. Photobiol.* **53**, 335 (1991).
13. R. B. Veenhuizen *et al.*, *Int. J. Cancer* **73**, 230 (1997).
14. K. A. Cengel, E. Glatstein and S. M. Hahn, *Cancer Treat. Res.* **134**, 493 (2007).
15. D. Mew *et al.*, *J. Immunol.* **130**, 1473 (1983).
16. M. Mitsunaga *et al.*, *Nat. Med.* **17**, 1685 (2011).
17. K. Sato *et al.*, *Sci. Transl. Med.* **8**, 352ra110 (2016).
18. C. T. Inglut *et al.*, *J. Clin. Med.* **8**, 1269 (2019).
19. H. C. Huang *et al.*, *Small* **2018**, e1800236 (2018).
20. B. J. Liang *et al.*, *J. Nanobiotechnol.* **18**, 1 (2020).
21. B. Q. Spring *et al.*, *Proc. Natl. Acad. Sci.* **111**, E933-E942 (2014).
22. M. D. Savellano and T. Hasan, *Photochem. Photobiol.* **77**, 431 (2003).
23. V. Almeida-Marrero *et al.*, *Chem. Soc. Rev.* **47**, 7369 (2018).
24. S. B. Tatter *et al.*, *J. Neurosurg.* **99**, 297 (2003).
25. J. S. Friedberg, *Ann. Cardiothorac. Surg.* **1**, 472 (2012).
26. C. B. Simone and K. A. Cengel, *Semin. Oncol.* **41**, 820 (2014).
27. M. T. Huggett *et al.*, *Br. J. Cancer* **110**, 1698 (2014).
28. W. F. Sindelar *et al.*, *Arch. Surg.* **126**, 318 (1991).
29. S. Xu *et al.*, *Cancers (Basel)* **12**, 2491 (2020).
30. Z. Xiao *et al.*, *J. Urol.* **178**, 308 (2007).
31. J. T. Abele *et al.*, *J. Vasc. Interv. Radiol.* **26**, 418 (2015).
32. M. P. Jenkins *et al.*, *Eur. J. Vasc. Endovasc. Surg.* **16**, 284 (1998).
33. R. B. Moore *et al.*, *Cardiovasc. Intervent. Radiol.* **31**, 164 (2008).
34. T. Osaki *et al.*, *Cancers (Basel)* **11**, 495 (2019).
35. Z. Huang *et al.*, *Technol. Cancer Res. Treat.* **7**, 309 (2008).
36. T. H. Foster *et al.*, *Transl. Oncol.* **3**, 135 (2010).
37. G. Shafirstein *et al.*, *Cancers (Basel)* **9**, 12 (2017).
38. J. M. DeWitt *et al.*, *Gastrointest. Endosc.* **89**, 390 (2019).
39. Y. Hanada *et al.*, *Gastrointest. Endosc.*, online ready (2021).
40. G. Obaid *et al.*, *Nanoscale* **8**, 12471 (2016).
41. H. C. Huang and T. Hasan, *Austin J. Nanomedicine Nanotechnol.* **2**, 1020 (2014).
42. M. R. Hamblin and E. L. Newman, *J. Photochem. Photobiol. B* **26**, 147 (1994).
43. E. Reddi *et al.*, *Br. J. Cancer*, **61**, 407 (1990).

44. M. A. D'Hallewin *et al.*, *Lasers Surg. Med.*, **40**, 543 (2008).
45. A. S. Derycke and P. A. de Witte, *Adv. Drug Deliv. Rev.* **56**, 17 (2004).
46. N. Zhang *et al.*, *Small* **12**, 5936 (2016).
47. O. M. Chepurna *et al.*, *J. Nanobiotechnology* **18**, 19 (2020).
48. M. K. Gnanasammandhan *et al.*, *Nat. Protoc.* **11**, 688 (2016).
49. W. Gao *et al.*, *Theranostics* **6**, 1131 (2016).
50. J. Peng *et al.*, *Biomaterials* **34**, 7905 (2013).
51. A. Ashkbar *et al.*, *Sci. Rep.* **10**, 21206 (2020).
52. G. Terentyuk *et al.*, *Nano Res.* **8**, 325 (2014).
53. H. C. Huang *et al.*, *Nano LIFE* **1**, 289 (2010).
54. D. Hu *et al.*, *Nanoscale* **10**, 17283–17292 (2018).
55. L. Luo *et al.*, *J. Control. Release* **298**, 99–109 (2019).
56. A. Bansal *et al.*, *Proc. Natl. Acad. Sci. USA* **115**, 1469 (2018).
57. H. C. Huang *et al.*, *Cancer Res.* **76**, 1066 (2016).
58. H. C. Huang *et al.*, *Cancer Res.* **78**, 558 (2018).
59. D. Luo *et al.*, *Biomaterials* **75**, 193 (2016).
60. C. T. Inglut *et al.*, *IEEE J. Sel. Top. Quantum Electron.* **27**, 7200311 (2021).
61. H. Saji *et al.*, *Clin. Cancer Res.*, **12**, 2568 (2006).
62. J. W. Kleinovink *et al.*, *Clin. Cancer Res.* **22**, 1459 (2016).
63. C. He *et al.*, *Nat. Commun.* **7**, 12499 (2016).
64. S. O. Gollnick and C. M. Brackett, *Immunol. Res.* **46**, 216 (2010).
65. S. M. Gallagher-Colombo *et al.*, *Cancer Res.* **75**, 3118 (2015).
66. B. Q. Spring *et al.*, *Photochem. Photobiol. Sci.* **14**, 1476 (2015).
67. S. Gupta *et al.*, *Technol. Cancer Res. Treat.* **3**, 295 (2004).
68. J. Ferlay *et al.*, *Int. J. Cancer*, **136**, E359 (2015).
69. J. Mariategui *et al.*, *Int J. Gynaecol. Obstet.* **100**, 24 (2008).
70. J. A. Cadeddu, *J. Urol.* **197**, 604 (2017).
71. M. Maza *et al.*, *J. Glob. Oncol.* **3**, 400 (2017).
72. C. Pusceddu *et al.*, *Breast Cancer: Targets and Therapy* **11**, 283 (2019).
73. L. Dolman *et al.*, *BJOG* **121**, 929 (2014).
74. M. Kuang *et al.*, *Radiology* **253**, 552 (2009).
75. M. Ebara *et al.*, *J. Hepatol.* **43**, 458 (2005).
76. G. T. Huang *et al.*, *Ann. Surg.* **242**, 36 (2005).
77. A. Heilo *et al.*, *J. Clin. Endocrinol. Metab.* **96**, 2750 (2011).
78. M. Koda *et al.*, *Gastrointest. Radiol.* **17**, 167 (1992).
79. A. Facciorusso, G. Serviddio and N. Muscatiello, *World J. Gastrointest. Pharmacol. Ther.* **7**, 477 (2016).
80. R. Morhard *et al.*, *Sci. Rep.* **7**, 8750 (2017).
81. R. Morhard *et al.*, *IEEE Trans. Biomed. Eng.* **67**, 2337 (2020).
82. S. Mallidi *et al.*, *J. Biomed. Opt.* **20**, 048003 (2015).

https://doi.org/10.1142/9789819809028_0013

Chapter 13

Nanoparticles in Joint Arthroplasties*

Rebecca J. Thomson[†], Afton K. Limberg[‡]
and Douglas W. Van Citters[§]

Thayer School of Engineering
Dartmouth College
15 Thayer Drive, Hanover, NH 03755, USA
[†]*rebecca.j.thomson.th@dartmouth.edu*
[‡]*afton.k.limberg.th@dartmouth.edu*
[§]*douglas.w.van.citters@dartmouth.edu*

Joint arthroplasty, specifically total knee arthroplasty (TKA) and total hip arthroplasty (THA), are two of the highest value surgical procedures. Over the last several decades, the materials utilized in these surgeries have improved and increased device longevity. However, with an increased incidence of TKA and THA surgeries in younger patients, it is crucial to make these materials more durable. The addition of nanoparticles is one technology that is being explored for this purpose. This review focuses on the addition of nanoparticles to the various parts of arthroplasty surgery comprising of the metallic, ceramic, or polyethylene components along with the bone cement used for fixation. Carbon additives proved to be the most widely studied, and could potentially reduce stress shielding, improve wear, and enhance the biocompatibility of arthroplasty implants.

Keywords: Total knee arthroplasty; total hip arthroplasty; polyethylene; carbon.

1. Introduction

Total joint arthroplasty is often described as one of the most successful elective surgical procedures when device longevity and patient

*To cite this article, please refer to its earlier version published in the *Nano LIFE*, Vol. 13, No. 1 (2023) 2330001 (12 pages), DOI: 10.1142/S1793984423300017
§Corresponding author.

satisfaction are concerned. The positive outcomes that come with a relatively low cost result in a high value operation for millions of patients annually. With an aging population, these procedures, specifically total knee arthroplasty (TKA) and total hip arthroplasty (THA) have become increasingly frequent. However, these surgeries are not faultless and can end in failure. The most common modes of failure include loosening of the implant, periprosthetic joint infection, wear, and pain.[1–3]

Traditionally total joint arthroplasty implants consist of a bearing couple of metal on polyethylene, metal on ceramic, metal on metal, or ceramic on ceramic.[4–6] Choosing the couple and the precise implant materials is an important consideration for surgeons when performing both TKA and THA. Each combination has advantages and disadvantages and can be chosen depending upon patient activity level, patient demographics, and material properties. The drawbacks associated with each of these materials have driven scientists and engineers to investigate the use of nanoparticles to improve their mechanical, tribological, and biological properties.

Nanoparticles, defined herein as materials with at least one dimension on the scale of 1–100 nm, are an evolving technology that are being incorporated into arthroplasty materials to improve on deficiencies leading to failure. The use of nanoparticles spans a wide range in arthroplasty, from improving antibiotic release in bone cement, to implant coatings for enhanced osteointegration, to carbon fiber composite implants to reduce stress shielding. The advancements in nanotechnology continue to push the boundaries in arthroplasty to improve patient outcomes. The present review shall focus on the use of nanoparticles in TKA and THA materials given the magnitude of these surgeries relative to other arthroplasty procedures. The objective is to orient the reader to the last decade of research directly related to these materials in arthroplasty, and identify key areas needed for progress in this field.

2. Methods

Two different databases, PubMed and Web of Science, were searched for articles relating to nanoparticles in joint arthroplasty. To ensure contemporary science was covered, only articles published from 1/1/2010 to 9/1/2022 were included in this review. All articles had to be available in English, and the full text had to be available. Articles studying wear particles coming from the implants were excluded.

The search terms relating to "nano-" were: nanoparticle, nanofiber, nanocomposite, nanostructure, nanocoating, carbon fiber, carbon-fiber, or metal nanoparticle. These terms were combined with arthroplasty specific search terms which included: bone cement, joint replacement, arthroplasty, unicondylar revision, implant, or joint arthroplasty. Finally, the search was limited by specifying the joint which for our search included shoulder, hip, knee, and ankle.

A total of 92 articles were reviewed. This included 12 review articles or book chapters relating to nanoparticles in the joint arthroplasty materials.

Additionally, it should be noted that carbon fiber, while not always on the nanoscale, was included for this review as this material has played a key role in the story of nanoparticles in joint arthroplasty materials. Moreover, the use of carbon fiber with smaller diameter continues to be investigated in the realm of orthopedics as it has promising mechanical and tribological properties.

3. Results

Literature review revealed that nanoparticles are incorporated into four classes of materials including coatings and lubricants, polymers, ceramics, and metals. Where found, biocompatibility results are highlighted though the reader will find that work remains to be done in this area.

3.1. *Coatings and lubricants*

Nanomaterials in coatings and lubricants for arthroplasty are dominated by reports on applications of carbon allotropes, titanium, and to a lesser extent degradable polymers.

Carbon is known to have many advantageous mechanical properties in the body as well as antibacterial characteristics. Additionally, diamond-like carbon coatings are being investigated for their use in orthopedics. These diamond-like coatings are proposed to reduce the wear of implants, hopefully leading to less loosening failures. The tribological properties of carbon coatings applied to both metal implants as well as polyethylene implants have been described.[7,8] These studies showed that the carbon coatings had no cytotoxic effects, and the addition of the coatings improved wear resistance compared to the traditional cobalt-chromium or titanium alloy and ultra-high molecular weight polyethylene (UHMWPE) interface. Total hip wear simulator tests have also shown decreased wear with nanocrystalline diamond coatings.[9] These authors also mention that the carbon coating could decrease the inflammation effects seen when wear particles are generated due to the bio-inertness of carbon. Furthermore, one study demonstrated the ability of nanodiamond particles to reduce the number of *Staphylococcus aureus* cultures *in vitro*, while also reducing friction at the metal–polymer implant interface.[10] Another study looking at the cytotoxicity of graphite nanoparticles that are generated by these diamond-like carbon coatings did notice significant dose-dependent effects *in vitro* when the wear particle biological load was over 30 μg/mL.[11] It will be important to keep this dose-dependent effect in mind as these coatings are further studied.

Kang *et al.* utilized finite element analysis (FEA) to evaluate weight loss under depth and kinematics under gait-loading conditions for four different surface properties including: nanostructured diamond, diamond-like carbon, titanium-nitride and oxidized zirconium.[12] From this analysis, the authors determined that oxidized zirconium had the lowest wear rate, weight loss, and wear depth of all the surface properties.

Other coatings that have been studied in the literature include hexavalent chromium electrolyte and C_{60} with the addition of fullerene nanoparticles both of which showed improved wear resistance but had limited literature sources.[13] Silver is another element that has been utilized as a coating material.[14,15] Silver has good antibacterial effects, however there is disagreement whether it can be toxic *in vivo*. Different methods for cytotoxicity studies have shown dissimilar results, and the toxicity may be related to the nanoparticle size.[16,17]

The addition of nanotubes to metallic implant surfaces is similarly being explored for improved bone interaction and infection treatment. First, nanotubes can promote osteointegration by providing an ingrowth surface for osteoblasts.[18,19] Both carbon and titanium nanotubes are being studied in this regard and several different implant materials have been analyzed including, ceramic, cobalt-chromium, and titanium. One study noted marginally better osteointegration with the titanium nanotubes over other candidates.[20] The authors hypothesized this could be due to the better organization of the titanium nanotubes compared to the carbon nanotubes. Titanium nanorods have also shown to promote osteointegration *in vitro*.[21]

With infection being one of the most complex and difficult to treat failure mechanisms in joint arthroplasty, the use of nanotubes for sensing, prevention, or treatment could provide new ways to approach this problematic complication. It is thought that severity of infection might be reduced if bacterial biofilms can be prevented. Carbon nanotubes have been shown to reduce the presence of these biofilms, specifically against methicillin-resistant *Staphylococcus aureus* biofilms.[22] After an infection sets in, the use of nanotubes has also been explored when integrated into a nanocomposite film for monitoring the pH of the joint via tomographic imaging to watch for pH changes that could relate to infection.[23] Finally, titanium nanotubes have been shown to assist with antibiotic release to treat periprosthetic joint infections [Fig. 1].[24]

Polymeric nanofiber coatings to treat infection are also being explored. Using a mouse model, one study looked at the effects of a PLGA coating that would provide local antibiotic delivery as well as prevent biofilm formation.[25] Electrospinning of PLGA and PCL to creates a lattice coating over the implant surface proved to have a significant antibiotic release over six weeks.[26]

3.2. *Structural polymers*

Polymers are a class of materials used in multiple aspects of arthroplasty procedures such as adhesion, bearings, and other structural components of the implants. Addition of nanoparticles to

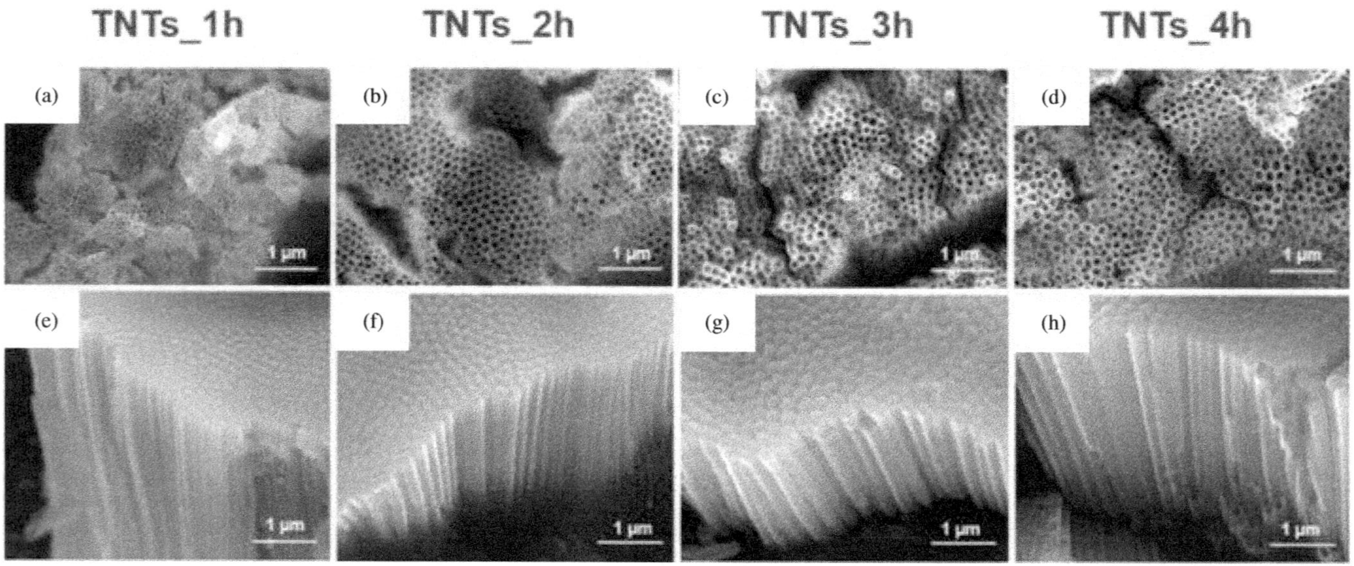

Fig. 1. FESEM micrographs of top and side views of titanium oxide nanotubes at 1 h, 2 h, 3 h, and 4 h from left to right. Pore diameters of nanotubes increased and length decreased when time of anodization increased.

Source: Adapted from Materials.[23]

polymers has been a continued effort to increase the strength, biocompatibility, and potential for application in human patients.

3.2.1. *Bone cement*

Poly-methyl methacrylate (PMMA) bone cement has been employed as a fixation material in joint arthroplasty since the very first total hip replacements. In addition to its ability to provide a stable union between the implant and surrounding bone, PMMA is employed as a delivery medium for antibiotics. This becomes particularly important during revision procedures for infected joints. Exploiting nanotechnology in bone cement has been studied in the context of its structural benefits and its drug-eluting character.

Wang *et al.* reported adding multiwalled carbon nanotubes (MWCNTs) to PMMA to increase osteointegration at the bone–cement interface. Both *in vitro* and *in vivo* animal studies have shown promising results wherein the weight percent of MWCNTs correlated with biocompatibility and osteointegration.[27] Positive outcomes are attributed to increased osteogenic differentiation of cells when exposed to the nanotubes as assessed at both the gene and protein levels. A notable benefit of this addition is that the PMMA composite density is decreased while mechanical properties such as hardness and elastic modulus increased.[28]

Antimicrobial nanoparticles such as gold and silver have also been considered as additives to bone cement. The main concern with this alternative to pharmaceuticals is whether the metals will affect the mechanical properties of the bone cement. One hypothesis is that the nanoparticles create weak points due to discontinuities in the cement structure. However, a lower weight percent of gold nanoparticles, on the order of 0.25 wt.%, did not significantly alter the compressive strength while exhibiting good antibacterial properties.[29] It should be noted that recent literature suggests that the antibacterial nature of silver is due more to the diffusive dynamics of the silver ions than the size of the particle itself. Instead, nanoparticles provide a very high surface area to volume ratio, maximizing the antibacterial activity.[30]

3.2.2. *Carbon fiber-reinforced polyether-ether-ketone*

Carbon fiber-reinforced polyether-ether-ketone (CFR-PEEK) has been investigated as an alternative to conventional UHMWPE and other bearing materials for many years. CFR-PEEK has many potentially beneficial characteristics such as reduction in wear particle volume, reduction in stress shielding, better bone-material mechanical property compatibility, and no risk of metal ion release. Many studies have investigated the biotribology, mechanical properties, wear particle biocompatibility, stress and strain distribution, and other properties of CFR-PEEK. Most contemporary articles revealed in the literature review focus on the wear properties and wear particle biocompatibility of CFR-PEEK compared to UHMWPE. Studies ranged from computational, to benchtop, to *in vivo* models.

In vivo testing for joint arthroplasties is expensive, time consuming, and inefficient. With increasing computational power, FEA models have increased in prevalence and accuracy for screening of new biomaterials in orthopedic applications. While computational wear prediction requires additional development, many validated models analyze von Mises and contact stresses. Despite fidelity of the models to experimental results, it should be warned that a limit of many of these models is the assumptions made about physiological parameters as well as the isotropy of materials and tissues.

CFR-PEEK has previously been reported to have higher wear resistance, hardness, and yield strength compared to standard UHMWPE, and this change can be attributed in part to the promotion of the thermoplastic matrix integration with the incorporated fibers.[31] Kwak *et al.* modeled the biomechanical effects of CFR-PEEK, PEEK, and UHMWPE on unicompartmental knee arthroplasties (UKAs) using von Mises stress evaluation to determine aseptic loosening and anteromedial pain in the tibia.[32] They concluded that CFR-PEEK could be used as an alternative to UHMWPE for tibial inserts due to it showing the lowest contact stress on lateral meniscus and tibial cartilage. Another study investigated the biomechanical effects of varus/valgus alignments of UHMWPE and CFR-PEEK from 9° of varus to 9° of valgus in UKAs.[33] For CFR-PEEK, the valgus condition should be avoided and varus conditions from 1° up to 6° showed similar biomechanical output and is recommended for UKA. A TKA FEA concluded that CFR-PEEK and PEEK could be used as alternate bearing materials but one should be cautious if planning to use either for a cruciate retaining TKA.[34]

In an alternative application for tumor-type distal-femoral prostheses, CFR-PEEK has the same stability as the CoCrMo but lower density, good light transmittance, and good mechanical fit which makes it a good alternative material for distal femur and extension rod for the distal femoral prosthesis.[35] Only limited FEA wear testing has been performed, with wear models built on mechanical properties of the material. These models have concluded that CFR-PEEK could be a good alternative, when looking at kinematics, wear depth, and volumetric wear, to UHMWPE for tibial inserts[33,36] [Fig. 2]. Such simulations failed to incorporate microscale and nanoscale interactions between the fibers and the matrix and the fibers and the counterface.

Owing to the complex motions and contact conditions associated with human joints, preclinical wear testing for eventual arthroplasty applications is more typically performed using pin-on-disk, ball-on-disk, and joint simulators. Grupp *et al.* looked at the *in vitro* biotribological behavior of CFR-PEEK as bushings and flanges in a rotating hinge knee with articulation on zirconium nitride (ZrN) multilayer surface coating.[37] At physiologic contact stresses, the wear rate was more than 10 times less with CFR-PEEK and ZrN compared to CFR-PEEK and CoCr. Given the significant metallic wear it was concluded that CFR-PEEK and CoCr should not be used in that

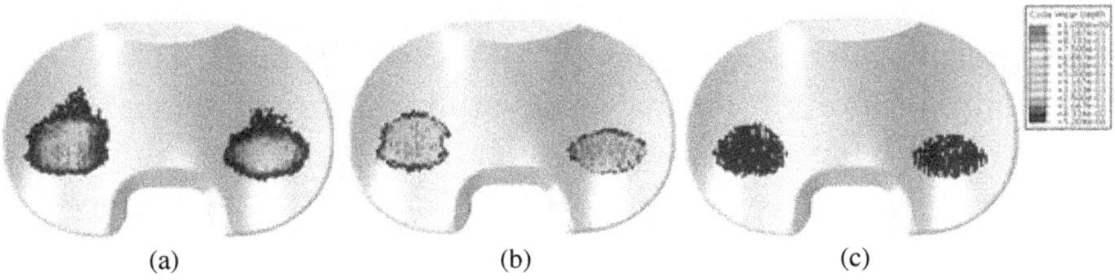

Fig. 2. FEA predicted wear depth for (a) UHMWPE, (b) PEEK, and (c) CFR-PEEK.

Source: Adapted from Lubricants.[36]

combination as an articular surface.[38] The higher wear rates were attributed to the enhanced hardness properties of the CFR-PEEK material, but the ZrN was sufficiently harder to guard against increased wear. Similarly, Grupp *et al.* conducted an *in vitro* wear simulation to determine suitability of CFR-PEEK materials for fixed bearing UKAs with low congruency. Wear rates between CFR-PEEK with two different carbon sources were not statistically different from one another but were high enough to conclude that they cannot be recommended for this application.[39] While the carbon fibers (diameter approximately 500–1000 nm) are cited as contributing to wear resistance of the composite material, the PEEK matrix could not be sufficiently protected during simulated walking.

Wear of the PEEK matrix in the prior studies may be related to the incomplete bonding of the matrix and the carbon fibers. Kyomoto *et al.* showed free radical production in PEEK under ultraviolet irradiation and the benzophenone (BP) units acted like photoinitiators that could control the "self-initiated" graft polymerization of poly(2-methacryloyloxyethyl phosphorylcholine) (PMPC).[40] Nanometer-scale photoinduced grafting of PMPC on both CFR-PEEK and neat PEEK improved frictional properties, wear resistance, and water wettability of surfaces and interfaces.[41] The wear resistance of PMPC-grafted CFR-PEEK hip liners was then tested against metal and ceramic heads. Similar to the prior studies, the authors showed that that zirconia-toughened alumina (ZTA) femoral heads revealed a significantly smoother surface compared to CoCrMo femoral heads after the hip simulator wear test. Again, the carbon filler served as a surface hard enough to abrade cobalt alloys typically used in arthroplasty. PMPC-grafted CFR-PEEK is a promising acetabular liner material and especially when combined with a ZTA femoral head.[42]

Despite promising results from studies like Kyomoto's, the significant metallic wear in other studies, high wear rates in pin-on-disc tests, and an increased likelihood of delamination failure suggest that CFR-PEEK is unlikely to see near-term use as a clinical bearing material in traditional articulation geometries.[38,43,44]

Many studies have explored the immunological reaction of *in vivo* models to CFR-PEEK wear particles. Lorber *et al.* analyzed the biological activity from wear particles of CFR-PEEK pitch and pan compared to UHMWPE in synovial fluid, bone marrow, and articular cartilage after injection into the joint.[45] There was an increased cytokine expression in adjacent bone marrow for both CFR-PEEK groups compared to UHMWPE and CFR-PEEK showed increased expression in articular cartilage. This resulted in proinflammatory potential of CFR-PEEK and was not recommended by the authors as a good alternative to UHMWPE for a bearing material. Grupp *et al.* also investigated *in vivo* biocompatibility with CFR-PEEK pitch and pan wear particles in mice to determine leukocyte or potential inflammatory tissue responses.[46] Synovial membrane thickening was caused after both CFR-PEEK were injected but no increased leukocyte activation or inflammatory tissue response compared to UHMWPE was seen. Another study showed similar results that CFR-PEEK wear particles did not increase the inflammatory response.[47] One study analyzed human synovial fluid with CFR-PEEK and UHMWPE wear debris in 10 patients undergoing rotating-hinge-knee implant revision surgery. CFR-PEEK was not the bearing material so there was a different wear mechanism that caused wear debris compared to the UHMWPE tibial insert. UHMWPE particles were scattered throughout the tissue while CFR-PEEK particles were agglomerated near various vessels but showed no giant-cell reactions [Fig. 3].[48]

Rotating-hinge-knee implants have become a more common use for CFR-PEEK in arthroplasty. An *in vitro* study showed that both CFR-PEEK composites had high polymeric wear rate compared to neat PEEK and UHMWPE, and CFR-PEEK pitch fibers had the worst wear resistance.[49] However, CFR-PEEK has been used *in vivo* as flexion bushings and flanges and studies have followed various retrieval analyses. Schierjott *et al.* examined the CFR-PEEK matrix worn out and fibers exposed both *in vitro* and in retrievals collected from revision surgeries.[50] However, EndRo, a new modular design using CFR-PEEK flanges and bushings resulted in good functional, radiologic, and clinical performances at a short-term follow-up.[51] Another study also showed positive results after looking at a longer-term clinical follow-up from complex primary and revision TKAs.[52]

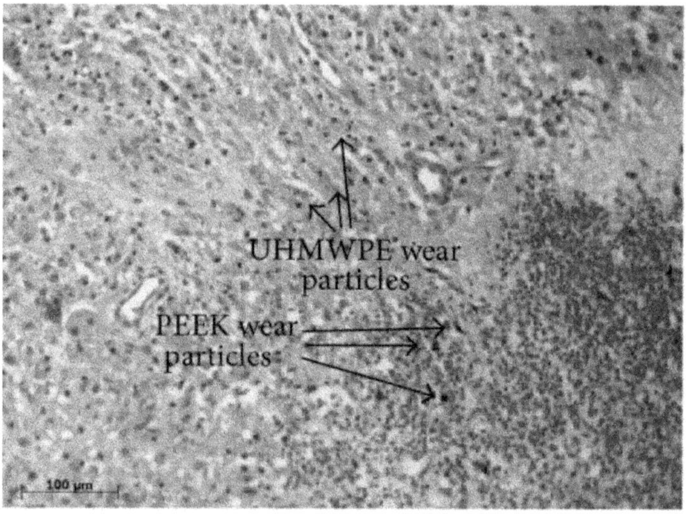

Fig. 3. UHMWPE and PEEK wear particles stained with hematoxylin and eosin.
Source: Adapted from BioMed Research International.[48]

Outside of bearing materials, CFR-PEEK has been indicated for structural applications including hip stems owing to a potentially better bone-implant compatibility and match in mechanical properties. Nakahara *et al.* observed, in an *in vivo* study, there was no obvious damage in the retrieved CFR-PEEK stem but saw corrosion and fretting in other stems; the taper connection between the CFR-PEEK and ceramic head was more secure.[53] Another *in vivo* model showed varying degrees of stress shielding on the hip stems and saw some bone ingrowth on the cementless cups.[54] Another study also saw stress shielding but concluded that a more flexible stem significantly lowers the stress shielding around the femoral bone.[55]

Similarly, FEA testing of acetabular components in total hip arthroplasties largely concluded that CFR-PEEK could be a potential as both a shell and acetabular liner.[31,56,57] All studies appeared preliminary and cautioned that more testing was needed to make full conclusions about CFR-PEEK as an alternative to UHMWPE or conventional metallic shells. However, results from the previously reported knee studies suggest that wear studies of hip articulations will not be successful in the absence of a hard femoral head that is either all ceramic or coated in some way.

3.2.3. *High-density polyethylene*

Although high-density polyethylene (HDPE) is not common in arthroplasty surgeries given inferior mechanical and tribological properties compared to UHMWPE, some scientists have hypothesized that the mechanical and tribological properties could be optimized with the addition of nanoparticles. The most widespread nanoparticle added to HDPE has been nanographene. There are several advantages of these polymer composite materials over neat UHMWPE including: moldability, low density, high corrosion resistance, and low cost.[58] The addition of graphene oxide powder to HDPE has exhibited improved wear and fatigue properties. All studies reviewed reported uniform distribution of the particles throughout the material up to 2.5 wt.%, with little to no agglomerations observed. Additionally, these nanoparticles also act against bacteria, are biocompatible, and can be sustainably produced.[58–60]

More recently, MWCNTs have been added to HDPE and aluminum oxide to create a nanocomposite hip stem. The authors reported low cytotoxicity and increased hardness with the inclusion of carbon nanotubes.[61] In addition, nanoparticles added to polyethylene utilized in shoulder joint arthroplasty to create bio-composite materials are also being studied with a rationale that these materials could improve soft tissue healing.[62]

3.2.4. *Ultra-high molecular weight polyethylene*

UHMWPE is currently the most used articular surface material for all joint arthroplasties. Carbon fibers have previously been combined with UHMWPE with detrimental results attributed to poor matrix integration, oxidation, and subsequent release of fibers.[63] Nanoparticles, most commonly MWCNTs and single-walled carbon nanotubes (SWCNTs), have been added to UHMWPE with the intention to improve tribological and mechanical properties. Other additives consist of biocompatible epoxies, chopped carbon fiber, and alumina.

SWCNTs have been investigated for arthroplasty application in combination with UHMWPE due to reported biocompatibility, corrosion resistance, and low wear debris. One study examined functionalized SWCNT-UHMWPE composite manufacturing and mechanical properties for the use in UKA.[64] Two composites were developed to enhance biocompatibility and mechanical properties when using single-point incremental forming (SPIF) process to manufacture unicompartmental knees. These composites had improved tensile properties, maintained 90% osteoblast viability, and promoted osteogenic differentiation more than neat.[64]

MWCNTs were used in one study to compare wear properties and biocompatibility against neat and cross-linked UHMWPE.[65] The MWCNT-UHMWPE composite was comparable in wear resistance to cross-linked UHMWPE and to noncross-linked UHMWPE in terms of impact resistance. The composite also showed no adverse biological effects and complied with requirements of biosafety testing. An additional study looked at the potential for a MWCNT-UHMWPE composite as a piezoresistive sensing material.[66] An analytical model was built to estimate the ideal depth from the tibio-femoral contact surface where an embedded sensor could attain the highest stress resolution and smallest distortion energy. The results showed resistance of MWCNT-UHMWPE composites exponentially decreased under applied stress and could be used as a piezoresistive sensing material.

Carbon fibers mixed into UHMWPE were investigated to understand the impact of the composite in lowering stress intensities and specific wear rates. Ramesh and Shashishekar used FEA to look at the design of flexion angle and sagittal radius of a tibial insert for prosthetic knees.[67] The goal was to minimize stresses at knee interfaces through chopped carbon fiber integration to ensure high performance knee joints. It was found that the alumina ceramic and UHMWPE-chopped carbon fiber combination had the lowest stress levels of the different variations. Additionally, Baliga *et al.* studied the synthesis and wear characterization of UHMWPE-carbon nanofiber (CNF) composites.[68] This showed composites mixed with paraffin processing improved the distribution of CNFs and lowered the specific wear rate compared to neat UHMWPE but not significant enough yet to be a competitor against the standard cross-linked polyethylene.

Ceramic-UHMWPE nanocomposites show promise in laboratory tests. UHMWPE-Al_2O_3 with 3 wt.% Al_2O_3 (20 nm) was compared to neat UHMWPE and UHMWPE-Al_2O_3 after mechanical activation in a ball mill for potential use for damaged cartilage replacement.[69] Mechanical properties such as compression and wear resistance were tested. UHMWPE-Al_2O_3 after activation showed improved mechanical properties, attributed to better interactions of the nanoparticles with the polymer matrix after mechanical treatment. UHMWPE-Al_2O_3 after activation was then implanted in rats which showed no signs of inflammation, cellular infiltration destruction of the material, or bone-cartilage defects.

3.2.5. *Polyamide*

Beyond bearing surfaces, composite materials are of interest in joint arthroplasty due to the ability to tune mechanical properties to be closer to bone than neat polymers or monolithic metals. One of the largest concerns with replacing a joint surface with high modulus materials is stress shielding of the underlying bone, leading to bone resorption and potentially mechanical failure. The suitability of polyamide in combination with carbon fiber as a support structure has been studied in a few computational models. These studies concluded that indeed the composite implants reduced stress shielding compared to their metal counterparts, which would theoretically lead to less bone loss over time.[70,71] The carbon fibers serve to create a more biomimetic implant, which is hypothesized to facilitate the load transfer at the bone–implant interface, and therefore reduce bone loss. Interestingly, one computational study found that there was more dense trabeculae near the implant when using a composite stem compared to both cobalt-chromium and titanium alloy stems.[72] However, dynamic-loading conditions will require further studies to ensure that the carbon fibers can also prevent fatigue crack propagation rather than provide pathways for crack travel along poorly integrated fibers.

3.3. *Ceramics*

Ceramic materials have long been utilized in arthroplasty surgeries, particularly as femoral heads in THA surgery and some femoral components in TKA surgery. The wettability and compression strength of ceramics make them well suited to serve as highly loaded bearings. Importantly, the high hardness of ceramics allows for creation of a durable surface with very low roughness. The surface itself doesn't wear, and when articulated against polymer bearings, it produces less wear particles, making it less likely to manifest osteolysis *in vivo*.[73]

Early ceramics demonstrated an increased risk of fracture *in vivo*, due in part to their decreased toughness in comparison to metals.[74] For nearly two decades, the most common ceramic in use in the USA has been an yttrium stabilized ZTA incorporating chromium oxide and strontium nanoparticles for additional resistance to crack propagation. More recently, different nanoparticles have been added to ceramic materials to further improve their biocompatibility and fracture toughness. Several studies have demonstrated decreased cytotoxicity and increased mechanical properties with the adjunct of these nanoparticles including zinc oxide and graphene.[75–77] A few studies have also explored the processing of ceramic nanomaterials including rapid sintering and CO_2 laser co-vaporization.[78,79] The theoretical hardness increase associated with the Hall–Petch relationship does not appear to be limited by increased brittleness owing to the nanomaterials' ability to prevent crack propagation.

3.4. *Other/Metals*

For decades most of the THA and TKA components that interact with bone (tibia and femur), have been made of titanium or cobalt alloys. Using nanoparticles to decrease the modulus of these metals could potentially reduce the aforementioned stress shielding and improve biocompatibility. For instance, composite hip stems combining a titanium alloy with carbon fiber exhibited good results at 10 years post-op in a randomized clinical trial in Northern Ireland.[80] The authors analyzed bone mineral density and found patients with the composite stem had retained more proximal femoral bone stock compared to the metal stem group. The carbon fibers serve to provide appropriate toughness to the otherwise notch-sensitive titanium. The addition of a graphene coating on titanium implants has also been explored to improve biocompatibility although the pathway of how graphene affects bone marrow cells warrants further investigation.[81]

3.5. *Biocompatibility concerns*

This review focused on the mechanical, tribological, antibiotic, and lubrication properties of nanoparticles in arthroplasties, however, biocompatibility is of paramount concern when considering implantation of these materials. By design, this review focused on intentional incorporation of nanoparticles into materials rather than their generation through wear or failure of a device. The biological impact of these unintentional particles on the human host is well characterized. However, most of the papers included in the review focused on material properties without considering cytotoxicity, endotoxicity, carcinogenicity, and teratogenicity.

Nonetheless, several reviewed articles did include biocompatibility tests as discussed in each section and summarized here. For coatings and lubricants, several of the studies included in this section examined a combination of cellular toxicity, cellular behavior, and/or biofilm resistance as it related to the nanoparticles of interest.[8,10,11,14,19–22,25,81] Additionally, a few of the articles dealing with nanoparticle additives to bone cement also addressed biocompatibility or antibacterial properties utilizing *in vitro* studies.[27,29] Fouad *et al.* evaluated the cytotoxicity of graphite nanoparticles added to HDPE.[60] Finally, for nanoparticle additives to ceramics, a few articles analyzed cytotoxicity and *in vitro* biocompatibility.[76,77,82] As discussed in Sec. 3.2.2, CFR-PEEK composite biocompatibility has been investigated through various *in vivo* studies. Lorber *et al.* discussed the cytotoxicity in the synovial joint fluid, bone marrow, and articular cartilage.[45] CFR-PEEK and UHMWPE particles have been injected as whole particles as well as wear particulates after an *in vivo* study has been completed.[45–52] To create a more holistic investigation, long-term carcinogenicity and endotoxicity studies must be completed. Additionally, degradation and the subsequent excretion pathways by which these nanoparticles are excised warrants further investigation.

In support of this work, an additional search for review articles concerning biocompatibility in the orthopedic space netted no new articles. However, biocompatibility of individual nanoparticles, not composites, was found. Carbon nanotube biocompatibility has been reviewed by Aoki and Saito and while there have been questions raised around possible carcinogenicity, there has been no clear evidence of neoplasms in mouse models other than inconclusive results with inhalation studies.[83] Similar to conclusions around biocompatibility in this review, varying results have been reported in other reviews and a continuation of such work must be performed before this nanotechnology could be employed in clinical settings. At larger scale, carbon in fiber form in orthopedics has been reported to exhibit good biocompatibility while the mechanical properties are still not matched for intended applications.[84] Overall, we conclude that the biological aspects of nanotechnology in knee and hip arthroplasty are insufficiently studied and reported.

4. Discussion

An aging population and increased acceptance of joint replacement as an early intervention for joint pain has led to a significant increase in the number of TKA and THA surgeries worldwide. More medical devices implanted at earlier life stages will require improvements in implant material durability realized through innovation in materials science. Nanoparticles are one avenue that have shown promise in several preliminary studies, although more holistic studies are needed prior to these technologies being adopted systematically. While no one material appears ready for clinical implementation, the present review reveals carbon additives to be at the forefront of the field. Multiple approaches showing promise appear to result in reduction in stress shielding, increased osteointegration, and the potential to reduce wear. The current literature review reveals that significantly more research should be performed before these materials can be advanced to human trials.

Despite the knowledge base incorporated in this review, scientific gaps remain. *In vivo* experiments, in animals and particularly in humans, are frequently referenced as the next necessary step of progression. Along with *in vivo* studies, the literature base is deficient with respect to (1) the impact of nanocarbon particles on bacterial infections, (2) expansion of FEA model parameters to address inclusion of nanoscale and microscale interactions in composites, and (3) experimental validation. Additionally, while the focus of most research works is knee and hip arthroplasty on account of their significant market share and societal expense, shoulder and ankle arthroplasty procedures are increasing in frequency but have different load and motion patterns than other joints. Biomaterials research for these applications is less mature and warrants more investigation.

4.1. *Limitations*

This study is not without limitations. First, this review was limited to investigating nanoparticles in joint replacement. This particular search strategy required cited materials to identify potential applications of a technology to joint arthroplasty. It is acknowledged that some materials at earlier technology readiness levels may well be positioned for use in human joints but not yet identified as such in the literature base. Further, because arthroplasty was specified, studies examining nanoparticles in joints, but related to ligaments, cartilage repair, or tissue regeneration were excluded. While studies investigating nanoparticles generated as wear debris were excluded, the authors recognize this is a large field of important research with potential to inform biological reaction to nanoparticles evolved from biomaterials outside of wear mechanisms. During the investigation into biocompatibility, holistic review articles on nanocomposite materials in orthopedics were lacking or outdated. Finally, nanoparticles for drug delivery applications were also not included.

Acknowledgements

All authors are supported in part by the NH EPSCoR NH BioMade Project awarded by the National Science Foundation's Research Infrastructure Improvement Award #1757371. Any opinion, findings, and conclusions or recommendations expressed in this material are those of the author(s) and do not necessarily reflect the views of the National Science Foundation. The authors would like to thank Jentry Campbell for assistance in conducting the holistic search in this review.

References

1. I. N. Ackerman, L. Busija, M. Lorimer, R. D. Steiger and S. E. Graves, *Bone Joint J.* **104-B**, 613 (2022), doi: 10.1302/0301-620x.104b5.Bjj-2021-1219.R1.
2. P. L. Lewis, A. W-Dahl, O. Robertsson, H. A. Prentice and S. E. Graves, *Acta Orthop.* **93**, 623 (2022), doi: 10.2340/17453674.2022.3512.
3. C. J. Wall, C. J. Vertullo, S. Kondalsamy-Chennakesavan, M. F. Lorimer and R. N. D. Steiger, *J. Bone Joint Surg. Am.* **104**, 1386 (2022), doi: 10.2106/jbjs.21.01491.
4. J. H. Currier, D. E. Anderson and D. M. V. Citters, *Wear* **269**, 782 (2010), https://doi.org/10.1016/j.wear.2010.08.006.
5. N. Kumar, G. N. Arora and B. Datta, *Med. J. Armed Forces India* **70**, 371 (2014), doi: 10.1016/j.mjafi.2014.04.015.
6. F. E. Kennedy, B. H. Currier, D. W. V. Citters, J. H. Currier, J. P. Collier and M. B. Mayor, *Tribol. Trans.* **46**, 111 (2003), doi: 10.1080/10402000 308982607.
7. B. Rothammer *et al.*, *Polymers (Basel)* **13** (2021), doi: 10.3390/polym13111880.
8. B. Rothammer *et al.*, *Polymers (Basel)* **13** (2021), doi: 10.3390/polym13121952.
9. M. M. Maru *et al.*, *J. Mech. Behav. Biomed. Mater.* **49**, 175 (2015), doi: 10.1016/j.jmbbm.2015. 05.005.
10. A. Shirani, Q. Hu, Y. Su, T. Joy, D. Zhu and D. Berman, *ACS Appl. Mater. Interfaces* **11**, 43500 (2019), doi: 10.1021/acsami.9b14904.
11. T. T. Liao *et al.*, *Biomed. Mater.* **12**, 015018 (2017), doi: 10.1088/1748-605X/aa52ca.
12. K. T. Kang, J. Son, H. J. Kim, C. Baek, O. R. Kwon and Y. G. Koh, *J. Mater. Sci. Mater. Med.* **28**, 105 (2017), doi: 10.1007/s10856-017-5916-5.
13. R. Sonntag, K. Feige, C. B. D. Santos and J. P. Kretzer, *Materials (Basel)* **10** (2017), doi: 10.3390/ma10121449.
14. N. Kose, A. Otuzbir, C. Pekşen, A. Kiremitçi and A. Doğan, *Clin. Orthop. Relat. Res.* **471**, 2532 (2013), doi: 10.1007/s11999-013-2894-x.
15. C. F. Alves, F. Oliveira, I. Carvalho, A. P. Piedade and S. Carvalho, *Mater. Sci. Eng. C, Mater. Biol. Appl.* **34**, 22 (2014), doi: 10.1016/j.msec.2013. 09.031.
16. E. M. Sussman, B. J. Casey, D. Dutta and B. J. Dair, *J. Appl. Toxicol.* **35**, 631 (2015), doi: 10.1002/jat.3104.

17. S. Castiglioni, A. Cazzaniga, L. Locatelli and J. A. M. Maier, *Nanomaterials (Basel)* **7** (2017), doi: 10.3390/nano7060124.
18. E. G. Zemtsova, N. M. Yudintceva, P. E. Morozov, R. Z. Valiev, V. M. Smirnov and M. A. Shevtsov, *Int. J. Nanomed.* **13**, 2175 (2018), doi: 10.2147/ijn. S161292.
19. C. J. Frandsen, K. Noh, K. S. Brammer, G. Johnston and S. Jin, *Mater. Sci. Eng. C, Mater. Biol. Appl.* **33**, 2752 (2013), doi: 10.1016/j.msec.2013. 02.045.
20. D. V. Portan, D. D. Deligianni, K. Deligianni, A. A. Kroustalli, M. Tyllianakis and G. C. Papanicolaou, *J. Biomed. Mater. Res. A* **106**, 621 (2018), doi: 10.1002/jbm.a.36265.
21. X. Lin *et al.*, *J. Nanosci. Nanotechnol.* **15**, 3893 (2015), doi: 10.1166/ jnn.2015.9275.
22. S. R. Morco, D. L. Williams, B. D. Jensen and A. E. Bowden, *J. Orthop. Res.* **40**, 1953 (2022), doi: 10. 1002/jor.25206.
23. S. Gupta and K. J. Loh, *Procedia Eng.* **188**, 110 (2017).
24. H. T. Chunate *et al.*, *Materials (Basel)* **14** (2021), doi: 10.3390/ma14216576.
25. A. G. Ashbaugh *et al.*, *Proc. Natl. Acad. Sci. USA* **113**, E6919 (2016), doi: 10.1073/pnas.1613 722113.
26. F. Jahanmard *et al.*, *J. Control. Release* **326**, 38 (2020), doi: 10.1016/j. jconrel.2020.06.014.
27. C. Wang *et al.*, *Mater. Sci. Eng. C, Mater. Biol. Appl.* **103**, 109823 (2019), doi: 10.1016/j.msec. 2019.109823.
28. S. Arun and S. Kanagaraj, *J. Mech. Behav. Biomed. Mater.* **50**, 33 (2015), doi: 10.1016/j.jmbbm. 2015.06.002.
29. T. Russo *et al.*, *Bioact. Mater.* **2**, 156 (2017), doi: 10.1016/j.bioactmat.2017.05.002.
30. A. A. Sadoon *et al.*, *Appl. Environ. Microbiol.* **86** (2020), doi: 10.1128/ aem.02479-19.
31. A. Abdal, R. Noorani and G. Cha, *J. Biomed. Phys. Eng.* **10**, 761 (2020), doi: 10.31661/jbpe.v0i0.2005-1123.
32. Y. H. Kwak, H. T. Hong, Y. G. Koh and K. T. Kang, *Appl. Sci. (Basel)* **10**, 6487 (2020), doi: 10.3390/app10186487.
33. Y. G. Koh, H. T. Hong and K. T. Kang, *Materials* **12**, 3345 (2019), doi: 10.3390/ ma12203345.
34. K. T. Kang, J. Son, S. K. Kwon, O. R. Kwon, J. H. Park and Y. G. Koh, *Compos. Struct.* **201**, 141 (2018), doi: 10.1016/j.compstruct.2018.06.036.
35. Y. Guo and W. Guo, *Comput. Methods Biomech. Biomed. Eng.* (2022), doi: 10.1080/10255842.2022. 2032681.
36. Y. G. Koh, J. A. Lee and K. T. Kang, *Lubricants* **7**, 30 (2019), doi: 10.3390/ lubricants7040030.
37. T. M. Grupp *et al.*, *Acta Biomater.* **9**, 7054 (2013), doi: 10.1016/j.actbio. 2013.02.030.
38. G. Kandemir, S. Smith and T. J. Joyce, *J. Mech. Behav. Biomed. Mater.* **97**, 117 (2019), doi: 10.1016/j.jmbbm.2019.05.022.
39. T. M. Grupp *et al.*, *Acta Biomater.* **6**, 3601 (2010), doi: 10.1016/j.actbio. 2010.04.003.

40. M. Kyomoto, T. Moro, S. Yamane, M. Hashimoto, Y. Takatori and K. Ishihara, *Biomaterials* **34**, 7829 (2013), doi: 10.1016/j.biomaterials.2013.07.023.
41. M. Kyomoto *et al.*, *Biomaterials* **35**, 6677 (2014), doi: 10.1016/j.biomaterials.2014.04.051.
42. S. Yamane *et al.*, *J. Biomed. Mater. Res. B, Appl. Biomater.* **106**, 1028 (2018), doi: 10.1002/jbm.b.33918.
43. D. Baykal, R. S. Siskey, R. J. Underwood, A. Briscoe and S. M. Kurtz, *Clin. Orthop. Relat. Res.* **474**, 2384 (2016), doi: 10.1007/s11999-016-4989-7.
44. H. Sakoda, M. Uematsu, Y. Okamoto and Y. Haishima, *Proc. Inst. Mech. Eng. H, J. Eng. Med.* (2022), doi: 10.1177/09544119211042992.
45. V. Lorber *et al.*, *J. Mater. Sci., Mater. Med.* **25**, 141 (2014), doi: 10.1007/s10856-013-5037-8.
46. T. M. Grupp *et al.*, Biotribology of alternativ bearing materials for knee arthroplasty, in *World Congress on Medical Physics and Biomedical Engineering*, September 7–12, 2009, Munich, Germany (Springer, Berlin, Heidelberg, 2009), pp. 353–355.
47. S. Utzschneider *et al.*, *Acta Biomater.* **6**, 4296 (2010), doi: 10.1016/j.actbio.2010.06.002.
48. A. C. Paulus *et al.*, *Biomed. Res. Int.* **2016**, 2198914 (2016), doi: 10.1155/2016/2198914.
49. S. Schroeder *et al.*, *J. Mech. Behav. Biomed. Mater.* **101**, 103434 (2020), doi: 10.1016/j.jmbbm.2019. 103434.
50. R. A. Schierjott *et al.*, *Biomed. Res. Int.* **2016**, 7032830 (2016), doi: 10.1155/2016/7032830.
51. A. Giurea *et al.*, *Biomed. Res. Int.* **2014**, 948520 (2014), doi: 10.1155/2014/948520.
52. K. Vertesich, K. Staats, C. Bohler, R. Koza, R. Lass and A. Giurea, *Front. Bioeng. Biotechnol.* **10**, 845859 (2022), doi: 10.3389/fbioe.2022.845859.
53. I. Nakahara, M. Takao, S. Bandoh and N. Sugano, *J. Artif. Organs* **17**, 358 (2014), doi: 10.1007/s10047-014-0789-6.
54. I. Nakahara, M. Takao, S. Bandoh, N. Bertollo, W. R. Walsh and N. Sugano, *J. Orthop. Res.* **31**, 485 (2013), doi: 10.1002/jor.22251.
55. M. Dworak and S. Błażewicz, *Acta Bioeng. Biomech.* **18**, 71 (2016).
56. D. Vogel, M. Klimek, M. Saemann and R. Bader, *Materials (Basel)* **13** (2020), doi: 10.3390/ma13061372.
57. D. Vogel, C. Schulze, H. Dempwolf, D. Kluess and R. Bader, *Proc. Inst. Mech. Eng. H* **232**, 1030 (2018), doi: 10.1177/0954411918797600.
58. K. Marimuthu and S. Rajan, *IOP Conf. Ser., Mater. Sci. Eng.* **346**, 012029 (2017).
59. N. Faisal, *Biointerface Res. Appl. Chem.* **10**, 7223 (2020), doi: 10.33263/briac106.72237233.
60. H. Fouad and R. Elleithy, *J. Mech. Behav. Biomed. Mater.* **4**, 1376 (2011), doi: 10.1016/j.jmbbm. 2011. 05.008.
61. S. Dabees, B. M. Kamel, V. Tirth and A. B. Elshalakny, *Bioengineered* **11**, 679 (2020), doi: 10.1080/21655979.2020.1775943.

62. K. Lu, C. Li, H. Z. Wang, Y. L. Li, Y. Zhu and Y. Ouyang, *J. Photochem. Photobiol. B* **197**, 111504 (2019), doi: 10.1016/j.jphotobiol.2019.05.001.
63. P. J. Hine, B. Brew, R. A. Duckett and I. M. Ward, *Compos. Sci. Technol.* **40**, 47 (1991).
64. J. M. D. Zavala *et al.*, *J. Mech. Behav. Biomed. Mater.* **120**, 104554 (2021), doi: 10.1016/j.jmbbm. 2021.104554.
65. A. Sobajima *et al.*, *ACS Biomater. Sci. Eng.* **6**, 7032 (2020), doi: 10.1021/acsbiomaterials.0c00916.
66. Q. Y. Do, S. O'Byrne, D. Perriman and P. Smith, Piezoresistive nanocomposite as an embedded stress sensor in instrumented knee prosthesis, *2015 37th Annual Int. Conf. IEEE Engineering in Medicine and Biology Society (EMBC)*, Milan, Italy, 2015, pp. 2677–2680, doi: 10.1109/EMBC.2015. 7318943.
67. C. S. Ramesh and C. Shashishekar, *Adv. Mater. Res.* **421**, 388 (2011).
68. B. R. Baliga, P. Reddy and P. Pandey, *Mater. Today, Proc.* **5**, 20842 (2018).
69. F. S. Senatov, A. N. Kopylov, N. Y. Anisimova, M. V. Kiselevsky and A. V. Maksimkin, *Mater. Sci. Eng. C, Mater. Biol. Appl.* **48**, 566 (2015), doi: 10.1016/j.msec.2014.12.050.
70. C. Caouette, L. H. Yahia and M. N. Bureau, *Proc. Inst. Mech. Eng. H* **225**, 907 (2011), doi: 10.1177/0954411911412465.
71. H. Bougherara, R. Zdero, A. Dubov, S. Shah, S. Khurshid and E. H. Schemitsch, *Med. Eng. Phys.* **33**, 121 (2011), doi: 10.1016/j.medengphy.2010. 09.011.
72. P. T. Avval, S. Samiezadeh, V. Klika and H. Bougherara, *J. Mech. Behav. Biomed. Mater.* **41**, 56 (2015), doi: 10.1016/j.jmbbm.2014.09.019.
73. J. E. Lang, D. R. Whiddon, E. L. Smith and A. K. Salyapongse, *J. Surg. Orthop. Adv.* **17**, 51 (2008).
74. B. S. Bal, J. Garino, M. Ries and M. N. Rahaman, *HIP Int.* **17**, 21 (2007), doi: 10.1177/112070000 701700105.
75. S. A. Basha, A. K. Agrawal and D. Sarkar, *J. Mech. Behav. Biomed. Mater.* **114**, 104178 (2021), doi: 10.1016/j.jmbbm.2020.104178.
76. A. Nieto, J. M. Zhao, Y. H. Han, K. H. Hwang and J. M. Schoenung, *J. Mech. Behav. Biomed. Mater.* **61**, 122 (2016), doi: 10.1016/j.jmbbm.2016.01.020.
77. Y. Zhu *et al.*, *Int. J. Nanomed.* **14**, 5977 (2019), doi: 10.2147/ijn.S202457.
78. J. F. Bartolomé, A. Smirnov, H. D. Kurland, J. Grabow and F. A. Müller, *Sci. Rep.* **6**, 20589 (2016), doi: 10.1038/srep20589.
79. D. G. Lee, J. K. Yoon, K. T. Hong and I. J. Shon, *J. Ceram. Process. Res.* **17**, 899 (2016).
80. D. B. Bennett *et al.*, *J. Bone Joint Surg. Am.* **96**, 2062 (2014), doi: 10.2106/jbjs.M.01542.
81. K. W. Li, J. H. Yan, C. H. Wang, L. Bi, Q. Zhang and Y. S. Han, *Biochem. Biophys. Res. Commun.* **489**, 187 (2017), doi: 10.1016/j.bbrc.2017.05.124.
82. A. Bagherifard *et al.*, *Med. Biol. Eng. Comput.* **58**, 1681 (2020), doi: 10.1007/s11517-020-02157-1.
83. K. Aoki and N. Saito, *Nanomaterials (Basel)* **10** (2020), doi: 10.3390/nano10020264.
84. J. S. Kawalec, Carbon in biomedical engineering, in *The Encyclopedia of Materials: Science and Technology*, 2nd edn. (Elsevier, 2001), pp. 922–926.

https://doi.org/10.1142/9789819809028_0014

Chapter 14

Iron Oxide Nanoparticles for Tissue Repair and Regeneration*

Tanya Nanda† and Mohammad Alobaid‡

School of Biological and Health Systems Engineering
Arizona State University
Tempe, Arizona 85281, USA
†*tnanda@asu.edu*
‡*malobaio@asu.edu*

Kaushal Rege

School for Engineering of Matter
Transport, and Energy
Arizona State University
Tempe, Arizona 85281, USA
kaushal.rege@asu.edu

Iron oxides are naturally occurring compounds, and several methods have been developed for generating iron oxide nanoparticles (IONPs) with a focus on precisely modulating their size and physicochemical properties. Facile synthesis approaches, narrow size distribution, ease of surface modification, tunable magnetic properties, and size-dependent elimination from blood circulation, make IONPs attractive for use in different biomedical applications. This review describes the use of IONPs for application in tissue repair and regeneration with a focus on neural and musculoskeletal tissues.

Keywords: Magnetic nanoparticles; tissue repair; regenerative medicine; tissue engineering; magnetic resonance imaging.

---

*To cite this article, please refer to its earlier version published in the *Nano LIFE*, Vol. 11, No. 1 (2021) 2030001 (10 pages), DOI: 10.1142/S1793984420300010
†Corresponding author.

1. Introduction

Nanoparticles (NPs) demonstrate unique material-, size-, and shape-dependent properties and have been investigated in biomedical applications including imaging, therapeutics, and sensing. Inorganic NPs have been developed from several elements including iron, silicon, carbon, gold, and silver and their compounds.[1,2] Of these, iron oxide NPs (IONPs), approximately 1–250 nm in dimension, are particularly attractive because of their unique physical, optical, and magnetic properties. Iron is one of the most abundant transition metals in the Earth's crust and forms iron oxides upon oxidation. At least sixteen different types of iron oxides including magnetite (Fe_3O_4), have been identified.[3] Favorable ferromagnetism (magnetic property of IONPs[4]), magnetic coercivity (ability to withstand high magnetic fields without losing magnetism), high saturation magnetization (condition at which magnetization does not vary with increasing magnetic fields that are applied externally), and Curie temperature (temperature at which magnetic properties are lost permanently) make IONPs attractive for biomedical applications. In addition, smaller IONPs (diameters < 10–20 nm) can exhibit superparamagnetism (known as superparamagnetic IONPs or SPIONPs) which refers to hysteresis-free reversible magnetization.[5] Moreover, the magnetic moment exhibited by SPIONPs can be much larger than what is observed with other metal NPs.[6]

Some IONP formulations have been approved by the Food and Drug Administration (FDA) for application in humans in the United States; additional formulations are in different stages of pre-clinical development or clinical trials.[7] For example, Feridex® (dextran-coated IONPs) is approved for imaging applications and Feraheme® (SPIONPs coated with carbohydrates) can be administered for anemia treatment in adult chronic kidney disease patients.[8,9] Here, we present a brief overview of IONPs and their applications in tissue repair and regeneration, with a focus on neural and musculoskeletal tissues. Cellular and tissue responses to IONPs are also discussed.

2. Synthesis of IONPs

Several methods have been developed for synthesizing IONPs with a focus on controlling particle size, shape, and properties for biomedical applications. A number of excellent reviews have detailed the methods for IONP synthesis and the reader is directed to those for further information.[10–12] Briefly, physical methods including crushing, milling, or grinding and chemical methods including thermal decomposition, microemulsion, solvothermal, sonochemical, microwave-assisted, co-precipitation, carbon arc discharge, chemical vapor deposition, and combustion syntheses have been developed for generating IONPs.[13–23] In addition, different shapes of IONPs including nanoscale rods, spheres, and cubes can be generated.[24] These protocols are fairly well established, cost-effective, and offer dimensional and shape control depending on the method employed.[25] Different surface modification methods including with polymeric[24,26–29] as well as small molecule and surfactant coatings[30–32] have also been investigated for enhancing the biocompatibility and stability of IONPs.

3. Applications of IONPs in tissue repair and regeneration

Considering their attractive magnetic properties and biocompatibility, IONPs have been investigated for various tissue engineering and repair applications,[33,34] including in neural and musculoskeletal repair and regeneration as discussed below.

3.1. *Neural repair and regeneration*

Several traumatic incidents can cause nerve injury, which can range from minimal damage to complete loss of function. Surgical repair of small nerve injuries and defects is likely possible, but regenerative technologies may be necessary in cases of more extensive damage and large defects. IONPs, in concert with externally applied magnetic fields, have been investigated for guiding mechanical tension in tissue repair as illustrated in Figure 1.[35] This approach has also been studied for guiding neural regeneration.[35]

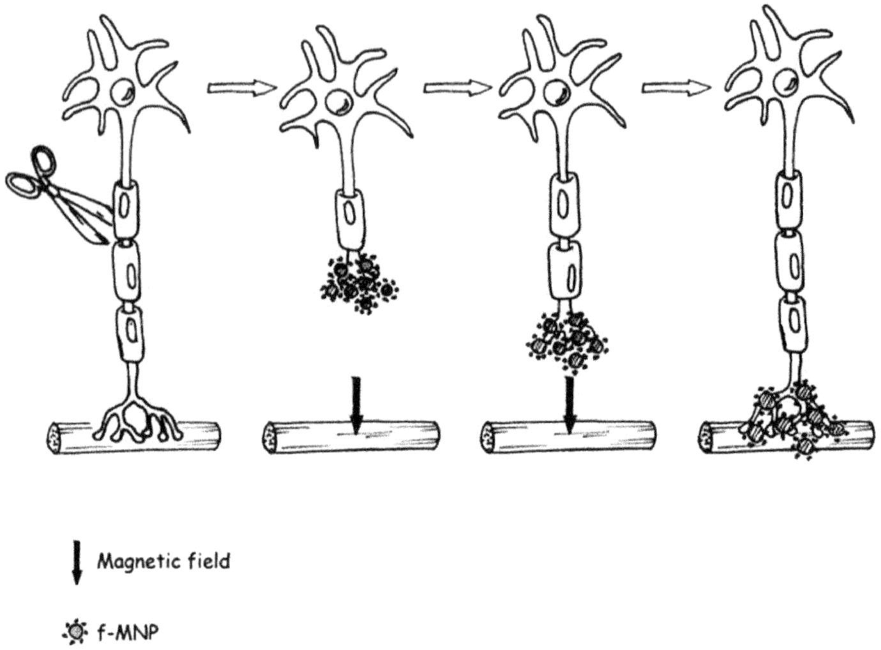

Fig. 1. IONPs, here, fluorescently labelled Nerve Growth Factor Beta-labeled (NGFfluor) Magnetic Nanoparticles (f-MNPs), were utilized for non-invasive physical regeneration of nerves using an externally applied magnetic field for guidance to the injury site.[35] Reprinted and adapted from Ref. 35 with permission.

Formulations consisting of IONPs with scaffolds have also been explored in nerve regeneration applications. A 15 mm defect in the sciatic nerve of Sprague Dawley rats was treated with a nanocomposite scaffold consisting of chitosan-glycerophosphate and IONPs (average diameter approximately 29 nm).[36] The IONP-containing magnetic scaffold (MG) was loaded with Schwann cells (SCs). External magnetic field application resulted in better outcomes for axon regeneration at 12 weeks with the MG-SC device compared to control groups.[36] Another study used SPIONPs in an anisometric micro-structured hydrogel (Anisogel), together with an external magnetic field to guide the regeneration and direction of neurite growth.[37] The dimensions of the hydrogel could be modulated to induce an ultrahigh magnetic response that played a role in reducing iron cytotoxicity.[37]

IONPs have also been used for cell tracking in neural applications. For example, the effect of SPIONP-mesenchymal stem cells (MSCs) on axon regeneration and neuronal survival was investigated in an optic nerve crush model in Lester Hood rats.[38] The labelled cells could be detected using magnetic resonance imaging (MRI) for up to 18 weeks, indicating that the cells remained at the site for this period. Survival studies of retinal ganglion cells (RGC) indicated that MSCs promoted regeneration of axons and also performed a protective function likely because of the production of soluble biochemical mediators (e.g., Fibroblast Growth Factor-2).[38]

Magnetic guidance of nerve growth factor (NGF) conjugated to 45 ± 17 nm IONPs (NGF-IONPs) was investigated in vivo.[39] The sciatic nerve of Balb/c mice was injected with NGF-IONPs (4 mg/mL, 100 μL for each mouse). A strong localized magnetic field was generated using a magnetic tip for 5 minutes, 0.5 cm away from the injection area and above the sciatic nerve. IONPs were found to be in proximity to the magnetic tip, likely indicating their transport along the sciatic nerve.[39] Nerve growth factor (NGF) and vascular endothelial growth factor (VEGF) were loaded on poly(ethyleneimine)-coated IONPs (core size $\sim 25 \pm 5$ nm) in a conduit that was sutured to two ends of a defect in a rat median nerve. These demonstrated improved motor function and nerve regeneration compared to that seen following delivery of free growth factors.[40]

Several in vitro studies that have investigated the fate of nerve cells following treatment with IONPs have demonstrated that exposure time, dosage, particle size, and concentration govern potential neurotoxicity of IONPs.[41,42] Table 1 presents additional studies that describe the use of different IONPs in nerve repair and regeneration and Table 2 summarizes studies involving neurotoxicity of IONPs. Applications of IONPs for imaging in neurosurgery are described elsewhere in a recent review.[43]

Table 1. Select examples of IONPs in neural cellular engineering and tissue repair.[35,44–50]

Particle type	Case(s) studied	Particle size	Particle dose	Contact duration	Outcomes
Polyethylenimine (PEI)-coated IONPs	Neurite outgrowth from PC12 cells	25 nm	10–100 μg/mL	24–72 h	Neurite outgrowth from PC12 cells was stimulated preferentially toward the direction of the applied magnetic field.[35]
Poly-l-lysine coated IONPs	Actuation of SH-SY5Y cell line and primary Schwann cell culture	73 ± 6 nm	0–100 μg/mL	1–7 days	Cells were actuated toward an injury site under the influence of an external magnetic field.[44]
Poly-L-lactic acid (PLLA) coated IONPs	Neurite outgrowth from dorsal root ganglia (DRG)	10–15 nm	3 mg of PLLA coated iron oxide composite NPs (cNPs)	7 days	Nerve growth factor-releasing PLLA-coated IONPs were guided via magnetic field and DRG was extended toward the direction of the magnetic field.[45]

Nerve Growth Factor (NGF)-functionalized SPIO-gold core shell NPs (NGF-SPIO-Au)	Neurite outgrowth and neuronal differentiation of PC 12 cells	20.8 nm	0–20 μg/mL	24 h	NGF-SPIO-Au NPs in PC 12 cells were irradiated with a low-intensity light emitting diode. This resulted in 51% of neurite outgrowth and 83% neuronal differentiation.[46]
SPIONPs	In vitro neuronal differentiation of murine neural stem cells (NSCs) and a neural stem cell line (C17.2)	30–150 nm	0, 25, 100, 250 μg/mL	5 and 10 days	Examination of Map2ab expression of labeled cells indicated that approximately 10% of the NSCs and C17.2 cells differentiated into mature neurons.[47]
SPIONPs	In vivo MRI tracking of primary murine neural stem cells (NSCs), and neural stem cell line (C17.2) in mice	30–150 nm	0, 25, 100, 250 μg/mL	2 h	MRI imaging results indicated that transplanted NSC and C17.2 cells were detectable at SPIONPs concentration of 100 and 250 μg/mL.[47]

(*Continued*)

Table 1. (*Continued*)

Particle type	Case(s) studied	Particle size	Particle dose	Contact duration	Outcomes
SPIONPs	Neuronal branching in PC 12 cells	100 nm	0–100 μg/mL	1–5 days	Treatment of PC12 cells with SPIONPs and quercetin resulted in neurite outgrowth and neuronal branching in presence of nerve growth factors.[48]
Superparamagnetic gold-coated monocrystalline IONs (Au-MION)	In vivo labeling of neural stem cells and tracking in rat spinal cord using MRI	20 nm	1–40 μg/mL	1 h, 48 h, and 1 month	Maximal cell labeling efficacy was obtained at 10 μg/mL and 24 h. Au-MIONs demonstrated MRI contrast. At a concentration of 30 μg/mL, the corresponding MRI signal was noticeably depleted.[49]
SPIONPs and ferumoxytol NPs (FNPs)	MRI labeling and tracking of human neural progenitor cells (hNPCs) that were transplanted into the spinal cord of porcine models	10 nm (FNPs)	0–1000 μg/mL (FNPs)	168 h	Labeling with SPIONPs facilitated conformation of cell engraftment, delivery, and injection accuracy.[50]

Table 2. Neurotoxicity studies with IONPs.[51–54]

Type of IONPs	Case(s) studied	Particle size	Particle dose	Exposure time	Outcomes
Maghemite NPs	Dopaminergic neural toxicity in SH-SY5Y cells	10 and 30 nm	2.5–10 μg/mL	24 h	Exhaustion of dopamine in cells led to the activation of oxidative stress pathways, which resulted in dopaminergic neurotoxicity.[51]
Silica coated-SPIONPs	In vitro cytotoxicity study: Viability of SH-SY5Y neuroblastoma and A172 glioblastoma cells	20.2 ± 2.9 nm	5–300 μg/mL	3, 6, and 24 h	Highest reduction in cell viability was obtained at a particle concentration between 200–300 μg/mL, and exposure time of 24 h.[52]
Maghemite NPs	Response of PC12 cells to NPs.	5–12 nm	0.15, 1.5, and 15 mM	2, 4, and 6 days	Noticeable reduction in the ability to form mature neurites and cell viability.[53]
Fe_3O_4-NPs	In vivo study: distribution and accumulation of intranasally instilled particles in brains of four-week-old male SD rats.	30 nm	25, 50, 100, 200 μg/mL	24 h	Regional distribution of particles was observed in brains, with highest concentration in rat striata and hippocampi. Particles may have caused oxidative damage to the striata at the end of 14 days.[54]

3.2. *Musculoskeletal repair and regeneration*

3.2.1. *Skin repair: Wound healing and infection control*

Skin wounds and injuries affect millions of people worldwide and can lead to high treatment costs.[55] Incisional wounds are common in surgical procedures and are approximated using sutures and staples but can be vulnerable to bacterial infections at the (surgical) site. Antibacterial drugs, including small-molecule antibiotics, enzymes, polymers, and/or nanomaterials have been investigated for wound repair.[55,56] In addition, IONPs have also been investigated for skin repair after wounding. For example, thrombin is a serine protease enzyme that regulates platelet aggregation and blood coagulation, which play a role in wound control and hemostasis.[57] As a potential approach to overcome limitations associated with stability,[58] thrombin was bound to bovine serum albumin (BSA) coated-maghemite NPs. Treatment with these particles resulted in the highest tensile strength at 28 days compared to free thrombin in 2.5 cm long incisional skin wounds created in Wistar rats.[58] Histological analysis showed that NP-thrombin treatment demonstrated better performance for scarring control compared to unbound thrombin and control (staples).[58] As summarized in Table 3, other studies have also used IONPs, in concert with or without other materials, for wound healing and infection control.

3.2.2. *Repair and regeneration of bone and cartilage*

Engineered tissues have several applications in musculoskeletal injuries and IONPs have been investigated for facilitating bone repair and regeneration. For example, polyglucose-sorbitol-carboxymethylether (PSC)-coated IONPs were incubated with primary human bone-derived mesenchymal stem cells (hBMSCs).[63] Cellular uptake studies indicated that these IONPs were internalized by hBMSCs in a "time- and dose-dependent manner" and an increase in alkaline phosphatase (ALP) activity was indicative of osteogenic potential. Treatment with IONPs resulted in approximately 20% increase in the formation of mineralized nodules, as quantified using Alizarin Red S (ARS). Microarray-based gene expression studies indicated

Table 3. Application of IONPs in incisional wound healing and infection control.[59–62]

Type of IONPs	Case(s) studied	Particle size	Particle dose	Exposure time	Outcomes
IONPs (Fe_2O_3) solution	Skin wound closure in Wistar rats	—	42 g/L Fe2O3 NPs in milli-Q water	7 days	A 1.5 cm long and 6 mm deep horizontal skin incision was made, and the treated wound demonstrated repair in seven days.[59]
SPIONPs	Anti–infection investigation of SPIONPs for prosthetic biofilm prevention in vitro	8 nm	10 μg/mL–2 mg/mL	12, 24, and 48 h	SPIONPs inhibited *Staphylococcus epidermidis* biofilm formation.[60]
Chitosan-coated IONPs	Reduction of biofilm bacterial infection *(Staphylococcus aureus)* in vitro	15–25 nm	200–4000 μg/mL	24 h	Bacterial growth was greatly reduced between 6–12 h at a concentration of 500 μg/mL. Chitosan NPs were used as control.[61]
SPIONPs	Anti-bacterial efficacy of SPIONPs against biomaterials associated-bacterial infections in vitro (Staphylococci)	14–18 nm	0.35 mg/mL	24 h	SPIONPs resulted in ablation of bacterial cells. No differences in cell spreading and morphology were observed in U2OS osteosarcoma cells in absence or presence of SPIONPs.[62]

Table 4. Brief summary of applications of IONPs in bone tissue engineering.[65–68]

Type of IONPs	Case(s) studied	Particle size	Particle dose	Exposure time	Outcomes
Magnetic NPs (MNPs) incorporated in poly (caprolactone) (PCL)	Tissue compatibility and efficacy for bone regeneration in male Sprague-Dawley rats	12 nm	5, 10, and 15 wt% MNPs in PCL	4–8 weeks	Minimal adverse impact on tissue and significant bone regeneration ability.[65]
SPIONP loaded Gelatin Sponge (SPIONPs GS)	Tissue repair effect in incisor sockets of Sprague-Dawley rats	9 nm	10 mg/mL	4 weeks	Compared to the control group, the group treated with SPIONPs-GS had more newly formed bone and "a better-preserved alveolar ridge."[66]
SPIONPs in an electrospun nanofibrous composite scaffold hydroxyapatite NPs and poly lactide acid (PLA)	New bone tissue formation in white rabbit models of lumbar transverse defects	18 nm	2.5 g γ-Fe_2O_3 in 100 mL N,N-dimethylacetamide	110 days	Acceleration of new bone tissue formation and remodeling in the rabbit defect under magnetic field.[67]
MNPs consisting of iron oxide core coated with branched polyethyleneimine, minicircle plasmid DNA encoding B-cell lymphoma-2 (Bcl-2), and poly-β-amino ester	Magnetofection for upregulating Bcl-2 expression in implanted adipose-derived stromal cells for bone regeneration in a calvarial defect model of adult male nude Crl:NU-*Fox1*^{v} CD-1 immuno-compromised mice.	4 mm (scaffold size)	20 μL NP solution in each hydroxyapatite-coated poly(lactic-coglycolic acid) (HA-PLGA) scaffold	8 weeks	Enhanced survival of adipose-derived stem cells and regeneration in the calvarial defect model compared to controls.[68]

upregulation of 2092 genes and downregulation of 1621 genes upon IONP treatment (100 μg/mL for 7 days) compared to the negative control.[63]

In a different study, SPIONPs did not result in significant loss of viability or proliferation activity of bone derived MSCs compared to cells not labeled with the NPs.[64] The labeled cells were injected into the knee joint cavity in an articular cartilage defect model in rabbits and tracked using MRI. The cells were able to persist in the synovial fluid for up to 12 weeks, indicating the use of SPIONPs — for tracking cells used in musculoskeletal tissue repair and regeneration in vivo.[64] Table 4 briefly describes additional studies where IONPs have been applied as tools for regeneration or repair of musculoskeletal tissues by facilitating osteogenesis-related cell function, stem cell/drug delivery, defect repair, and/or in vivo labelling and tracking.

4. Cellular and tissue responses to IONPs

Iron is involved in several natural processes including metabolism, proliferation, and oxygen transport in the human body, and is generally bound to transferrin or ferritin proteins.[69] Transferrin transports iron to cells following uptake by receptor-mediated endocytosis in clathrin-coated pits,[70] and ferritin typically stores iron in the cytoplasm of cells.[71] Free iron may also be present in cytoplasm and may participate in the formation of reactive oxygen species (ROS).[72] Considering the essential role of iron in the human body, it is important to elucidate the biodistribution and cellular or tissue toxicity following the delivery or use of IONPs for tissue repair and regeneration.

Systemic delivery of NPs, including IONPs, is followed by their opsonization and subsequent clearance by reticuloendothelial system.[73] Physicochemical characteristics of NPs including hydrodynamic size, surface charge (zeta potential), and shape can act as primary factors to determine cellular and tissue toxicity of IONPs. It is likely that smaller SPIONPs can be more effectively cleared via renal clearance compared to larger sized IONPs.[72–75] It is also likely that generation of ROS following IONP delivery can contribute to potential loss in cell viability because ROS generation can damage biomolecules, including DNA, in cells.

Although studies that describe short-term, acute toxicities of IONPs have led to significant insights, more information on long-term effects and multiple dosing of these NPs is warranted. Biodistribution studies in mice indicated presence of IONPs in the blood, heart and kidney tissues after three months of intravenous administration.[76] In male Wistar rats, biodistribution studies following intravenous administration of IONPs (once a week for four weeks) showed presence of IONPs in the spleen and liver, with the least presence in the brain.[77] Studies in vertebrate animals and humans were indicative of the utility of Ferumoxtran-10, which is an ultrasmall ($\sim$30 nm) formulation of NPs, for MRI, including of lymph.[78] As new IONP formulations continue to be developed for different applications, it is important to note that some transport mechanisms may be relevant across species, but detailed biodistribution and toxicity studies in humans will eventually be needed to determine the potential for translation to the clinic.

5. Conclusions

Use of engineered IONPs can have transformative impact in tissue repair and regeneration, including in neural and musculoskeletal tissues. IONPs and their formulations have demonstrated potential applications in nerve guidance, wound healing, infection control, and cell labeling. Furthermore, the ability to image IONPs has particular relevance in implantable scaffolds and other devices used in tissue repair. Detailed analyses of short- and long-term toxicities of different IONP formulations and related nanomaterials, in small and large vertebrate animals, will be necessary for obtaining comprehensive insights into formulation-dependent biocompatibility, toxicity and performance, prior to translation to human patients.

Acknowledgements

TN is grateful to Master's Opportunity for Research in Engineering (MORE), Kern Entrepreneurial Engineering Network (KEEN), and

Graduate and Professional Student Association — Graduate Research Support Program awards from Arizona State University.

Conflict of interest

KR is affiliated with Synergyan, LLC.

References

1. H.-C. Huang, S. Barua, G. Sharma, S. K. Dey and K. Rege, *J. Control Release.* **155**(3), 344 (2011).
2. R. Urie, D. Ghosh, I. Ridha and K. Rege, *Annu. Rev. Biomed. Eng.* **20**, 350 (2018).
3. R. M. Cornell and U. Schwertmann, *The Iron Oxides: Structure, Properties, Reactions, Occurrences and Uses*, 2nd Edn. (Wiley, USA, 2003).
4. C. Kittel, *Phys. Rev.* **70**, 965 (1946).
5. C. P. Bean and J. D. Livingston, *J. Appl. Phys.* **30**(4), S120 (1959).
6. H. Danan, A. Herr and A. J. P. Meyer, *J. Appl. Phys.* **39**(2), 669 (1968).
7. D. Bobo, K. J. Robinson, J. Islam, K. J. Thurecht and S. R. Corrie, *Pharmaceut Res.* **33**(10), 2373 (2016).
8. J. W. M. Bulte, *Am. J. Roentgenol.* **193**(2), 314 (2009).
9. Y.-X. J. Wang, *World J. Gastroentero.* **21**(47), 13400 (2015).
10. M. Faraji, Y. Yamini and M. Rezaee, *J. Iran. Chem. Soc.* **7**(1), 1 (2010).
11. A. Ali, H. Zafar, M. Zia, Haq I ul, A. R. Phull, J. S. Ali *et al.*, *Nanotechnol. Sci. Appl.* **9**, 49 (2016).
12. A. Tavakoli, M. Sohrabi and A. Kargari, *Chem. Pap.* **61**(3), 151 (2007).
13. E. Flahaut, F. Agnoli, J. Sloan, C. O'Connor and M. L. H. Green, *Chem. Mater.* **14**(6), 2553 (2002).
14. H. Karami, *J. Clust. Sci.* **21**(1), 11 (2010).
15. T. Hyeon, *Chem. Commun.* 927 (2002).
16. K. Woo, H. J. Lee, J.-P. Ahn and Y. S. Park, *Adv. Mater.* **15**(20), 1761 (2003).
17. P. Tartaj, S. Veintemillas-Verdaguer, T. Gonzalez-Carreño and C. J. Serna, *Magnetic Nanoparticles in Biosensing and Medicine*, N. J. Darton, A. Ionescu and J. Llandro, Cambridge University Press (2019).
18. S. Giri, S. Samanta, S. Maji, S. Ganguli and A. Bhaumik, *J. Magn. Magn. Mater.* **285**(1–2), 296 (2005).
19. J. Wang, F. Ren, R. Yi, A. Yan, G. Qiu and X. Liu, *J. Alloy. Compd.* **479**(1–2), 791 (2009).
20. T. J. Mason and J. P. Lorimal, *Applied Sonochemistry* (Wiley, New York, 2002).
21. H. O. Pierson, *Handbook of Chemical Vapor Deposition: Principles, Technology and Applications* (William Andrew Inc., USA, 1999).
22. Z. H. Wang, C. J. Choi, B. K. Kim, J. C. Kim, Z. D. Zhang, *Carbon.* **41**(9), 1751 (2003).

23. C. F. Wang, J. N. Wang and Z. M. Sheng, *J. Phys. Chem. C.* **111**(17), 6303 (2007).
24. F. N. Sayed and V. Polshettiwar, *Sci. Rep-uk.* **5**(1), 9733 (2015).
25. S.-N. Sun, C. Wei, Z.-Z. Zhu, Y.-L. Hou, S. S. Venkatraman and Z.-C. Xu, *Chinese Phys. B.* **23**(3), 037503 (2014).
26. M. Anbarasu, M. Anandan, E. Chinnasamy, V. Gopinath and K. Balamurugan, *Spectrochimica. Acta. Part Mol. Biomol. Spectrosc.* **135**, 536 (2015).
27. E. A. Osborne, T. M. Atkins, D. A. Gilbert, S. M. Kauzlarich, K. Liu and A. Y. Louie, *Nanotechnology.* **23**(21), 215602 (2012).
28. A. Mohammadi, H. Daemi and M. Barikani, *Int. J. Biol. Macromolecules.* **14**, 447 (2014).
29. P. B. Shete, R. M. Patil, N. D. Thorat, A. Prasad, R. S. Ningthoujam, S. J. Ghosh *et al.*, *Appl. Surf. Sci.* **288**, 149 (2014).
30. D. Li, D. Jiang, M. Chen, J. Xie, Y. Wu, S. Dang *et al.*, *Mater Lett.* **64**(22), 2462 (2010).
31. K. Yang, H. Peng, Y. Wen and N. Li, *Appl. Surf. Sci.* **256**(10), 3093 (2010).
32. G. Wang, Y. Ma, Y. Tong and X. Dong, *Smart Mater. Struct.* **25**(3), 035028 (2016).
33. X. Li, J. Wei, K. E. Aifantis, Y. Fan, Q. Feng, F. Cui *et al.*, *J. Biomed. Mater. Res. A.* **104**(5), 1285 (2016).
34. A. Hasan, M. Morshed, A. Memic, S. Hassan, T. J. Webster, H. E.-S. Marei, *Int. J. Nanomed.* **13**, 5637 (2018).
35. C. Riggio, M. P. Calatayud, M. Giannaccini, B. Sanz, T. E. Torres, R. Fernández-Pacheco *et al.*, *Nanomed. Nanotechnol. Biology. Medicine.* **10**(7), 1549 (2014).
36. Z. Liu, S. Zhu, L. Liu, J. Ge, L. Huang, Z. Sun *et al.*, *Int. J. Nanomed.* **12**, 7815 (2017).
37. J. C. Rose, M. Cámara-Torres, K. Rahimi, J. Köhler, M. Möller and L. D. Laporte, *Nano Lett.* **17**(6), 3782 (2017).
38. L. A. Mesentier-Louro, C. Zaverucha-do-Valle, A. J. Silva-Junior da, G. Nascimento-dos-Santos, F. Gubert, A. B. P. Figueirêdo de *et al.*, *Plos One.* **9**(10), e110722 (2014).
39. M. Marcus, A. Smith, A. Maswadeh, Z. Shemesh, I. Zak, M. Motiei *et al.*, *Nanomaterials-basel.* **8**(9), 707 (2018).
40. M. Giannaccini, M. P. Calatayud, A. Poggetti, S. Corbianco, M. Novelli, M. Paoli *et al.*, *Adv. Healthc. Mater.* **6**(7), 1601429 (2017).
41. C. R. Carvalho, J. Silva-Correia, J. M. Oliveira and R. L. Reis, *Adv. Drug. Deliver Rev.* **148**, 308 (2019).
42. A. Karmakar, Q. Zhang and Y. Zhang, *J. Food Drug. Anal.* **22**(1), 147 (2014).
43. A. Meola, J. Rao, N. Chaudhary, G. Song, X. Zheng, S. D. Chang, *World Neurosurg.* **125**, 261 (2019).
44. C. Riggio, M. P. Calatayud, C. Hoskins, J. Pinkernelle, B. Sanz, T. E. Torres *et al.*, *Int. J. Nanomed.* **7**, 3155 (2012).
45. J. M. Zuidema, C. Provenza, T. Caliendo, S. Dutz and R. J. Gilbert, *Acs. Chem. Neurosci.* **6**(11), 1781 (2015).
46. M. Yuan, Y. Wang and Y.-X. Qin, *Nanomed Nanotechnol Biology Medicine.* **21**, 102052 (2019).

47. S. Magnitsky, R. M. Walton, J. H. Wolfe and H. Poptani, *Acad. Radiol.* **15**(10), 1269 (2008).
48. S. Katebi, A. Esmaeili, K. Ghaedi and A. Zarrabi, *Int. J. Nanomed.* **14**, 2157 (2019).
49. F. H. Wang, I. H. Lee, N. Holmström, T. Yoshitake, D. K. Kim, M. Muhammed *et al.*, *Nanotechnology.* **17**(8), 1911 (2006).
50. J. J. Lamanna, 1 corresponding author, Gutierrez 2 Juanmarco, Urquia 1 N. Lindsey, Hurtig 1 C. Victor, E. Amador *et al.*, *Stem. Cells Transl. Med.* 139 (2017).
51. S. Z. Imam, S. M. Lantz-McPeak, E. Cuevas, H. Rosas-Hernandez, S. Liachenko, Y. Zhang *et al.*, *Mol. Neurobiol.* **52**(2), 913 (2015).
52. C. Costa, F. Brandão, M. J. Bessa, S. Costa, V. Valdiglesias, G. Kiliç *et al.*, *J. Appl. Toxicol.* **36**(3), 361 (2016).
53. T. R. Pisanic, J. D. Blackwell, V. I. Shubayev, R. R. Fiñones, S. Jin, *Biomaterials.* **28**(16), 2572 (2007).
54. J. Wu, T. Ding and J. Sun, *Neurotoxicology.* **34**, 243 (2013).
55. M. Parani, G. Lokhande, A. Singh and A. K. Gaharwar, *ACS Appl. Mater. Inter.* **8**(16), 10049 (2016).
56. S. K. Nethi, S. Das, C. R. Patra and S. Mukherjee, *Biomater. Sci-uk.* **7**(7), 2652 (2019).
57. N. R. Goldsack, R. C. Chambers, K. Dabbagh, G. J. Laurent, *Int. J. Biochem. Cell. Biology.* **30**(6), 641 (1998).
58. O. Ziv-Polat, M. Topaz, T. Brosh and S. Margel, *Biomaterials.* **31**(4), 741 (2010).
59. A. Meddahi-Pellé, A. Legrand, A. Marcellan, L. Louedec, D. Letourneur and L. Leibler, *Angew. Chem. Int. Ed.* **53**(25), 6369 (2014).
60. T. Webster, *Int. J. Nanomed.* **4**, 145 (2009).
61. S. Shi, J. Jia, X. Guo, Y. Zhao, D. Chen, Y. Guo *et al.*, *Int. J. Nanomed.* **11**, 6499 (2016).
62. G. Subbiahdoss, S. Sharifi, D. W. Grijpma, S. Laurent, Mei HC van der, M. Mahmoudi *et al.*, *Acta Biomater.* **8**(6), 2047 (2012).
63. Q. Wang, B. Chen, M. Cao, J. Sun, H. Wu, P. Zhao *et al.*, *Biomaterials.* **86**, 11 (2016).
64. X. Jing, L. Yang, X. Duan, B. Xie, W. Chen, Z. Li *et al.*, *Joint Bone Spine.* **75**(4), 432 (2008).
65. R. K. Singh, K. D. Patel, J. H. Lee, E.-J. Lee, J.-H. Kim, T.-H. Kim *et al.*, *PLOS One.* **9**(4), e91584 (2014).
66. S. Hu, Y. Zhou, Y. Zhao, Y. Xu, F. Zhang, N. Gu *et al.*, *J. Tissue Eng. Regen. M.* **12**(4), e2085 (2018).
67. J. Meng, B. Xiao, Y. Zhang, J. Liu, H. Xue, J. Lei *et al.*, *Sci. Rep-uk.* **3**(1), 2655 (2013).
68. E. Brett, E. R. Zielins, A. Luan, C. C. Ooi, S. Shailendra, D. Atashroo *et al.*, *Stem. Cell Transl. Med.* **6**(1), 151 (2017).
69. N. Abbaspour, R. Hurrell and R. Kellshadi, *J. Res. Med. Sci.* **14**, 164 (2014).
70. P. Ponka, C. R. Beaumont and D. R. Richardson, *Seminars in Hematology.* **14**, 35 (1998).

71. P. Arosio and S. Levi, *Free Radical Biology & Medicine.* **14**, 457 (2002).
72. Y. Kohgo, K. Ikuta, T. Ohtake, Y. Torimoto and J. Kato, *Int. J. Hematol.* **88**(1), 7 (2008).
73. H. H. Gustafson, D. Holt-Casper, D. W. Grainger and H. Ghandehari, *Nano. Today.* **10**(4), 487 (2015).
74. H. S. Choi, W. Liu, P. Misra, E. Tanaka, J. P. Zimmer, B. I. Ipe *et al.*, *Nat. Biotechnol.* **25**(10), 1165 (2007).
75. M. E. Conrad, J. N. Umbreit, *Blood Cells Mol. Dis.* **29**(3), 336 (2002).
76. R. Mejías, L. Gutiérrez, M. P. Morales and D. F. Barber, *Adv. Theranost. Mater.* 131 (2015).
77. U. S. Gaharwar, R. Meena, P. Rajamani, *Int. J. Nanomed.* **14**, 9677 (2019).
78. K. Leung, *Molecular Imaging and Contrast Agent Database* (National Center for Biotechnology Information, USA), 2004).

https://doi.org/10.1142/9789819809028_0015

Chapter 15

Adverse Outcome Phenomena and Toxicity Mechanisms of Micro and Nanoplastics in Human Health*

Fei He [†,‡,§], Xiaohan Wu [†,‡,¶] and Sijie Lin [†,‡,||]

[†]*College of Environmental Science and Engineering*
Biomedical Multidisciplinary Innovation Research Institute
Shanghai East Hospital Tongji University
Shanghai 200092, P. R. China
[‡]*Key Laboratory of Yangtze River Water Environment*
Shanghai Institute of Pollution Control and Ecological Security
Tongji University, Shanghai 200092, P. R. China
[§]*2310149@tongji.edu.cn*
[¶]*2111069@tongji.edu.cn*
[||]*lin.sijie@tongji.edu.cn*

The ubiquitous presence of micro and nanoplastics (MNPs) in the environment has become a pressing global concern, particularly regarding the potential impacts on human health. This review underscores the urgent need for an integrative research framework that bridges the gap between epidemiological observations and toxicological insights. Human exposure to MNPs occurs predominantly through ingestion, inhalation and dermal contact pathways. Epidemiological findings have consistently demonstrated the presence of MNPs in diverse human tissues, signaling a broad exposure and emphasizing the imperative to explore potential health risks. Population surveys have shown that the concentration of MNPs in the feces of people using disposable plastic tableware reaches 24.65 items/g. These results are associated with changes in microbiota composition and metabolite levels relevant to central nervous system disorders, energy metabolism and inflammatory responses. The detectable abundance of MNPs in the

*To cite this article, please refer to its earlier version published in the *Nano LIFE*, Vol. 14, No. 4 (2024) 2440003 (19 pages), DOI: 10.1142/S1793984424400038
[||]Corresponding author.

nasal mucus of individuals wearing N95 masks was measured to be 10.6 ± 2.3 items/mg. Moreover, population-based studies have linked MNP exposure to adverse health outcomes, suggesting correlation relationships between exposure levels and specific diseases such as inflammatory bowel disease (IBD) and human pulmonary ground-glass nodules (GGN). These associations underscore the necessity for in-depth toxicological investigations to elucidate the toxicity mechanisms of MNPs. Meanwhile, laboratory-based toxicological studies have the potential to reveal causative relationships and various *in vitro* and *in vivo* models have been used to explore the mechanisms of the toxicity of MNPs in the gastrointestinal tract, lungs and cardiovascular system. However, early studies failed to reflect on the complexity of the real environment. To foster interdisciplinary collaborations, this paper aims to reconcile the disparities between exposure risks and human health impacts. By critically reviewing recent advancements in understanding the exposure risks of MNPs, epidemiological observations and organ-specific toxicity, this work furnishes a comprehensive perspective on the health implications of MNPs.

Keywords: Micro and nanoplastics; toxicity mechanisms; human health; disease model; epidemiology.

1. Introduction

Human's reliance on plastics in daily life has led to an extraordinarily high annual production and usage of plastics. Presently, the global annual production of plastics has reached 400 million metric tons.[1] However, plastic mismanagement the limited efficiency in recycling, with less than 10% of plastic products being recycled, and consumer habits have led to a substantial amount of plastic waste entering the environment causing plastic pollution.[2] In the environment, most of the plastic waste undergoes weathering subjected to environmental factors such as mechanical abrasion, ultraviolet radiation and biodegradation.[3] These processes would lead to a reduction in size, resulting in the formation of minuscule plastic fragments or particles. Among these, plastic fragments with a maximum equivalent diameter of less than 5 mm are designated as microplastics (MPs), while those achieving nanoscale dimensions are referred to as nanoplastics (NPs).[4] The definition for NPs has been proposed,[5] distinguishing between two main types: those synthetically produced, measuring 1–100 nm, and those generated from the degradation of MPs, with sizes between 1 nm and 1000 nm. This classification seeks to encompass the variety of NP origins and dimensions, offering a detailed basis for assessing their implications on health and the environment.

Micro and nanoplastics (MNPs) have attracted great attention as an emerging pollutant in recent years. Accumulating evidence suggests a widespread of MNPs in the atmosphere, terrestrial environment and aquatic systems. The concern of MNPs posing toxic effects and health risks on both living organisms and humans is continuously rising.[6] To date, studies on the toxic effects and corresponding mechanisms caused by MNPs remain inclusive, particularly regarding human health. Existing literature suggests that humans are exposed to MNPs through ingestion, inhalation and dermal contact.[7,8] Evidence of the presence of MNPs includes human feces,[9–12] lung tissues,[13–16] placental tissues[17] and blood samples,[18] which underlines the urgency of understanding the risks associated with MNP exposure.[19] Although recent epidemiological studies indicate the associations between MNPs exposure and certain human diseases such as inflammatory bowel disease (IBD),[12] human pulmonary ground-glass nodules (GGN)[20] and chronic interstitial hepatitis,[21] the causative relationships remain unclear and the underlying toxicological mechanisms require further investigations.

Given the related health risks and adverse outcomes posed by MNPs, toxicology studies require a comprehensive understanding of their heterogeneity in the human body, including characteristics such as size, shape and plastic-type.[22] The current research gap is mostly due to the disconnect between epidemiological observations and laboratory investigations. Population-based studies focus on different exposure pathways and aim to understand the correlation relationship between exposure patterns and health outcomes. In contrast, toxicology studies in controlled laboratory environments have the potential to reveal causative relationships but fail to reflect on the complexity of the real environment. Epidemiological studies highlight the links between MNPs exposure and health outcomes, focusing on chronic and cumulative exposure scenarios. This approach enables a deeper understanding of the temporal dimensions and lasting effects of MNPs. In contrast, toxicology research often uses higher concentrations of MNPs in controlled environments, potentially overlooking the more subtle, long-term effects associated with lower, environmentally relevant doses. Furthermore, toxicology studies with short exposure times may have limited ability to capture delayed and chronic effects, leading to gaps in the understanding of the prolonged health effects of MNPs. While various*in vitro* and *in vivo* models exist for toxicology experiments, population-based studies provide insights into a wide range of responses and susceptibilities, while laboratory studies may not fully reflect the diverse responses observed in populations, particularly in disease scenarios.

Currently, there are some known mechanisms for the toxic effects of MNPs, such as cell membrane rupture, oxidative stress, immune response, inflammatory response, altered gene expression and disruption of intestinal and alveolar fluid flora,[23] but knowledge gaps about possible toxic effects and health hazards remain. Laboratory-based toxicology studies often disregard the disparity between MNPs present in the environment and commercially acquired model plastics. These distinctions manifest in the inherent physical and chemical properties of the particles, encompassing size, polarity, surface roughness and functional groups.[24,25] Such alterations significantly impact the physical harm inflicted by MNPs during interactions with organisms. Moreover, environmental stresses may induce the release of toxic substances and deleterious factors within MNPs, including the leaching of plastic additives and the formation of polymer intermediates, which can exacerbate the intrinsic toxic effects of MNPs. Changes in the physicochemical properties of MNPs can influence their vector effect on other organic pollutants, thereby increasing associated environmental risks. In this review, we aim to foster a meaningful integration between epidemiological studies and laboratory investigations by reviewing the current progress of each part: the human exposure risks to MNPs (through ingestion, inhalation and dermal contact), epidemiological investigations on corresponding human biological components and the toxicological studies elucidating organ toxicity. Then, it provides a theoretical basis for the human health risk of MNPs and suggests the future research direction of MNPs.

2. Exposure risks & adverse outcome phenomenon of MNPs

Human exposure to MNPs comes from various sources, including air, water, food and products like personal care products and cosmetics with plastic microbeads as well as the release of MNPs during the use or heating of plastic products. In essence, human exposure to MNPs can be categorized into three pathways, i.e., ingestion, inhalation and dermal contact [Fig. 1] (Table 1). As to the exposure levels of MNPs in the human body and the health risks of MNPs, this necessitates research focusing on epidemiological investigations to delve into the potential health risks and their associations with human diseases arising from MNPs. Hence, this review summarizes the adverse outcomes examined from four vantage points: gastrointestinal (colon and fecal), respiratory (lung and alveolar fluid), dermal (skin and hair) and cardiovascular (blood and heart).

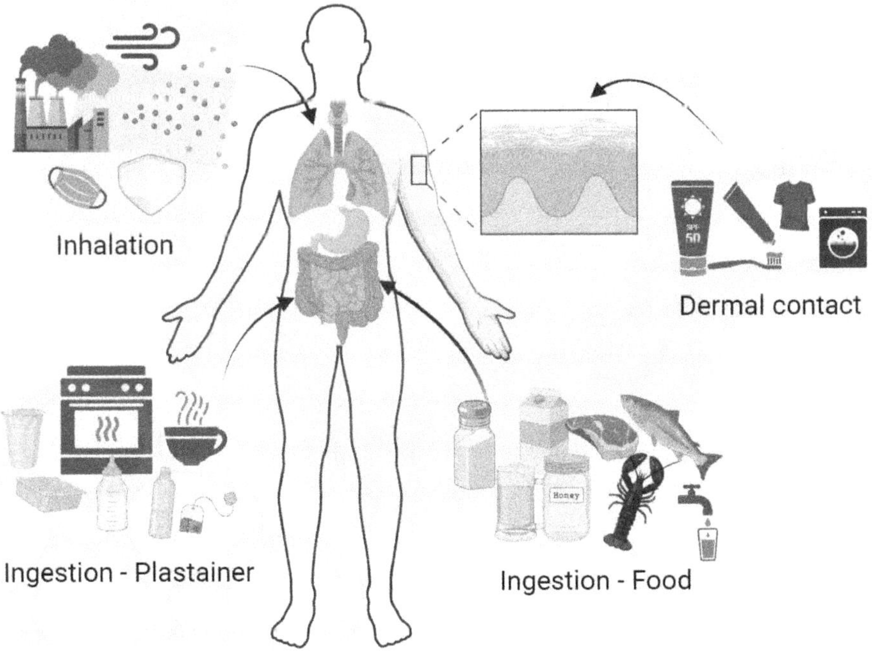

Fig. 1. Various exposure pathways of MNPs to humans.

Table 1. The occurrence and exposure scenarios of various MNPs in different matrices.

Type	Sample	Polymer type	Size	Concentration	Reference
Ingestion-plastic container	Plastic containers and reusable food pouches	PP, PE	1–14 μm 10–100 nm	Human burden: 20.3–22.1 ng/(kg · day)	26
	Beverage storage bottles	PE, PP, PET	<30 μm <1 μm	Release concentration: 68–4.66×10^8 items/L	27
	Tea bags	PP	50–100 μm 10–400 nm	Human burden: 11.68–29.20 mg/(individual · year)	28
	Baby bottles	PP	2–5 μm	Human burden: 1.58 million items per baby per day	29
	Cutting Boards	PP, PE	<100 μm	Human burden: 14.5–71.9 million items per person per year 7.4–50.7 g per person per year	30
	Plastic food containers	PP	<50 nm	Release concentration: 38 ± 5.29 mg per disposable plastic cup	31
Ingestionfood	Salt	PET, PP, PE	515 ± 171 μm	Containing concentration: 0.007–0.68 particles/g	33
		PET, PE, cellophane	<200 μm	Containing concentration: 0.550–0.681 particles/g	34
	Honey	PET, Resin	10–20 μm	Containing concentration: 166 ± 147 fibbers/kg 9 ± 9 fragments/kg	35

	PET, Resin	500 μm	Containing concentration: 1760–8680 items/kg (black particles) 132–728 items/kg (white fibers) 60–172 items/kg (white particles) 60–172 items/kg (white particles) 32–108 items/kg (colored fibers)	36
Beer	—	—	Containing concentration: Fibers: 2–79 items/L Fragments: 12–109 items/L Particles: 2–66 items/L	37
Milk	PSF	11–5000 μm	Containing concentration: 6.5 ± 2.3 items/L	38
Fish	EVA, PP, PET, PVC, PVA, PA	80–3400 μm	—	39
	PAN, PEVA, PP, PET	147–479 μm	Containing concentration: 0.16 items/g	
	—	22–4986 μm	Containing concentration: 0.2–0.5 items/individual	
	PA, PE, PET, PMMA	—	—	

(*Continued*)

Table 1. (*Continued*)

Type	Sample	Polymer type	Size	Concentration	Reference
		PE, PP, PET	<5000 μm	Containing concentration: 0.69 ± 1.25 items/individual	
		—	<100 μm	Containing concentration: 0.16–0.59 items/g	
	Bivalves	PE, PET, PA	10–5000 μm	Containing concentration: 0.2–2.2 items/g	
		PP, PS, PA	—	Containing concentration: 0.07–5.47 items/g	
		PES, PP, PE	5–5000 μm	Containing concentration: 0.7–2.9 items/g	
	Bottle water	PA, PP, PE, PMMA, PVC, PS, PET	<100 nm	Containing concentration: $2.4 \pm 1.3 \times 10^5$ particles/L	40
	Drinking water	PET, PE, PP	1–100 μm	Containing concentration: 6.7×10^3 items/L	
		PET, PE, PP	1–100 μm	Containing concentration: 9.3×10^2 items/L	
		PES, PVC, PA, epoxy resin, PE	50–150 μm	Containing concentrations: 0.7 items/m^3	
	Tap water	PE, PS, PET, rayon, PP, PMP, PA	10–5000 μm	Containing concentration: 0.3–1.6 items/L	

		PS, PVC, PA, epoxy resin, PE	$>20\,\mu m$	Containing concentration: 0–0.0007 items/L	
		Synthetic polymers	$0.1–5\,\mu m$	Containing concentration: 5.45 items/L	
		PET, PP, PE	$<10\,\mu m$	Containing concentrations. 469.6 items/L (mean)	
		PE, PP, PET	$3–4453\,\mu m$	Containing concentration: 0–1247 items/L	
	Bottle water	PET	$0–10\,\mu m$	Containing concentration: 2.6×10^3 (PET bottle) 4.9×10^3 (reusable PET bottle) 6.3×10^3 (glas bottle) items/L	
Inhalation	Outdoor air	Cotton, PET, PA, polyolefin, PTFE, PE	$40–3000\,\mu m$	132 items/($m^2 \cdot d$)	44
		PP	$50–4850\,\mu m$	0.3–1.5 fibers/m^3	45
		PP	$50–4850\,\mu m$	1.0–60.0 fibers/m^3	45
	Air	—	—	Human burden: 53,700 items per year per person	46
	N95 Mask	PP	$5\,nm–600\,\mu m$	Containing concentration: 10.6 ± 2.3 items/mg (nasal discharge)	48

(Continued)

Table 1. (*Continued*)

Type	Sample	Polymer type	Size	Concentration	Reference
Dermal contact	Shower Fonam	PE, PET, PP, PMMA, PA	26 μm–11 mm	—	54
	Shampod, face creams, hand washes, and sunscreens	PE, PET, PP	—	—	55
	Toothpaste	Cellophane, PP, PVC, PA	100–399 μm	Emission concrntration: 1.4 billion g per year	56
	Textile (Household detergent)	PET, PMMA	<5000 μm	Emission concentration: 0.5–6 million items per wash	57
	Mobile phone protective covers	PC, PU	28 μm 32 μm	Release concentration: 1122 items/cm^2 (mobile phone protective cowers) 314 items/cm^2 (palm)	58

2.1. *Exposure through ingestion and the gastrointestinal tract-related adverse outcomes*

Human ingestion of MNPs can come from two main sources. First, it arises from the utilization of food containers and kitchen utensils, such as takeaway boxes, cups, spoons and bowls made of plastic. During the cooking process and under high-temperature conditions, plastic containers and packaging[26] can release MNPs particles, which can subsequently enter the body through the consumption of food. Additionally, repeated freezing and thawing of plastic beverage bottles,[27] and routine brewing of plastic tea bags[28] and baby bottles[29] can result in significant releases of MNPs. This risk may also exist with other plastic kitchen utensils due to mechanical abrasion during use, such as plastic cutting boards,[30] knives and forks.[31] The risk associated with the release of MNPs particles from these sources is conspicuously apparent. Diverse studies indicate that the release of MNPs particles ranges from tens of millions to hundreds of millions of particles per liter. A prevailing consensus across most studies underscores that NPs exhibit a notably higher propensity for release compared to MPs particles. Noteworthy evidence from a specific study focusing on beverage bottles[27] reveals a significant difference, reaching up to five orders of magnitude higher for NPs. Regarding plastic types,[26–31] many studies consistently indicate that polypropylene (PP) exhibits an elevated propensity for release when contrasted with other plastic variants such as polyethylene terephthalate (PET) and polyethylene (PE).

Another major source of ingestion exposure to MNPs is through food, beverages and drinking water. Some food production processes may also entail MPs contamination, giving rise to potential risks to human health.[32] MNPs have been reported in food such as salt,[33,34] honey,[35,36] beer,[37] milk[38] and seafood.[39] Concerning salt, MPs concentrations range from 0.007 to 0.68 particles/g, and the three types of polymers (PET, PP, PE) constitute many of all particles.[33,34] The average content of MPs in honey is 0.166 fibers/g and 0.009 fragments/g. Most of the polymer types for fibers are PET.[35,36] Similarly, beer exhibits MPs contamination, with fiber, fragment and particle contents of 0.025, 0.033 and 0.017/mL, respectively.[37] Mexican brand milk has been found to contain plastic fragments and fibers at a rate of 0.0065/mL.[38] Existing data from various seafood species, including fish, shrimp, bivalves and other food items, reveals an average particle count ranging from 1 to 7 per fish, 0.75 particles/g in shrimp and an average of 0.2–4 particles/g in bivalves.[39] Lastly, our drinking water safety is impacted by the presence of MNPs. Various sources, including drinking water treatment plants, tap water and bottled water, contribute to the exposure risk of ingestion. Bottled water can pose unexpected risks,[40] as a quantified study indicates it contains over 10^5 particles/L, predominantly comprised of NPs. In addition, emerging technologies like hyperspectral stimulated Raman scattering (SRS) are made possible by the less complex matrix of bottled water, which makes such research frequently intersect with advances in analytical detection techniques. Statistical data reveals that the human body burden of MNPs through drinking water can be $(0\text{–}4.7) \times 10^3$ items/person/year.[41]

Hence, the sources contributing to ingestion exposure to MNPs are remarkably diverse, thereby significantly elevating the exposure risks. Subsequently, these MNPs will enter the human body, potentially undergoing enrichment within the human digestive system. Currently, MNPs have been detected in various biological components of the human body, including regularly in human feces.[9–12] A study of fecal samples from eight healthy adults from several Asian and European countries found that, on average, every 10 grams of human feces contained about 20 MPs (ranging in size from 50 μm to 500 μm).[9] This study represents the first detection of MNPs in human feces and demonstrates the potential gastrointestinal burden of MPs due to ingestion.

As the release of MNPs from plastic use poses a risk of ingestion, a two-month fecal survey,[42] where participants exclusively utilized disposable plastic tableware for three daily meals for one mouth, found a delayed impact on the disturbance of the intestinal microbiota. Compared to the control group, fecal samples from the post-exposure group, which used plastic products for one month and then abstained for another month, showed an increased MPs detection rate, reduced microbial diversity and a change in microbial community distribution.

Specifically, variations in the abundance of *Actinomycetes*, *Proteobacteria*, *Firmicutes* and *Bacteroides* were observed. These results indicate that ingestion exposure induces changes in intestinal microbiota and metabolites, particularly implicating the central nervous system, energy metabolism and inflammatory processes. Considering the developmental stage of the exposed individuals, one study in fecal samples from infants and adults revealed the presence of PET and polycarbonate (PC) MPs. Calculations based on estimated daily exposure levels suggest that infants are significantly more exposed to MPs compared to adults, with PET concentrations an order of magnitude higher.[10] This clearly shows that plastic products that young children come into frequent contact with (e.g., PC bottles and pacifiers) pose some risk of exposure. Simultaneously, disparities in exposure between infants and adults underscore variations in exposure levels across distinct stages of human development. As to ingestion exposure from air, water and food, another study focused on young people in Beijing, China, found that water consumption could be one of the factors affecting MPs levels in the gastrointestinal tract.[11] In addition to the investigation of human feces, existing research has confirmed the widespread presence of MPs in the human colon.[43]

In the context of gastrointestinal diseases, a study on fecal samples from IBD patients indicated a higher MPs content in the feces of individuals with IBD compared to healthy subjects.[12] Furthermore, 15 types of MPs were identified, signifying a positive correlation between MPs content in feces and the presence of IBD. These findings concerning the detection of MNPs in feces, along with diagnostic research, elucidate that ingestion exposure leads to the entry of MNPs into the human digestive system, potentially bearing relevance to associated IBD.

2.2. *Exposure through inhalation and respiratory-related adverse outcomes*

Inhalation exposure to MNPs is often associated with air pollution and occupational exposure. In terms of air pollution, the environmental exposure of airborne MPs depends on their widespread distribution from various sources.[44] Erosion of synthetic textiles, synthetic rubber tires and urban dust are considered primary contributors to airborne MPs. A study has indicated indoor concentrations ranging from 1.0 fibers/m^3 to 60.0 fibers/m^3, while outdoor concentrations are notably lower, ranging from 0.3 fibers/m^3 to 1.5 fibers/m^3.[45] Moreover, these plastic particles in the atmosphere often undergo chemical transformations (such as nucleation and condensation), significantly amplifying the risk to human health. Regarding to human body burdens of MPs through inhalation, with an air concentration averaging 9.8 MPs/m^3 and an inhalation rate of 15 m^3/day, the annual exposure to inhaled particles was estimated at 53,700/person.[46] As for occupational exposure, it is largely associated with aerosolized NPs and commonly occurs in industries involving synthetic textiles, flocking and the production of vinyl chloride (VC) and polyvinyl chloride (PVC).[47] Lastly, due to the COVID-19 pandemic, the use of masks, a plastic product, can also lead to human exposure through the release of MNPs. Research indicates that each surgical or N95 mask can release over a billion MNPs particles, leading to inhalation exposure during usage. The concentration of MNPs detected in the nasal mucus of individuals subjected to brief mask-wearing periods can attain a level of 10.6 ± 2.3 items/mg.[48]

As for inhalation exposure to MNPs, numerous epidemiological investigations have been conducted on MNPs levels in the human pulmonary system. As early as 1998, a study observed the presence of synthetic fibers in lung tissue samples obtained from patients undergoing lung tumor resection.[13] However, the detection of MNPs in the human pulmonary system was not confirmed until 2021, when an investigation of postmortem lung tissue samples in humans was conducted.[14] In the context of living human lungs, one study found MPs in surgically removed lung tissue samples.[15] The most abundant types of MPs detected were PP, PET, resin and PE. MPs were primarily present in the form of fibers (49%) and fragments (43%). Notably, the observed size of MNPs in various lung tissues, such as bronchoalveolar lavage fluid14 (BALF) could range from several tens to hundreds of micrometers, contradicting the prevailing notion that only particles with a physical diameter smaller than 3 μm can enter the alveolar region of the lungs. This underscores the complexity of the MNPs exposure.

To explore MNPs exposure disparities between healthy individuals and those with respiratory diseases, a study investigated BALF samples from patients with respiratory conditions.[16] This study confirmed the inhalation of MPs into the deepest areas of the lungs and established correlations between MPs concentrations and pathological outcomes. These outcomes included radiological abnormalities, pathological microbial growth and decreased lung function. Additionally, a correlation was noted between MNPs exposure in the human pulmonary system and blood indicators,[49] with positive associations observed with human platelets (PLT), platelet crit (PCT) and fibrinogen (FIB), along with negative correlations with direct bilirubin (DB). In another study of sputum samples from patients with various respiratory diseases, 21 types of MPs were identified, with PU (polyurethane) and PET accounting for the majority and found a connection between MPs exposure and personal smoking habits and the performance of invasive tracheal examinations.[50]

Regarding specific pulmonary diseases, epidemiological evidence highlighted that workers in the plastics and textile industries, exposed to significant amounts of plastic fiber dust, were susceptible to lung injuries,[51] including inflammation, fibrosis and allergies. Notably, one study explored the link between MPs exposure and human pulmonary GGN, detecting various microfibers in tumor and normal lung tissue samples.[20] Among them, the detection rate of microfibers in tumors was 58%, higher than in normal tissues (46%), Moreover, the quantified amount of MPs ($>20\,\mu$m) identified in tumors was twice that found in normal lung tissue samples. Individuals with a history of higher MPs exposure exhibited a significantly higher tumor detection rate, indicating a potential association between MPs inhalation and GGN formation. In addition to lung diseases, the emerging concern about the potential link between occupational exposure to MNPs and the risk of cancer diseases. A review of 34 studies revealed a critical link between occupational exposure to MPs, particularly PVC, and an increased incidence of liver diseases, particularly liver cancer such as angiosarcoma and hepatocellular carcinoma.[52] This research highlights the urgent need for in-depth research into the different health threats posed by various MPs, particularly PVC, in work environments and highlights their carcinogenic potential compared to other MPs.

2.3. *Exposure through dermal contact and the dermal-related adverse outcomes*

Skin exposure sources often occur through contact with personal care products and clothing in our daily lives. Cosmetics and personal care products in our daily routines, such as face washes and toothpaste, often incorporate plastic microbeads during production to enhance scrubbing effectiveness and augment their cleansing or exfoliating functionalities. These MPs constitute a significant source of environmental plastic pollution.[53] They encompass various polymer types, including PE, PET, PP, PMMA (polymethyl methacrylate) and PA (polyamide/nylon).[54] Studies indicate that shampoo, face creams, hand washes and sunscreens contain 71%, 60%, 80% and 83% MPs, respectively.[55] Commercial toothpaste sold in India consistently contains MPs of different size categories, distributions and polymer forms.[56] The content of MPs particles in toothpaste is between 0.2% and 0.9% by weight, with fibers and fragments often occurring. During the laundering of clothing, both the presence of MNPs in detergents and the washing process itself generate corresponding MNPs fibers. Statistics show that washing synthetic garments can release from 500,000 to over 6 million microfibers per wash while washing cotton garments can release up to 13 million microfibers.[57] Polyester fibers dominate (constituting approximately 80%) among them. These microfibers also have the potential to pose exposure risks to the human body during the clothing usage process. Additionally, the utilization of mobile phone protective covers (PMPC) represents an overlooked potential source of MPs.[58] It can generate MPs, which are transferred to human hands.

The human skin, oral cavity and hair serve as passive receptors for human exposure to MNPs. A study conducted in Iran investigated the aspect of human contact exposure to MNPs.[59] It examined the presence of MNPs in the skin of individuals' hands and faces, saliva and hair. This research has already demonstrated the ubiquity of contact exposure to MNPs, and it also pointed out the high heterogeneity of exposure among different individuals. These pieces of evidence collectively underscore the inevitability of human exposure to MNPs. Therefore, it is imperative to pay attention to the health risks posed by MNPs to the human body. Additionally, further research is needed to ascertain whether these exposures entail risks related to human diseases.

2.4. *Cardiovascular-related adverse outcomes*

In addition to investigating the background of human exposure to MNPs through ingestion, inhalation and skin contact, current epidemiological studies have also discovered MNPs in various biological components and organs of the human body, including blood,[18] placenta,[17] breast milk,[60] liver[21] and heart.[61] This suggests that after entering the human body through exposure routes, MNPs may undergo internalization and transformation, entering other biological components and organ tissues. In the first study to find MPs in human blood for the first time, quantifiable MPs were detected in 77% of samples, with an average frequency of 1.6 μg/mL of blood.[18] The proportions of PET, polystyrene (PS) and PE were 50%, 36% and 23%, respectively. The duration of MPs presence in the blood is unknown, necessitating further research into their transportation and mechanisms of action within the human body. Another study detected the presence of MNPs in five different cardiac tissue samples from cardiac surgery patients and pre- and post-operative venous blood samples.[61] The largest MPs diameter found in cardiac tissue samples was 469 μm, while in blood samples, the maximum diameter was 184 μm. This study indicates the existence of MPs not only due to inadvertent exposure during surgery but also from nonsurgical factors. Moreover, the size distribution variations between different tissue and blood samples suggest potential impacts of MNPs on visceral organs and human health. Therefore, the evidence from these studies suggests that MNPs may have more complex toxicity mechanisms and health risks for the human body. Further investigation is urgently needed to address scientific questions regarding whether MNPs are associated with human diseases such as cancer and cardiovascular disorders.

In summary, as to the exposure pathways of MNPs, contemporary research suggests that ingestion and inhalation are two major routes of human exposure. Conversely, dermal contact does not pose a significant health risk. The complexity of human exposure to MNPs becomes apparent through the integration of exposure sources with epidemiological studies of human biological components. This intricacy is potentially linked to the diverse array of exposure sources, but correlations can be discerned by juxtaposing MNPs detected in specific biological components of the human body. Figure 2 provides a comprehensive summary of the MNPs detected in the human body. A comparative analysis of the polymer type of MNPs during epidemiological studies of human biological components and specific plastic products can illuminate the potential MNPs exposure risks associated with the utilization of plastic products. Simultaneously, epidemiological research data on population stratification reveals individual variations in the exposure to MNPs within the human body, with personal habits and occupational factors emerging as prominent determinants. Regardless of the exposure pathways, specific plastic types of MNPs, notably PET, PP and PE plastics, manifest elevated exposure, and detection proportions. This occurrence is ascribed not solely to their widespread environmental contamination but also to their incorporation as raw materials in distinct formulations of plastic products. Simultaneously, the identification of MNPs in human blood and cardiac tissues underscores the pressing human health risks, intricately linked to the internalization risk of MNPs upon entering the human body. Notably, size-related investigations into MNPs detection in various human body components consistently reveal the presence of larger-sized MPs. It challenges the conclusions derived from conventional toxicology experiments regarding the interplay between particle size and biological barriers.[62] Consequently, it becomes imperative to employ

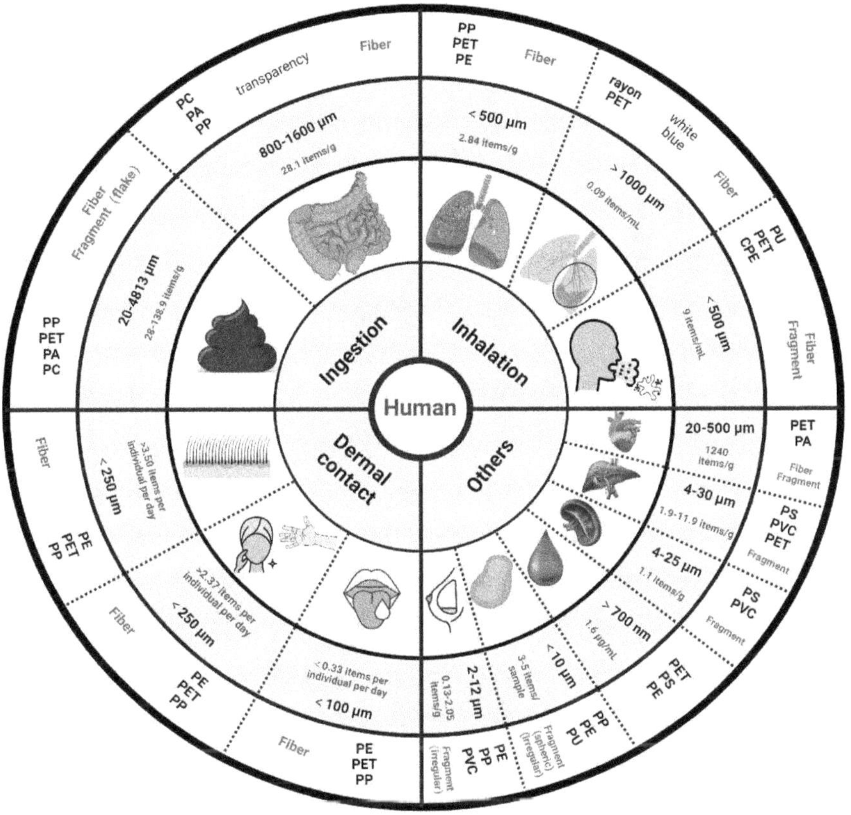

Fig. 2. A summary of MNPs detected in the human body.

epidemiological investigations as a guiding framework to probe into the toxicology of MNPs.

3. Toxicity mechanisms of MNPs revealed by laboratory investigations

Thanks to advancements in nanomaterial and nanotoxicology,[63] laboratory studies on MNPs have improved, leading to methods and results that may show causative relationships between exposure patterns and health outcomes. In addition, current research in the toxicology of model organisms concerning various target organs has made progress in elucidating the toxic mechanisms of the effects of MNPs on the gastrointestinal tract, lungs and cardiovascular system.

3.1. *Gastrointestinal toxicity*

Current toxicity research suggests that MNPs pose potential risks to human health when ingested. And the mechanisms of toxicity often manifest in two distinct aspects, on one hand, MNPs directly enter the gastrointestinal tract, leading to increased intestinal permeability, alterations in gut microbiota composition, and metabolic changes, among other adverse effects. On the other hand, once NPs particles are absorbed through the intestine, they can be transported *via* the circulatory system to reach other organs, resulting in internalization and biotransformation. Moreover, high concentrations of MNPs can elevate oxidative stress, leading to the production of inflammatory cytokines, cell apoptosis, cytotoxicity and disrupted gene expression, among other effects, the related toxicity of MNPs can be shown in Fig. 3.

As to the direct impact, extensive *in vivo* studies in zebrafish and mice have demonstrated that MPs can alter the composition of human gut microbiota, characterized by an increased abundance of taxa like *Chlamydiae*, *Firmicutes* and *Proteobacteria*.[64] Moreover, gut microbiota can adhere to the surface of MPs, inducing biofilm formation. Exposure to MPs leads to increased intestinal permeability and expression of inflammation-related immune features, such as interleukin-6(IL-6), interleukin-1α(IL-1α), interleukin-1β(IL-1β), tumor necrosis factor-α(TNF-α) and interferon-γ(IFN-γ). This effect may be the result of a consequence of MPs capturing and stimulating inflammatory infiltration in the intestines. Another *in vivo* study indicates that micron-sized (25 μm) polylactic acid (PLA) plastic particles, upon entering the intestines, are enzymatically catalyzed by intestinal enzymes, releasing oligomer nanoparticles and triggering acute inflammation.[65] It has been demonstrated that PLA MPs in the gastrointestinal process undergo enzymatic degradation by competing for triglycerides and forming nanoparticles, potentially posing a health risk. Furthermore, another *in vitro* study suggests that

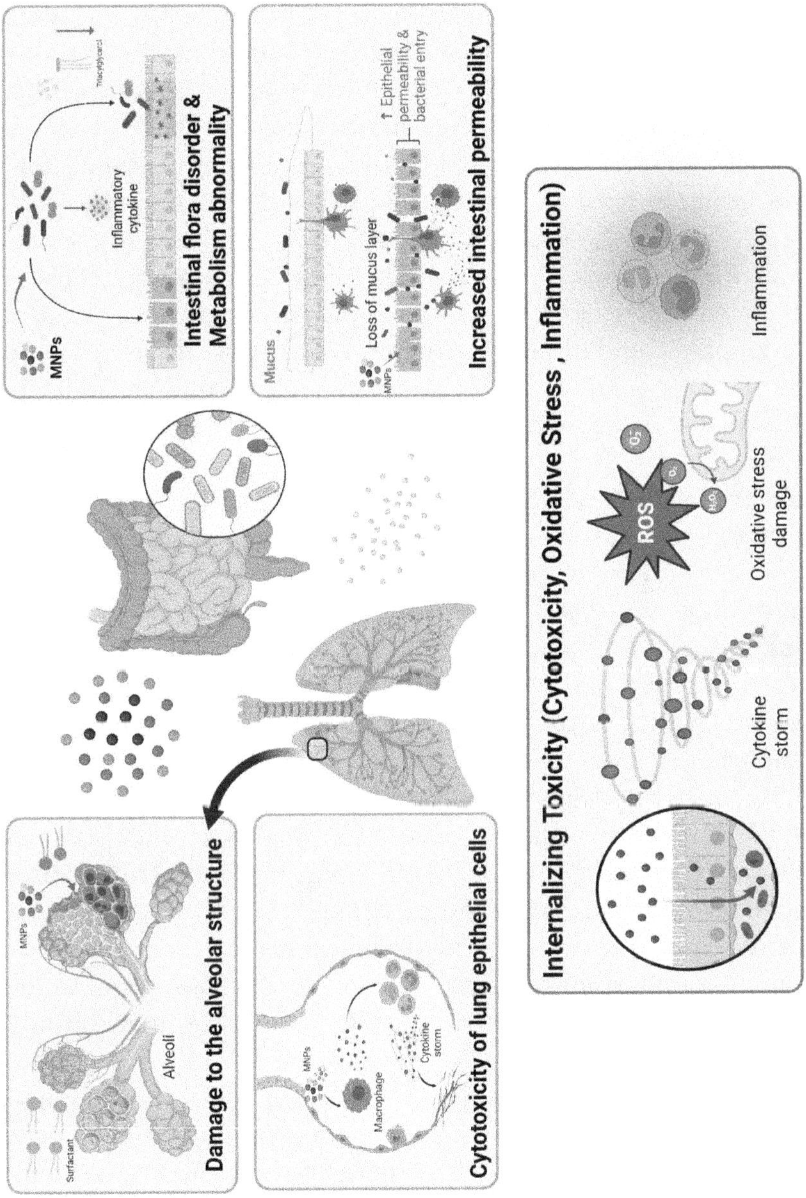

Fig. 3. Toxicity mechanisms of MNPs to the intestine and lung.

large-sized (millimeter-scale) PLA MPs may have a potential impact on human colonic microbiota composition and metabolism.[66] MPs initially induce noticeable changes, followed by colonic fermentation, leading to an increased proportion of Bifidobacterium. MPs entering the intestines through ingestion also adversely affect lipid digestion. An *in vitro* study indicates that five types of MPs, PS, PET, PE, PVC and polylactic acid-co-glycolic acid (PLGA) significantly inhibit lipid digestion in an *in vitro* gastrointestinal system.[67] Among these, PS exhibits the highest level of inhibition (12.7%), and as the concentration of PS increases, lipid digestion capacity decreases. This is attributed to MPs forming large lipid-MP hetero-aggregates, adsorbing lipases, and altering enzyme secondary structure, thereby reducing the bioavailability of lipid droplets. These findings indicate that MPs have a detrimental impact on lipid digestion, posing a risk to human health.

As to another toxicological mechanism, for MPs, those larger than 150 μm in size cannot be absorbed.[68] Instead, they adhere to the intestinal mucosal layer, making direct contact with the apical portion of intestinal epithelial cells. This can lead to intestinal inflammation and has a localized impact on the immune system. However, for smaller particles (less than 150 μm), both MPs and NPs can pass through the mucous barrier. They are absorbed through processes such as endocytosis of intestinal epithelial cells, transcellular uptake by microfold cells, barrier penetration (permeation), and paracellular uptake by adjacent cells. This could potentially lead to systemic toxicity, penetrating deep into organs. For instance, in a study conducted in rats, oral ingestion of PS (0.87 μm) resulted in 6% reaching the circulatory system after 15 min, whereas oral ingestion of PS (50 nm) led to 34% absorption.[69] These may be transported to the circulatory system through the mesenteric lymph and preferentially accumulate in the liver. In the case of zebrafish embryos,[70] exposure to PS MPs caused the particles to migrate to the heart, resulting in a decrease in heart rate. Furthermore, some *in vitro* studies suggest that PS nanospheres can be passively translocated through cell membranes, internalized, and released by human colonic fibroblasts.[71,72] After internalization by human gastric adenocarcinoma cells, 44 nm

PS particles can alter gene expression, reduce cell viability, and trigger pro-inflammatory responses and morphological changes. Moreover, chemicals present in MNPs may potentially be released, enter the bloodstream, and affect the endocrine, immune and nervous systems.[73]

3.2. *Pulmonary toxicity*

MNPs can enter the human respiratory tract and lungs through inhalation exposure. A substantial body of research on model organisms has indicated that MNPs exert detrimental effects on the lungs through various toxic mechanisms. Upon entry into the alveolar environment, MNPs interact with pulmonary surfactants. This interaction disrupts the epithelial barrier function, causing MNPs to transition *via* vesicle fusion to the air-water interface of the alveoli. This disrupts the ultrastructure and flow of pulmonary surfactants, leading to the collapse of the pulmonary surfactant film.[74] Additionally, plastic particles in this process adsorb phospholipids and proteins from the lung surfactant material, altering the behavior of pulmonary surfactants. This process also generates hydrogen peroxide and reactive oxygen species, which adversely affect the lungs.[75]

Furthermore, after MNPs enter the pulmonary environment, their small size allows them to be internalized into epithelial cells, resulting in cytotoxicity. Exposure to PS NPs can induce the upregulation of pro-apoptotic proteins such as A549DR5, caspase-3, caspase-8, caspase-9 and cytochrome c in pulmonary epithelial cells, indicating that MNPs can induce cell apoptosis.[76] A study employing PP NPs to investigate their toxic effects on murine and human lung epithelial cells (A549) found that *in vivo*, PP induces lung inflammation and ROS generation in mice, activating p38 and NF-κB signaling pathways.[77] *In vitro*, PP causes mitochondrial depolarization and reduced levels of adenosine triphosphate (ATP) within cells, leading to organelle dysfunction. A study focusing on PS nanoparticles reached similar conclusions, and metabolomics further demonstrated that NPs induce mitochondrial damage in human lung cells (BEAS-2B).[78] Regarding MPs, *in vitro* experiments also discovered that MPs disrupt intercellular adhesive proteins of lung cells and induce cytotoxicity through the generation of ROS.[79]

Finally, the epithelial cells of the respiratory system not only serve as physical barriers but also possess immunological functions. They actively participate in the immune response to allergens, MPs and other stimuli by releasing numerous signaling molecules.[80] Therefore, a wealth of research suggests that exposure to MNPs can trigger inflammation in epithelial cells. MNPs stimulate pulmonary epithelial cells to produce pro-inflammatory cytokines such as TNF-α, IL-6, IL-1β and TGF-β.[51,76,81] Furthermore, contact with MNPs leads to a significant decrease in the activity of oxidative stress-related enzymes like GSH-Px, CAT and SOD, inducing the production of ROS and disrupting redox balance. Intratracheal injection of PS MPs increases the expression of pro-inflammatory cytokines TNF-α, IL-6 and IL-1β in rat BALF. Inhalation exposure may also compromise the integrity of the respiratory epithelial barrier, leading to lung injury and inflammation.[82]

3.3. *Cardiovascular toxicity*

The detection of MNPs in various biological components of the human body has significantly deepened our understanding of their exposure risks. This is particularly evident when detected in the blood and heart, where several toxicological model organism studies may indicate that MNPs are a major factor in human cardiovascular disease. Research shows that the toxicity of MNPs is mainly manifested by hemolysis, thrombosis and blood clotting. In the case of the heart, symptoms include pericardial edema, abnormal heart rate and myocardial fibrosis [Fig. 4].[83]

Regarding vascular toxicity, the harmful effects of MNPs are primarily seen in hemolysis, thrombosis and vascular structural damage. The hemolytic capacity of MNPs has been confirmed *in vitro* in human cells. Both PS and PE MPs cause hemolysis in human peripheral blood mononuclear cells (PBMCs), often due to physical damage from plastic particles leading to membrane disruption.[84,85] Thrombosis is considered a major cardiovascular risk factor leading to

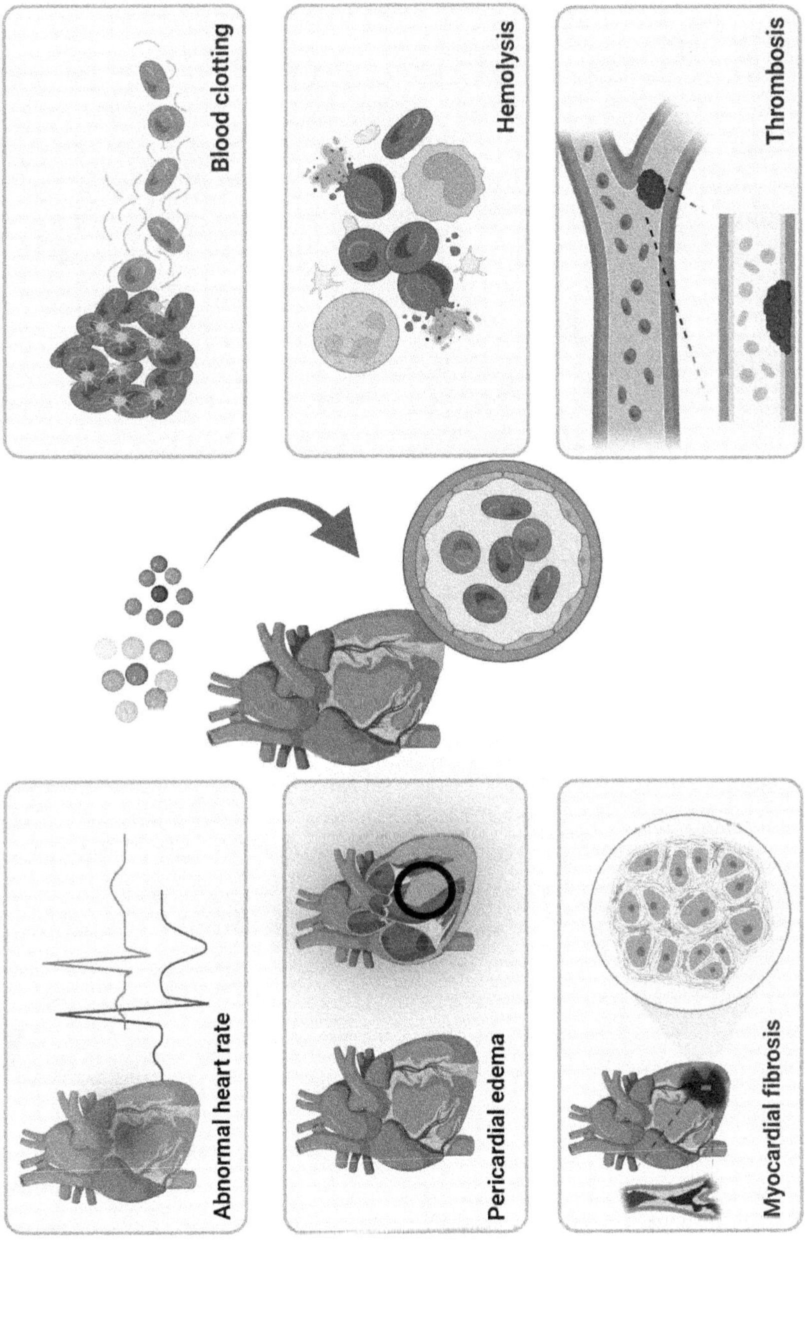

Fig. 4. Toxicity mechanisms of MNPs to the cardiovascular system.

vascular occlusion. NPs can inhibit subintestinal vessel development in zebrafish embryos,[86] causing endothelial cell dysfunction, and simultaneously inhibiting CO_2 and blood flow rates, ultimately affecting thrombosis. Blood coagulation, which leads to clot formation through a series of cascade effects, has been shown in studies to be affected by differently sized and modified PS nanoparticles.[87] Amination nanoparticles can reduce the formation of coagulants in human plasma, as they interact with human coagulation factors. Conversely, carboxylation and sulfonation nanoparticles increase the conversion of prothrombin to thrombin through intrinsic pathways, resulting in coagulation dysfunction. Endothelial damage may produce the toxic effect of atherosclerosis. Studies have shown that oral exposure to PS nanoparticles exacerbates atherosclerosis in ApoE −/− mice fed a high-fat diet for 19 weeks.[88] This is primarily characterized by reduced aortic elasticity, increased plaque area in the aortic intima, and accelerated progression of atherosclerotic plaque lesions. The toxic mechanism is attributed to the combined action of MNPs with endogenous metabolites (long-chain acylcarnitine), which exacerbate atherosclerosis in mice by upregulating macrophage receptors with collagenous structure (MARCO) induced by NPs.

Regarding cardiac toxicity, MNPs mainly manifest as pericardial edema, abnormal heart rate and myocardial fibrosis. Exposure to PE NPs causes cardiac toxicity in zebrafish embryos.[86] NPs can induce pericardial edema in zebrafish embryos, and with increasing exposure dose, chemotaxis and recruitment of neutrophils become more pronounced in the tail vein of zebrafish embryos, suggesting that the induced pericardial edema may be related to inflammation. In another study, particles and fibers made of PET (p-PET, diameter approximately 150 μm) and fibers (f-PET, length approximately 3–5 mm, diameter 20 μm) were used to expose zebrafish embryos.[89] It was found that the presence of these MPs accelerated the heart rate of zebrafish embryos and suppressed hatching due to the barrier effect on the embryonic chorionic canal. Myocardial fibrosis is one of the important pathways leading to cardiac dysfunction or even heart failure. Studies have shown that PS MPs induce oxidative stress in rat hearts, leading to cardiomyocyte apoptosis and activating the

Wnt/-catenin protein, ultimately leading to cardiac fibrosis.[90] Exposure to MNPs increases serum cardiac troponin I and creatine kinase MB (CK-MB) levels, causing structural damage and apoptosis of myocardial cells and leading to cardiac collagen proliferation. Cardiac organoids (CO) are currently a new model for studying MPs cardiac toxicity. Studies have shown that exposure to PS MPs at a low dose of 2.5 μg/mL significantly increases the volume of cardiac organoids, along with collagen accumulation and disrupted cell arrangement.[91] This indicates that exposure to MNPs at environmental doses leads to cardiac hypertrophy.

Here, diverse toxicological studies on model organisms can illustrate the varying exposure outcomes and consequent toxicity mechanisms of MNPs. Current research has elucidated two primary toxic mechanisms of MNPs [Fig. 3]. The first mechanism is characterized by direct interaction, where MNPs directly engage with biological structures within the gastrointestinal tract, lungs, or broader human body environment, inducing toxicity. The second mechanism involves MNPs facilitating further damage upon internalization, either through cellular uptake or transport mechanisms, leading to their entry into the human circulatory system and causing cytotoxic effects. Notably, these mechanisms are often influenced by the interaction between the particulate matter and the bio-barrier of an organism, with the size, shape, hydrophilicity and surface potential of MNPs playing a pivotal role.

4. The key factors — physicochemical property of MNPs

In various biological systems such as the gastrointestinal tract, lung and cardiovascular system, MNPs exhibit specific toxicity mechanisms in different target organ environments. This phenomenon has been extensively documented through empirical research. However, the interaction between MNPs and the biological interface remains a focus in the field of toxicology. Given the different environmental conditions of different biological systems, such as: B. Variations in pH, lipophilicity and charge potential, MNPs can trigger a range of biological reactions. The physicochemical properties of MNPs often play a decisive role. For MNP particles of the same polymer type, toxicity mechanisms vary with size, and smaller particles may have higher reactivity and a greater potential to penetrate biological barriers, thus posing different levels of risk to organisms.[92–94] In addition, fibrous MPs often pose a greater threat to organisms in terms of shape and charge than spherical or fragmentary MPs,[95] and positively charged MPs have greater toxic effects than negatively charged or neutral ones.[96]

Furthermore, the physicochemical properties of MNPs in the environment may change after aging, thereby altering their toxicity and environmental hazards. First, the inherent resistance of MNPs to biodegradation, in addition to their particle shape, poses physical damage to living organisms. Aging leads to significant changes in surface morphology, particularly an increase in surface roughness, which is directly linked to increased cytotoxic and inflammatory reactions.[85,97] In addition, the aging process increases the ability of MPs to act as vectors for environmental pollutants due to changes in their surface properties. This enhanced "Trojan horse" phenomenon potentially increases the chemical toxicity of these particles.[98] A crucial component of aging is photooxidation, which generates environmentally persistent free radicals (EPFRs) and reactive oxygen species (ROS) and triggers oxidative stress, leading to cellular and systemic damage.[99,100] The aged MPs exhibit altered physicochemical properties, including increased amounts of conjugated carbonyls and ROS, which increase their cytotoxicity. The vector effect is further increased by aging, which means that the MNPs can act as a mediator for pollutants and as a promoter of microbial colonization, thus changing its ecological toxicity.[101,102] Interactions with other pollutants and biofilms significantly alter the combined toxicity of these plastics and increase their potential.[103]

However, these toxic results caused by the physicochemical property of MNPs still need to be unified, often due to limitations in characterization techniques for the physicochemical properties of MNPs and differences in experimental research.[104] For example, one study used microvibration technology and Fourier transform infrared spectroscopy (FTIR) to identify MPs. However, due to the spatial resolution limited by the optical diffraction limit, only micrometer-sized MPs could be detected. Photothermal infrared heterodyne imaging (IR-PHI), on the other hand, enables the detection of NP particles and can analyze aging-related changes in their physicochemical properties.[105,106] Therefore, there is an urgent need for future standardization of characterization techniques for MNPs.

5. Summary and outlook

There are associations found between the presence of MNP and adverse outcomes. As evidenced by numerous studies investigating MNP exposure sources. Humans are primarily exposed to MNPs through ingestion, inhalation and dermal contact. In the field of epidemiological research, it is time to look more deeply into the exposure and health issues associated with MPs, rather than just focusing on detecting and analyzing their exposure levels. It seems that the widespread presence of MNPs in the human body has already found consensus. What requires greater attention is research into the connection between MPs and human health. This endeavor will contribute to subsequent toxicology studies involving *in vitro* and *in vivo* experiments with MNPs. Identifying and tracing sources does not seem to be a primary concern. The key focus is on investigating the connection between health risks and MPs. Therefore, epidemiological investigations and toxicological studies on model organisms reinforce each other. They represent two aspects that must confirm and reinforce each other. Studies on the detection of MPs in human blood, for example, suggest that from a biological-toxicological point of view, it is conceivable that MNPs can be internalized and transported through the body.[23]

Current research on the mechanisms of MNP toxicity has advanced, primarily through extensive toxicological studies using model plastics.[107] However, challenges persist in this research approach. Commercially available model plastics, often used as initial exposure solutions, commonly contain suspension additives. The potential toxicity of these additives may introduce confounding factors in toxicological evaluations.[108] Additionally, the use of model plastics embedded with fluorescent agents in toxicological studies has raised concerns about the induced toxicity from these agents, potentially obscuring the assessment of the inherent toxicity. Despite the frequent use of commercial PS microspheres and nanospheres in research, their environmental abundance is relatively low, and there is a significant gap in studies using model microspheres made from other polymer types.[109] The diversity of MNP particulates noted in epidemiological studies indicates the need for more varied models in future toxicological research. These models should account for the simultaneous detection of MNPs of various sizes and types in biological matrices. A recent study[110] has reported on mixed-size MNPs exposure *in vivo*, underscoring the importance of considering different plastic types and shapes in future toxicological investigations. Additionally, using MNPs that have undergone environmental aging in experiments would yield more ecologically relevant results.

A gap exists between mechanism-oriented research and epidemiological studies on MNPs. Epidemiological studies concentrate on the exposure levels and risks of MNPs in the human body and their correlation with diseases. These studies assess the health effects of variable and usually low-dose exposures in populations, linking actual exposure levels to health outcomes, including chronic and cumulative exposure scenarios. Conversely, mechanistic toxicity studies often employ high MNP concentrations to elicit measurable effects in controlled environments. This approach leads to gaps in understanding the subtle, long-term effects at lower, environmentally relevant doses. Thus, epidemiological data could be instrumental in redesigning exposure doses for future toxicity studies.

Population surveys offer insights into varied responses and vulnerabilities across different age groups, demographics and health statuses. Findings from these studies, especially those concerning specific human diseases, can inform and enhance the study of MNP toxicity mechanisms in disease models and individuals with pre-existing conditions, providing detailed insights into disease processes. For instance, exploring the enteric toxicity of MNPs *in vivo* using mouse and zebrafish models of IBD can be enlightening.[111] Longitudinal population studies are valuable for understanding the temporal aspects of MNP exposure and its long-term effects, capturing the cumulative nature of environmental exposures and the delayed manifestation of toxicity effects. An example of this is a study on plastic lunch boxes, which demonstrated greater variability in intestinal flora distribution in the post-exposure group compared to the exposed and control groups.[42] These findings can guide the direction of toxicity mechanism studies.

Establishing an adverse outcome pathway (AOP) framework for MNPs should be a primary focus of future research. It is important to note that a comprehensive AOP framework relies on a close collaboration between epidemiological studies and toxicological investigations. Given the varieties of MNPs, diverse physicochemical characteristics, exposure scenarios, etc., linking adverse outcomes to toxicity mechanisms requires significant interdisciplinary effort. The comprehensive analysis of MNP exposure, human epidemiology, disease-related research and model toxicology studies will open new avenues and provide significant insights into understanding the effects and risks of MNPs on human health.

Conflict of interest

Sijie Lin declares that, as an Associate Editor of this journal, there is a conflict of interest regarding this paper. However, Sijie Lin confirms that he was not involved in the peer review procedure of this paper, which was handled by another Associate Editor of the journal, and therefore, he did not influence the editorial decision making process. The conflict of interest was disclosed to the editorial team, and appropriate steps were taken to ensure that the peer review and decision-making process for this paper were handled impartially and transparently.

All authors declare that they have no known competing financial interests or personal relationships that could have appeared to influence the work reported in this paper.

Author contributions

Fei He: Investigation, Data curation, Formal analysis, Writing — original draft, Writing — review & editing. Xiaohan Wu: Validation, Writing — original draft, Writing — review & editing. Sijie Lin:

Funding acquisition, Writing — review & editing, Writing — original draft, Supervision, Conceptualization.

Data availability

Data will be made available on request.

Statement of usage of artificial intelligence

This article does not employ artificial intelligence, language models, machine learning, or similar technologies to create, assist in creating, or edit any content (such as text and graphics) within the manuscript.

Funding information

This work received financial support from the National Natural Science Foundation of China (No. 22176150), Shanghai Pilot Program for Basic Research and the Fundamental Research Funds for the Central Universities.

ORCID

Fei He https://orcid.org/0009-0003-7810-7254
Xiaohan Wu https://orcid.org/0009-0002-1993-3639
Sijie Lin https://orcid.org/0000-0002-6970-8221

References

1. PlasticsEurope, *Plastics — The Facts 2022 — An analysis of European plastics production, demand and waste data* (PlasticsEurope, Belgium, 2023). https://plasticseurope.org/knowledge-hub/plastics-the-facts-2022/.
2. OECD, *Plastic Pollution is Growing Relentlessly as Waste Management and Recycling Fall Short, Says OECD* (Newsroom Paris, France, 2022). https://www.oecd.org/environment/plastic-pollution-is-growing-relentlessly-as-waste-management-and-recycling-fall-short.htm.
3. J. Duan, N. Bolan, Y. Li, S. Ding, T. Atugoda, M. Vithanage, B. Sarkar, D. C. Tsang and M. Kirkham, *Water Res.* **196**, 117011 (2021).
4. R. C. Thompson, Y. Olsen, R. P. Mitchell, A. Davis, S. J. Rowland, A. W. John, D. McGonigle and A. E. Russell, *Science* **304**, 838 (2004).

5. J. Gigault, A. Ter Halle, M. Baudrimont, P.-Y. Pascal, F. Gauffre, T.-L. Phi, H. El Hadri, B. Grassl and S. Reynaud, *Environ. Pollut.* **235**, 1030 (2018).
6. C. M. Rochman and T. Hoellein, *Science* **368**, 1184 (2020).
7. R. Lehner, C. Weder, A. Petri-Fink and B. Rothen-Rutishauser, *Environ. Sci. Technol.* **53**, 1748 (2019).
8. C. Wang, J. Zhao and B. Xing, *J. Hazard. Mater.* **407**, 124357 (2021).
9. P. Schwabl, S. Köppel, P. Königshofer, T. Bucsics, M. Trauner, T. Reiberger and B. Liebmann, *Ann. Intern. Med.* **171**, 453 (2019).
10. J. Zhang, L. Wang, L. Trasande and K. Kannan, *Environ. Sci. Technol. Lett.* **8**, 989 (2021).
11. N. Zhang, Y. B. Li, H. R. He, J. F. Zhang and G. S. Ma, *Sci. Total Environ.* **767**, 144345 (2021).
12. Z. Yan, Y. Liu, T. Zhang, F. Zhang, H. Ren and Y. Zhang, *Environ. Sci. Technol.* **56**, 414 (2021).
13. J. L. Pauly, S. J. Stegmeier, H. A. Allaart, R. T. Cheney, P. J. Zhang, A. G. Mayer and R. J. Streck, *Cancer Epidemiol. Biomarkers Prev.* **7**, 419 (1998).
14. L. F. Amato-Lourenço, R. Carvalho-Oliveira, G. R. Júnior, L. dos Santos Galvão, R. A. Ando and T. Mauad, *J. Hazard. Mater.* **416**, 126124 (2021).
15. L. C. Jenner, J. M. Rotchell, R. T. Bennett, M. Cowen, V. Tentzeris and L. R. Sadofsky, *Sci. Total Environ.* **831**, 154907 (2022).
16. C. Baeza-Martínez, S. Olmos, M. González-Pleiter, J. López-Castellanos, E. García-Pachón, M. Masiá-Canuto, L. Hernández-Blasco and J. Bayo, *J. Hazard. Mater.* **438**, 129439 (2022).
17. A. Ragusa, A. Svelato, C. Santacroce, P. Catalano, V. Notarstefano, O. Carnevali, F. Papa, M. C. A. Rongioletti, F. Baiocco and S. Draghi, *Environ. Int.* **146**, 106274 (2021).
18. H. A. Leslie, M. J. Van Velzen, S. H. Brandsma, A. D. Vethaak, J. J. Garcia-Vallejo and M. H. Lamoree, *Environ. Int.* **163**, 107199 (2022).
19. G. Kutralam-Muniasamy, V. Shruti, F. Pérez-Guevara and P. D. Roy, *Sci. Total Environ.* **856**, 159164 (2023).
20. Q. Chen, J. Gao, H. Yu, H. Su, Y. Yang, Y. Cao, Q. Zhang, Y. Ren, H. Hollert and H. Shi, *Environ. Sci. Eur.* **34**, 25 (2022).
21. T. Horvatits, M. Tamminga, B. Liu, M. Sebode, A. Carambia, L. Fischer, K. Püschel, S. Huber and E. K. Fischer, *EBioMedicine* **82**, 104147 (2022).
22. F. Dang, Q. Wang, Y. Huang, Y. Wang and B. Xing, *Eco-Environ. Health* **1**, 11 (2022).
23. Y. Li, L. Tao, Q. Wang, F. Wang, G. Li and M. Song, *Environ. Health* **1**, 249 (2023).
24. H. Luo, C. Liu, D. He, J. Xu, J. Sun, J. Li and X. Pan, *J. Hazard. Mater.* **423**, 126915 (2022).
25. A. A. Koelmans, P. E. Redondo-Hasselerharm, N. H. M. Nor, V. N. de Ruijter, S. M. Mintenig and M. Kooi, *Nat. Rev. Mater.* **7**, 138 (2022).
26. K. A. Hussain, S. Romanova, I. Okur, D. Zhang, J. Kuebler, X. Huang, B. Wang, L. Fernandez-Ballester, Y. Lu and M. Schubert, *Environ. Sci. Technol.* **57**, 9782 (2023).

27. Y. Chen, H. Xu, Y. Luo, Y. Ding, J. Huang, H. Wu, J. Han, L. Du, A. Kang and M. Jia, *Water Res.* **242**, 120243 (2023).
28. L. M. Hernandez, E. G. Xu, H. C. Larsson, R. Tahara, V. B. Maisuria and N. Tufenkji, *Environ. Sci. Technol.* **53**, 12300 (2019).
29. D. Li, Y. Shi, L. Yang, L. Xiao, D. K. Kehoe, Y. K. Guńko, J. J. Boland and J. J. Wang, *Nat. Food* **1**, 746 (2020).
30. H. Yadav, M. R. H. Khan, M. Quadir, K. A. Rusch, P. P. Mondal, M. Orr, E. G. Xu and S. M. Iskander, *Environ. Sci. Technol.* **57**, 8225 (2023).
31. J.-L. Hu, Y. Duan, H.-N. Zhong, Q.-B. Lin, T. Zhang, C.-C. Zhao, S. Chen, B. Dong, D. Li and J. Wang, *Food Addit. Contam. Part A Chem. Anal. Control Expo. Risk Assess.* **40**, 305 (2023).
32. M. Jin, X. Wang, T. Ren, J. Wang and J. Shan, *J. Food Sci.* **86**, 2816 (2021).
33. A. Karami, A. Golieskardi, C. Keong Choo, V. Larat, T. S. Galloway and B. Salamatinia, *Sci. Rep.* **7**, 46173 (2017).
34. D. Yang, H. Shi, L. Li, J. Li, K. Jabeen and P. Kolandhasamy, *Environ. Sci. Technol.* **49**, 13622 (2015).
35. G. Liebezeit and E. Liebezeit, *Food Addit. Contam. Part A Chem. Anal. Control Expo. Risk Assess.* **30**, 2136 (2013).
36. P. Mühlschlegel, A. Hauk, U. Walter and R. Sieber, *Food Addit. Contam. Part A Chem. Anal. Control Expo. Risk Assess.* **34**, 1982 (2017).
37. G. Liebezeit and E. Liebezeit, *Food Addit. Contam. Part A Chem. Anal. Control Expo. Risk Assess.* **31**, 1574 (2014).
38. G. Kutralam-Muniasamy, F. Pérez-Guevara, I. Elizalde-Martínez and V. Shruti, *Sci. Total Environ.* **714**, 136823 (2020).
39. EFSA Panel on Contaminants in the Food Chain (CONTAM), *EFSA J.* **14**, e04501 (2016).
40. N. Qian, X. Gao, X. Lang, H. Deng, T. M. Bratu, Q. Chen, P. Stapleton, B. Yan and W. Min, *Proc. Natl. Acad. Sci. U.S.A.* **121**, e2300582121 (2024).
41. Q. Zhang, E. G. Xu, J. Li, Q. Chen, L. Ma, E. Y. Zeng and H. Shi, *Environ. Sci. Technol.* **54**, 3740 (2020).
42. X. Zhang, X. He, D. Pan, L. Shi, Y. Wu, Y. Yang, Y. Zhu, Y. Wang, H. Wang and L. Pu, *J. Hazard. Mater.* **462**, 132800 (2024).
43. Y. S. Ibrahim, S. Tuan Anuar, A. A. Azmi, W. M. A. Wan Mohd Khalik, S. Lehata, S. R. Hamzah, D. Ismail, Z. F. Ma, A. Dzulkarnaen and Z. Zakaria, *JGH Open* **5**, 116 (2021).
44. J. Gasperi, S. L. Wright, R. Dris, F. Collard, C. Mandin, M. Guerrouache, V. Langlois, F. J. Kelly and B. Tassin, *Curr. Opin. Environ. Sci. Health* **1**, 1 (2018).
45. J. C. Prata, *Environ. Pollut.* **234**, 115 (2018).
46. K. D. Cox, G. A. Covernton, H. L. Davies, J. F. Dower, F. Juanes and S. E. Dudas, *Environ. Sci. Technol.* **53**, 7068 (2019).
47. M. A. Bhat, K. Gedik and E. O. Gaga, *Air Qual. Atmos. Health* **16**, 233 (2023).
48. J. Ma, F. Chen, H. Xu, H. Jiang, J. Liu, P. Li, C. C. Chen and K. Pan, *Environ. Pollut.* **288**, 117748 (2021).
49. S. Wang, W. Lu, Q. Cao, C. Tu, C. Zhong, L. Qiu, S. Li, H. Zhang, M. Lan and L. Qiu, *Toxics* **11**, 759 (2023).

50. S. Huang, X. Huang, R. Bi, Q. Guo, X. Yu, Q. Zeng, Z. Huang, T. Liu, H. Wu and Y. Chen, *Environ. Sci. Technol.* **56**, 2476 (2022).
51. K. Lu, D. Zhan, Y. Fang, L. Li, G. Chen, S. Chen and L. Wang, *Front. Toxicol.* **4**, 958414 (2022).
52. G. M. Zarus, C. Muianga, S. Brenner, K. Stallings, G. Casillas, H. R. Pohl, M. M. Mumtaz and K. Gehle, *Am. J. Ind. Med.* **66**, 1033 (2023).
53. V. Zitko and M. Hanlon, *Mar. Pollut. Bull.* **22**, 41 (1991).
54. S. M. Bashir, S. Kimiko, C.-W. Mak, J. K.-H. Fang and D. Gonçalves, *Front. Mar. Sci.* **8**, 683482 (2021).
55. H. Lynn, S. Rech and M. Samwel, Plastics, gender and the environment. European Commission Framework Agreement 'Women2030', (WECF, Netherlands, 2017).
56. C. T. Madhumitha, N. Karmegam, M. Biruntha, A. Arun, A. A. Al Kheraif, W. Kim and P. Kumar, *Chemosphere* **296**, 133976 (2022).
57. F. S. Cesa, A. Turra and J. Baruque-Ramos, *Sci. Total Environ.* **598**, 1116 (2017).
58. Q. Li, M. Yuan, Y. Chen, X. Jin, J. Shangguan, J. Cui, S. Chang, M. Guo and Y. Wang, *J. Hazard. Mater.* **441**, 129911 (2023).
59. S. Abbasi and A. Turner, *J. Hazard. Mater.* **403**, 123799 (2021).
60. A. Ragusa, V. Notarstefano, A. Svelato, A. Belloni, G. Gioacchini, C. Blondeel, E. Zucchelli, C. De Luca, S. D'Avino and A. Gulotta, *Polymers* **14**, 2700 (2022).
61. Y. Yang, E. Xie, Z. Du, Z. Peng, Z. Han, L. Li, R. Zhao, Y. Qin, M. Xue and F. Li, *Environ. Sci. Technol.* **57**, 10911 (2023).
62. J. Rong, Y. He, J. Tang, R. Qiao and S. Lin, *Nanoscale* **13**, 5954 (2021).
63. S. Lin, T. Yu, Z. Yu, X. Hu and D. Yin, *Adv. Mater.* **30**, 1705691 (2018).
64. T. G. de Souza-Silva, I. A. Oliveira, G. G. da Silva, F. C. V. Giusti, R. D. Novaes and H. A. de Almeida Paula, *Life Sci.* **294**, 120366 (2022).
65. M. Wang, Q. Li, C. Shi, J. Lv, Y. Xu, J. Yang, S. L. Chua, L. Jia, H. Chen and Q. Liu, *Nat. Nanotechnol.* **18**, 403 (2023).
66. C. Jiménez-Arroyo, A. Tamargo, N. Molinero, J. Reinosa, V. Alcolea-Rodriguez, R. Portela, M. Bañares, J. Fernández and M. Moreno-Arribas, *Sci. Total Environ.* **902**, 166003 (2023).
67. H. Tan, T. Yue, Y. Xu, J. Zhao and B. Xing, *Environ. Sci. Technol.* **54**, 12285 (2020).
68. Z. Yuan, R. Nag and E. Cummins, *Sci. Total Environ.* **823**, 153730 (2022).
69. J. Eyles, H. Alpar, W. Field, D. Lewis and M. Keswick, *J. Pharm. Pharmacol.* **47**, 561 (1995).
70. J. A. Pitt, R. Trevisan, A. Massarsky, J. S. Kozal, E. D. Levin and R. T. Di Giulio, *Sci. Total Environ.* **643**, 324 (2018).
71. I. Fiorentino, R. Gualtieri, V. Barbato, V. Mollo, S. Braun, A. Angrisani, M. Turano, M. Furia, P. A. Netti and D. Guarnieri, *Exp. Cell Res.* **330**, 240 (2015).
72. M. Forte, G. Iachetta, M. Tussellino, R. Carotenuto, M. Prisco, M. De Falco, V. Laforgia and S. Valiante, *Toxicol. In Vitro* **31**, 126 (2016).

73. C. Campanale, C. Massarelli, I. Savino, V. Locaputo and V. F. Uricchio, *Int. J. Environ. Res. Public Health* **17**, 1212 (2020).
74. L. Li, Y. Xu, S. Li, X. Zhang, H. Feng, Y. Dai, J. Zhao and T. Yue, *J. Hazard. Mater.* **427**, 127872 (2022).
75. W. Shi, Y. Cao, X. Chai, Q. Zhao, Y. Geng, D. Liu and S. Tian, *J. Hazard. Mater.* **429**, 128109 (2022).
76. M. Xu, G. Halimu, Q. Zhang, Y. Song, X. Fu, Y. Li, Y. Li and H. Zhang, *Sci. Total Environ.* **694**, 133794 (2019).
77. J.-H. Woo, H. J. Seo, J.-Y. Lee, I. Lee, K. Jeon, B. Kim and K. Lee, *Part. Fibre Toxicol.* **20**, 1 (2023).
78. S. Lin, H. Zhang, C. Wang, X.-L. Su, Y. Song, P. Wu, Z. Yang, M.-H. Wong, Z. Cai and C. Zheng, *Environ. Sci. Technol.* **56**, 12483 (2022).
79. C.-D. Dong, C.-W. Chen, Y.-C. Chen, H.-H. Chen, J.-S. Lee and C.-H. Lin, *J. Hazard. Mater.* **385**, 121575 (2020).
80. B. C. Barros, B. R. Almeida, D. T. Barros, M. S. Toledo and E. Suzuki, *J. Fungi* **8**, 548 (2022).
81. K. E. Goodman, J. T. Hare, Z. I. Khamis, T. Hua and Q.-X. A. Sang, *Chem. Res. Toxicol.* **34**, 1069 (2021).
82. Z. Fan, T. Xiao, H. Luo, D. Chen, K. Lu, W. Shi, C. Sun and Q. Bian, *Environ. Int.* **163**, 107223 (2022).
83. X. Zhu, C. Wang, X. Duan, B. Liang, E. G. Xu and Z. Huang, *Environ. Int.* **171**, 107662 (2022).
84. D. Choi, J. Bang, T. Kim, Y. Oh, Y. Hwang and J. Hong, *J. Hazard. Mater.* **400**, 123308 (2020).
85. D. Choi, J. Hwang, J. Bang, S. Han, T. Kim, Y. Oh, Y. Hwang, J. Choi and J. Hong, *Sci. Total Environ.* **752**, 142242 (2021).
86. M. Sun, R. Ding, Y. Ma, Q. Sun, X. Ren, Z. Sun and J. Duan, *Chemosphere* **282**, 131124 (2021).
87. C. Oslakovic, T. Cedervall, S. Linse and B. Dahlbäck, *Nanomedicine* **8**, 981 (2012).
88. B. Wang, B. Liang, Y. Huang, Z. Li, B. Zhang, J. Du, R. Ye, H. Xian, Y. Deng and J. Xiu, *Adv. Sci.* 2205876 (2023).
89. H. Cheng, Y. Feng, Z. Duan, X. Duan, S. Zhao, Y. Wang, Z. Gong and L. Wang, *Chemosphere* **269**, 128677 (2021).
90. Z. Li, S. Zhu, Q. Liu, J. Wei, Y. Jin, X. Wang and L. Zhang, *Environ. Pollut.* **265**, 115025 (2020).
91. Y. Zhou, Q. Wu, Y. Li, Y. Feng, Y. Wang and W. Cheng, *Environ. Int.* **179**, 108171 (2023).
92. W. Shi, Y. Han, S. Sun, Y. Tang, W. Zhou, X. Du and G. Liu, *J. Hazard. Mater.* **396**, 122603 (2020).
93. G. Liu, R. Jiang, J. You, D. C. Muir and E. Y. Zeng, *Environ. Sci. Technol.* **54**, 1782 (2019).
94. C.-B. Jeong, E.-J. Won, H.-M. Kang, M.-C. Lee, D.-S. Hwang, U.-K. Hwang, B. Zhou, S. Souissi, S.-J. Lee and J.-S. Lee, *Environ. Sci. Technol.* **50**, 8849 (2016).

95. K. Park, W.-S. Kim, J. W. Park, T. H. Kim and I.-S. Kwak, *J. Hazard. Mater.* **462**, 132691 (2024).
96. M. Kang, D. Gong, Y. Weng, Y. Huang, Y. Chen, F. Li and X. Bai, *Environ. Sci.: Nano* **10**, 1244 (2023).
97. B. Xia, Q. Sui, Y. Du, L. Wang, J. Jing, L. Zhu, X. Zhao, X. Sun, A. M. Booth and B. Chen, *J. Hazard. Mater.* **424**, 127421 (2022).
98. M. Zhang and L. Xu, *Crit. Rev. Environ. Sci. Technol.* **52**, 810 (2022).
99. A. Das, *Sci. Total Environ.* **895**, 165076 (2023).
100. K. Zhu, H. Jia, S. Zhao, T. Xia, X. Guo, T. Wang and L. Zhu, *Environ. Sci. Technol.* **53**, 8177 (2019).
101. W. Qiongjie, Z. Yong, Z. Yangyang, L. Zhouqi, W. Jinxiaoxue and C. Huijuan, *J. Hazard. Mater.* **424**, 127340 (2022).
102. X. Fan, Y. Zou, N. Geng, J. Liu, J. Hou, D. Li, C. Yang and Y. Li, *J. Hazard. Mater.* **401**, 123363 (2021).
103. Q. Chen, X. Zhang, Q. Xie, Y. H. Lee, J.-S. Lee and H. Shi, *Ecotoxicol. Environ. Saf.* **228**, 112991 (2021).
104. M. A. Mallah, Z. Yu, Z. Qu, M. Ali and N. Liu, *Environ. Sci. Pollut. Res.* **31**, 11428 (2024).
105. O. Nwachukwu, K. Kniazev, A. Abarca Perez, M. Kuno and K. Doudrick, *Environ. Sci. Technol.* **58**, 1312 (2024).
106. K. Kniazev, I. M. Pavlovetc, S. Zhang, J. Kim, R. L. Stevenson, K. Doudrick and M. Kuno, *Environ. Sci. Technol.* **55**, 15891 (2021).
107. R. Qiao, M. Mortimer, J. Richter, B. Rani-Borges, Z. Yu, M. Heinlaan, S. Lin and A. Ivask, *Sci. Total Environ.* **853**, 158560 (2022).
108. K. J. Groh, T. Backhaus, B. Carney-Almroth, B. Geueke, P. A. Inostroza, A. Lennquist, H. A. Leslie, M. Maffini, D. Slunge and L. Trasande, *Sci. Total Environ.* **651**, 3253 (2019).
109. V. N. de Ruijter, P. E. Redondo-Hasselerharm, T. Gouin and A. A. Koelmans, *Environ. Sci. Technol.* **54**, 11692 (2020).
110. B. Liang, Y. Zhong, Y. Huang, X. Lin, J. Liu, L. Lin, M. Hu, J. Jiang, M. Dai and B. Wang, *Part. Fibre Toxicol.* **18**, 20 (2021).
111. Q. Zhao, H. Chang, J. Zheng, P. Li, L. Ye, R. Pan, D. Li, J.-Z. Shao, R. C. Zhao and Y. Chen, *Signal Transduct. Target. Ther.* **8**, 86 (2023).

https://doi.org/10.1142/9789819809028_0016

Chapter 16

Exploiting the Electrical Nature of Biofilms for Long-Term Monitoring of Quiescent Aquatic Environments via Open-Circuit Microbial Potentiometric Sensors: Evidence of Long-Distance Electrical Signaling*

Scott R. Burge[†], Kiril D. Hristovski[‡,||], Russell G. Burge[†], Ljupco Pejov[‡,§], Dragan Boscovic[¶], Evan Taylor[†] and David A. Hoffman[†]

[†]*Burge Environmental Inc., 6100 South Maple Avenue Tempe, Arizona 85283, USA*
[‡]*Environmental and Resource Management The Polytechnic School, Ira A. Fulton Schools of Engineering Arizona State University, Mesa, Arizona 85281, USA*
[§]*Institute of Chemistry, University of Ss. Cyril and Methodius Skopje 1000, North Macedonia*
[¶]*School of Computing and Augmented Intelligence Ira A. Fulton Schools of Engineering Arizona State University Tempe, Arizona 85281, USA*
[||]*kiril.hristovski@asu.edu*

This study was based on the hypothesis that spatial–temporal characterization of contaminant-affected redox gradients in a quiescent system could be measured by microbial potentiometric sensor (MPS) arrays incorporated in large, natural biofilm networks. Two experimental chambers, each containing at least 48 equidistantly located MPS electrodes, were fabricated to examine reproducibility of the patterns. The MPS electrodes were

*To cite this article, please refer to its earlier version published in the *Nano LIFE*, Vol. 13, No. 4 (2023) 2350014 (13 pages), DOI: 10.1142/S1793984423500149
||Corresponding author.

exposed to biofilm growth conditions by introducing high dissolved organic carbon (DOC) and dechlorinated tap water at the bottom of the experimental chamber; and the spatial–temporal changes in the MPS array signals were recorded, which showed that signal trends were correlated to the induced changes in DOC. The results indicated that MPS arrays measured the spatial–temporal changes in the aqueous solution caused by an influx of carbon rich water, which could not be detected by conventional oxidation-reduction potential (ORP) electrodes. Interestingly, the experiments conducted over long time periods revealed unusual behaviors like electrical signaling and possible potentiometrically driven communication within the biofilm. These observed behaviors suggest that biofilms may create a large network through which communication signals can be generated and propagated by inducing changes in electric potentials similar to a sophisticated electronic device.

Keywords: Sensor, biofilm, monitoring, signaling, electrical.

1. Introduction

Commonly used descriptions in the literature describe biofilms as consortia of different microorganisms organized in a communal structure, which promotes symbiotic functions and protection against adverse external influences.[1–3] In a broader sense, however, biofilms have many of the characteristics of a primitive lifeform that is capable of interacting with the surrounding environment and communicating information throughout the biofilm structure and microorganisms.[4,5] Chemical communication among the different cells within a biofilm has been documented in the literature.[1–5] Recent evidence suggests that biofilm microorganisms may be capable of communicating via electrical signaling pathways using cytochromes and specialized nanosized organelles to transfer charge and thus information within and beyond the biofilm boundary.[6–8]

Much of the evidence suggesting electrical or electrochemical communication originates from the work conducted on fuel cell technology, which explores electrochemically active biofilms.[9–16] These biofilms can funnel the excess electrons to an electrode, while protons flux out of the biofilm.[17–21] The overall electron fluxes could be generally organized into two categories: Soluble electron transfers and bound electron transfers. Soluble electron transfers could be envisioned as electrons exchanged between the solution and the biofilm surface.[22] In contrast, bound electron transfers are modeled as electrons exchanged in the biofilm matrix or at the cell membrane.[23–25] The magnitude of these electron fluxes correlates strictly with the metabolic processes of the biofilm.[26–30] Regardless of the specific types of metabolic and electron transfer pathways, the overall electron fluxes control the establishing of electric potential gradients on a microscale (or even nanoscale) as determined by the local redox and nutrient conditions.[31–33]

Under equilibrium conditions, a steady state exists between the soluble electron transfers and bound electron transfers, which is characterized by a steady-state open-circuit electric potential.[34–36] Because no electric current is flowing in an open-circuit system, the electric potential is precisely dependent on the local equilibrium conditions that are driven by both the biochemical processes in the biofilm and the redox conditions outside the biofilm, such as nutrient concentration.[26–33] Any biochemical changes in the local environment surrounding the biofilm will inherently induce changes in the biochemical rates and types of processes within the biofilm, which will change the open-circuit potential (OCP). Such biochemical changes in the local environment cannot be readily detected by the oxidation-reduction potential (ORP) sensors, which represent the golden standard in measuring the oxidizing and reducing conditions in water bodies.[37,38] Although the ORP sensors measure open-circuit potential, this golden standard is flawed when it comes to long-term measurements of naturally existing water matrices, which exhibit heterogeneous redox conditions and may require high activation energies for redox reactions or dilute concentrations of redox species.[39]

In a closed-circuit scenario, like in a fuel cell, an induced electric current is flowing through the biofilms enabling them to transfer the electrons to a preferential electron acceptor (typically oxygen), which is kept at a gradient to maximize the flow of electrons.[40–42] While closed-circuit scenarios create a steady-state flow of electrons, this electron flow does not reflect the normal metabolic pathways that are typical of equilibrium conditions.[34–36] This flow of electrical current deviates the system from its normal metabolic paradigm, so it no longer describes the state of the natural, endemic biofilm, which proliferates in undisturbed local redox and nutrient conditions. As such, using a closed-circuit approach to monitor biofilm behavior and correlating that behavior to comprehensively understand biofilms and their local environments has limitations because it does not permit observing behavior in normal equilibrium conditions, and thus is a representative of the natural processes (e.g., exoelectrogens proliferation increased compared to undisturbed conditions). In brief, closed-circuit approaches do not enable observation of biofilm behavior under equilibrium conditions, which represent the most prevalent scenarios in a life of a biofilm. Similar to Heisenberg's Uncertainty Principle, one cannot observe a system in a natural state when the natural state is disturbed by the observation tool. By inducing a flow of electric current to observe the biofilm behavior, one is disturbing the natural state of the biofilm. The subsequent question then becomes how can one observe the behavior of biofilms without changing the system or their natural states. Developing such a tool or methodology has the potential to open new perspectives on understanding how biofilms communicate and interact with their local environment.

In this study, we propose an alternative approach to monitoring the behavior of biofilms via an open-circuit method. Monitoring of the behavior of a biofilm and its local environment with an open-circuit approach eliminates the drawbacks associated with inducing external changes in the bioelectrochemistry of the biofilm and enables temporal characterization of a system undisturbed by a flow of externally introduced electrons. Consequently, all the changes in the electric potential are directly related only to the local environmental conditions and the biofilm characteristics and its biochemical processes.

Figure 1 illustrates a simplified depiction of an open-circuit measurement sensor array through which the electric potentials of biofilms can be measured. Rooted in simple electronics, the open-circuit system comprises a reference electrode (an electrode with a constant electric potential (e.g., Ag/AgCl reference electrode) and an electrode comprising a nonoxidizable conductive surface upon which

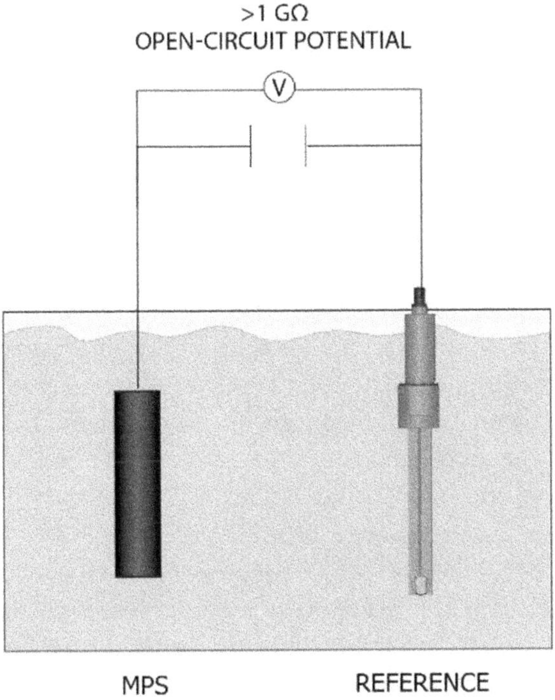

Fig. 1. Simplified depiction of an OCP measurement system (microbial potentiometric electrode and reference electrodes) connected to a high impedance OCP measuring device.

endemic microorganisms can establish biofilm populations. The two electrodes are connected to high impedance ($>1\,\text{G}\Omega$) measurement circuitry capable of measuring OCP (voltage). Because OCPs are measured, multiple biofilm electrodes (an array) could be referenced against a single reference electrode.[43] The described open-circuit measurement system is dubbed microbial potentiometric sensor (MPS) system because the biofilm microorganisms represent the actual electrode whose OCP is measured against the reference electrode.

Considering the advantage of using a single reference, an MPS array system comprising multiple biofilm electrodes, which are placed at different locations through an environmental system, can be used to provide real-time spatial–temporal monitoring and visualization of contaminant mass transport or other changes in quiescent systems.[38,39,44–47] Consequently, an overarching hypothesis was postulated that spatial–temporal characterization of contaminant affected redox gradients in a quiescent system could be obtained by creating an MPS array system comprising multiple equidistant biofilm electrodes.

To validate the hypothesis, four task-oriented objectives were completed. Specifically, two experimental chambers, each containing at least 48 equidistantly located MPS electrodes, were fabricated to examine reproducibility of the patterns. The MPS electrodes were exposed to biofilm growth conditions and monitored following a methodology described by Burge *et al.*[38] Upon biofilm growth stabilization, the experimental chambers were filled with dechlorinated tap water and monitoring of the MPS potentials was conducted by introducing high dissolved organic carbon (DOC) and dechlorinated tap water at the bottom of the experimental chamber. Spatial–temporal changes in the MPS array signals were recorded and signal trends were correlated to the induced changes in DOC water quality.

2. Methodology

2.1. *Fabrication of experimental chambers and biofilm growth*

Two experimental chambers were fabricated for the purposes of this study. As illustrated in Fig. 2, the experimental chambers were fabricated using clear polycarbonate tubes with inner diameter of $d_I = 15.25\,\text{cm}$ and length of $l = 152\,\text{cm}$. These vertically orientated chambers were sealed at the bottom and the top, with the top containing ports enabling exchange with atmospheric oxygen as needed. Ports were fabricated at several vertical locations along the wall of the chambers to enable introduction and removal of solutions. The total volume of the chambers was 28.1 L.

Each chamber contained a vertical array of 48 graphite (MPS) electrodes with diameter of $d_E = 0.64\,\text{cm}$ mounted in a PVC threaded fitting. The MPS electrodes were spaced at 1 inch (2.54 cm) center-to-center distance from each other. The surface of the graphite rod

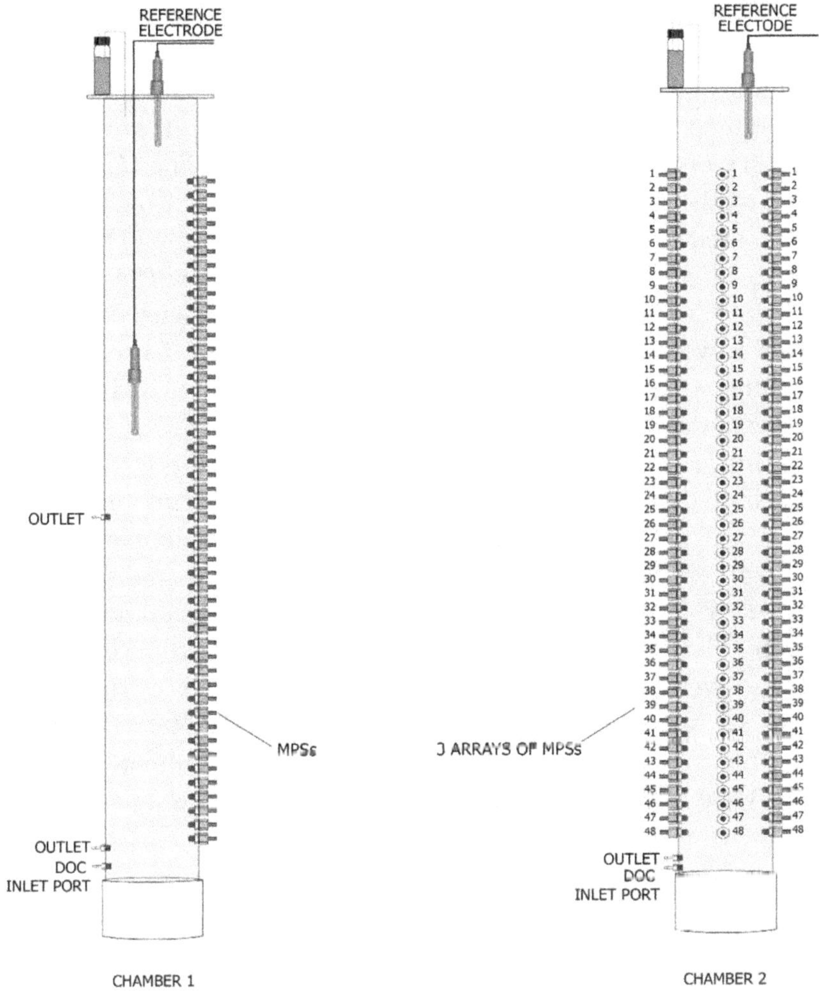

Fig. 2. Schematic representations of the chamber arrays containing 48 MPS electrodes (left) and 3 × 48 MPS (right) electrodes, respectively.

exposed to the environment was flush with the terminal end of the fitting and enabled sufficient surface for biofilm proliferation.[38] The opposite end of the graphite electrode was fitted with an electrical wire/cabling for connection with the signal acquisition tools. An Ag/AgCl electrode was placed on the top of each chamber so as to serve as a reference for the MPS electrodes.

Chambers 1 and 2 were fabricated identically to examine data reproducibility and repeatability, except that chamber 2 comprised 144 MPS sensors in three vertical arrays, organized in the same equidistance pattern as experimental chamber 1, to examine variability of the sensor signal at the same height. The three sensors located at the same height were located at 90° angles from each other as illustrated in Fig. 2. Additionally, chamber 1 contained three ORP electrodes located at 30 cm, 67.5 cm and 95 cm below the top of the chamber. Chamber 2 contained two ORP electrodes. The ORP electrodes were installed in the systems to observe if there are any deviations in signal difference between the ORP and the MPS sensors as the experimental conditions changed.

To initiate biofilm growth, the chambers were filled with dechlorinated tap water (City of Tempe) and kept at temperature of $T = 24 \pm 1°C$ in the dark to prevent the development of any photosynthetic microorganisms. The system was left undisturbed for a period of several weeks to promote biofilm development on the graphite electrode surfaces. The OCP signals from each MPS electrode were measured against the reference electrode at least once a day with a high-impedance voltmeter (>1 GΩ). The biofilm development on the electrodes was considered complete once the signals were stable, exhibiting signal variability of ±3 mV between daily measurements.

2.2. *Spatial–temporal monitoring of the MPS potentials under high DOC and dechlorinated tap water conditions*

Chamber 1. Upon completion of the biofilm stabilization period, chamber 1 was filled with dechlorinated water, and anaerobic water (DOC > 100 mg/L) was slowly gravity-fed through a port located at the bottom of the chamber at a rate of 450 ± 150 mL/day. This rate of anaerobic water introduction allowed the visual observation of the interface between the dark brown anaerobic solution and the overlying clear water. Once the anaerobic water reached a height between MPS 40 and MPS 41, the introduction of the anaerobic water was stopped and ORP electrodes were installed. The ORP electrodes were installed later to minimize the disruption of any diffusive processes by a free hanging electrode during the high DOC water injection period. The chamber was left undisturbed and exposed to atmospheric air for a period of approximately four months to monitor any changes resulting from oxygen diffusion. After this period, the chamber was sealed off to eliminate any atmospheric influences. Any headspace was removed by adding <1 L aerobic (atmospheric oxygen containing) water. The monitoring of chamber 1 was continued for a period of six months before the experiment was terminated. Three months after the capping, a small pinhole opening in the system was created that enabled small diffusion of oxygen.

Chamber 2. To validate the observations from chamber 1 and obtain better understanding of the spatial variability of the signals, chamber 2 was constructed with three times more sensors allowing for examination of the horizontal changes in the OCPs. Upon completion of biofilm stabilization and the conditioning period, anaerobic water was slowly gravity-fed through a port located at the bottom of the chamber at a rate of 600 ± 100 mL/day until the anaerobic water interface solution reached MPS 34. Approximately two weeks later, the column was bleached three times (using a 1% bleach solution) and rinsed with tap water before filling the chamber with aerobic water. Four days after filling the chamber with aerobic water, aerobic water was introduced through the bottom port at the same rate. Once the anaerobic water interface reached the height between MPS 30 and MPS 31, the introduction of anaerobic water was terminated and the ORP electrodes were installed. The chamber was left undisturbed and exposed to atmospheric air for a period of about three months. The chamber was then capped and any headspace was removed by adding <1 L aerobic water, so that no atmospheric oxygen could enter the system until the experiment was completed several days later.

3. Results and discussion

3.1. *Spatial–temporal monitoring of the MPS potentials in Chamber 1*

Figure 3 illustrates the average OCPs for several nine-consecutive-day durations as generated by each of the 48 MPS sensors against the

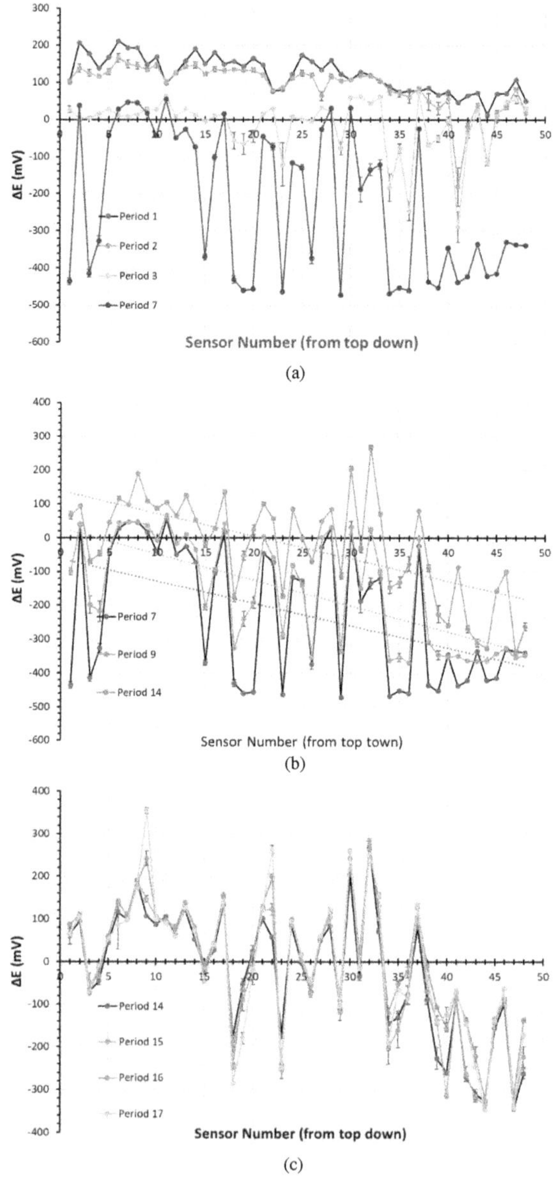

Fig. 3. The average OCPs for several 17 periods as generated by each of the 48 MPS sensors in chamber 1 against the reference electrode. Each period consists of 9 ± 1 days. The error bars represent 95% confidence intervals. The dotted lines illustrate the linear trend illustrating the overall charge gradient in the system shifting up with respect to time.

reference electrode. Only periods 1, 2, 3 and 9 are illustrated in Fig. 3(a) to minimize the data crowding in this figure (Figs. S1 and S2 contain the additional seven nine-day periods). Period 1 illustrates the OCP pattern generated by the MPS sensors before the injection of high DOC water. During this period, the signals generated by each MPS sensor were very stable as characterized by very small 95% confidence intervals of $\sim 1\,\text{mV}$. However, once the high DOC water was introduced (period 2), the stability of each of the 48 MPS sensors decreased as their OCPs started declining. Interestingly, the introduction of the high DOC water caused unexpected drop in potential of almost all MPS sensors, and not only of the MPS sensors located near the bottom of the chamber where the high DOC water was introduced. While the OCP changes in MPS sensors located near the injection port where the high DOC water was introduced were expected, they could not only be attributed to the diffusion of the DOC. Diffusion of the DOC from the bottom upwards was slow and created a clear potential gradient slowly moving from the bottom up as evidenced in Fig. 3(a); these gradients in potential cannot be explained if only diffusion was at work. By the end of period 7, most of the sensors above the visible gradient boundary between MPS 40 and MPS 41 responded to the change in OCP corresponding to high DOC, for example, the biofilm in the sensors near the bottom of the chamber was communicating an electrical information about an incoming influx of DOC. Interestingly, not all MPS sensors above the DOC gradient boundary responded equally. Some exhibited a greater change in their OCP, and some hardly changed as illustrated in OCP change and the depicted 95% confidence intervals.

When the introduction of the high DOC water ceased and oxygen was allowed to diffuse from the top, the OCP of all MPS sensors started increasing, which was followed by the shifting of the entire pattern of the potential gradient vertically upward in the chamber as illustrated in Fig. 3(b). The form of the pattern, however, maintained its general shape as the oxygen could enter and diffuse the column from the end of period 7 to the end of period 14. When the chamber was capped at the top to prevent diffusion of oxygen, the changes in the OCP in all MPS sensors started decreasing and eventually stopped by the end of periods 16 and 17 as illustrated in Fig. 3(c). This behavior was expected considering that additional oxygen was prevented from entering the system, which led to the microorganisms in the chamber (both biofilm and solubilized) to utilize the remaining dissolved oxygen and stabilize the redox potentials. This type of behavior implies that microorganisms in biofilms may be able to temporarily store the potential energy of the electrons, generated from the biochemical decomposition of organic carbon, in their networks of temporary electron acceptors when the energy harnessing conditions are unfavorable, and release them under more favorable conditions when the electron acceptor is present, which could provide with more energy. In brief, when oxygen is present, the microorganisms could extract most of the energy from the carbon; however, if oxygen is not present, they may decide to store the electrons by conserving their potential energy in the temporary electron acceptors, which would manifest the exhibited patterns.

The temporal changes in the overall bioelectrochemical conditions of the system during these 17 periods are illustrated in Fig. 4 which shows the daily changes of the average OCP in the chamber as detected by the 48 MPS sensors referenced against the Ag/AgCl electrode. The average OCP in the system decreased when the introduction of high DOC water commenced. Interestingly, however, the average OCP continued to decrease until it reached a minimum approximately 900 h after the injection had stopped. Once the minimum was reached, the ORP sensors were introduced, which showed stable but highly reducing conditions with an average ORP < -430 mV. As the average MPS potential started to increase, the ORP stayed relatively stable at < -430 mV for another 400 h, and then exhibited severe electric potential fluctuations, which stopped shortly after the chamber was capped. The MPS sensors detected the chamber capping by registering a small signal “dip” in the average signal. Once the chamber was capped, the ORP fluctuation subsided and the ORP remained generally < -400 mV regardless of the changes exhibited in the average MPS OCP. In contrast, the average MPS OCP stabilized and remained relatively stable for over 2000 h after the capping with a slight decreasing tendency as illustrated in

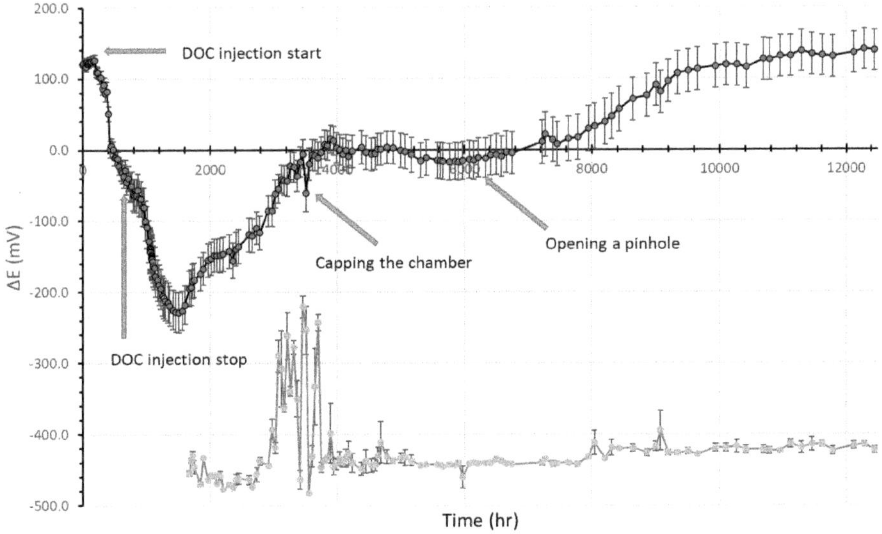

Fig. 4. Temporal changes in the overall bio-electrochemical conditions of the system during these 17 periods. Each data point represents an average of all the MPS or ORP generated OCP signals. Black symbols represent the average OCP signals from the 48 MPS electrodes in chamber 1. The gray symbols represent the average signals from the three ORP electrodes. The error bars represent 95% confidence intervals.

Fig. 4. Once the pinhole was created, the miniscule amount of diffusive atmospheric gas (oxygen) caused the average MPS OCP to start slowly increasing until it reached the levels at the beginning of the experiment at $t > 12\,000$ h.

3.2. *Spatial–temporal monitoring of the MPS potentials in Chamber 2*

Figure 5(a) illustrates the overall bioelectrochemical conditions of the system during a period of over 4000 h as revealed by the OCPs of the three different columns, each containing 48 sensors. Once the system was stabilized as shown in Video 1 (Supplemental Materials), the average OCPs of columns did not deviate from each other. The average value for each column was <15 mV and 95% confidence intervals showed that there is no statistical difference among the average values. The variance, as depicted through the 95% confidence intervals, started to increase as more high DOC water was introduced

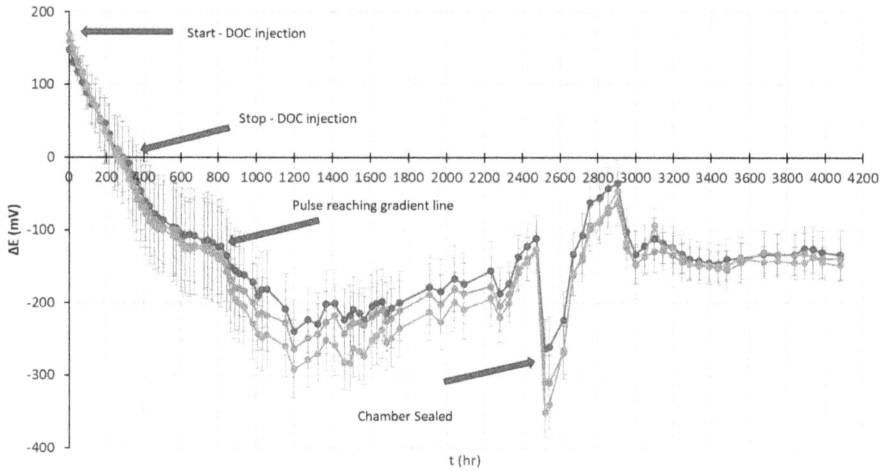

(a)

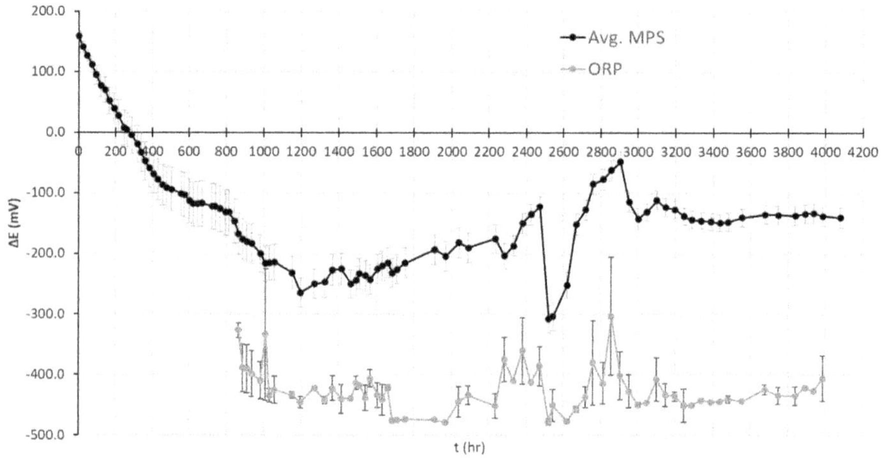

(b)

Fig. 5. Temporal changes in the overall bio-electrochemical conditions of the system during a period of $t > 4000$ h. (a) Each color represents the average signals from one of the three vertical arrays comprising 48 sensors in chamber 2. (b) Each data point represents an average of all the MPS or ORP generated OCP signals. Black symbols represent the average OCP signals from the 144 MPS electrodes in chamber 2. The gray symbols represent the average signals from the three ORP electrodes. The error bars represent 95% confidence intervals.

at the bottom of the chamber. This was expected considering that the sensors at the bottom started to identically respond to the presence of high DOC and created a well-defined gradient that reflected the DOC influx. This is well illustrated in Video 2 (Supplemental Materials), where the stability of the sensors and change of the OCP with the incoming flux is shown through time. At time $t \approx 318$ h, the injection of high DOC water was stopped, and the system stabilized as a result of which each sensor showed very little divergence from the main signal trend. Interestingly, however, a specific pulse is registered by all the MPSs near the bottom as illustrated in Video 2. The pulse is characterized by $\sim$50 mV drop in the potential, and it subsequently moved up toward the gradient, although the high DOC water injection was terminated. All MPSs at a specific height generated OCP signals in concert. Apparently, the MPSs at the bottom were sending an electrical signal that the influx of high DOC water was terminated, and the system needed to readjust. This behavior could not be attributed to diffusion because diffusion would have already perturbed the established gradient characterized by a difference of about 400 mV. The upward movement of this pulse is also evident in Fig. 4, where a decrease in the average OCP continued to occur after the DOC injection had stopped. As more and more sensors from the bottom register the pulse, the average OCP signal variance increases, which is illustrated through the increasing 95% confidence intervals. The extensive overlap of these intervals shows that the probability of the average OCP signals being statistically different is significantly lower than 5%.

At $t \approx 815$ h, the pulse reaches the already established gradient, which causes the entire signal pattern to start shifting down. It appears like the pulse reached its designated destination and signaled the system to start decreasing its overall bio-electrochemical potential above the established $\sim$400 mV gradient, while the shape of the pattern remains the same. This behavior could not be attributed to any bulk mass transport mechanism because there was no advective transport of DOC; and diffusion would not cause translational movement without changing the shape of the pattern. While it is documented that biofilms use nanovesicles to communicate and signal across distances, these represent mass transport mechanisms occurring over short distances.[48–54] Here, the communication occurred across distances exceeding 0.6 m and was exhibited by all sensors located at corresponding levels. Logically, there must have been a different mechanism that induced this type of behavior. Considering the velocity of signaling across all sensors, the nature of the signal (e.g., voltage), and the distance involved, it could be postulated that the pulse signal was electrical in nature. If so, this signal could only travel at this speed and distance only if there is some kind of interconnected network that enabled rapid transfer of electrons. If such a network exists, it is possible to imagine that the sensors in the MPS array could represent nothing more than nodes in this large biofilm network that would probably extend across the length of the system.

In addition to the translational shift of the pattern, once the OCP signals of the upper sensors approach 0 mV, their OCPs began to diverge, even though some of these MPSs were located at the same column height. As illustrated in Video 2, this divergence occurred among the sensors above the 400 mV gradient line, but it also causes this gradient to start dissolving. Interestingly, once almost all OCPs reached $\Delta E < 0$, the sensors below the gradient line started to diverge until each sensor located at the same height position signal differed in OCP. By $t \approx 2300$ h, a new highly disordered gradient emerged, which slowly began to shift toward more positive potentials. Although this behavior could be attributed to diffusive processes occurring over a period of >1500 h which aimed to reduce the concentration gradient across the three-dimensional space, the difference in OCPs of sensors located at the same height position in the column suggested that the biofilms were actively engaged in influencing the local environment surrounding them. Considering that electrons flow in the presence of an electric potential (voltage gradient), it is reasonable to postulate that the biofilms have mechanisms that generate and modulate these local gradients to enable transfer of electrons and communication across the entire biological network.

When the chamber was capped, the entire system responded to this externally induced change. As shown in Fig. 5, the average OCP of the system decreased. This is evident in Video 2 at $t \approx 2500\,\text{h}$. Interestingly, the entire array of sensors responded in the same manner; the OCP of all sensors decreased, which shifted the pattern toward lower potentials, yet the pattern shape remained relatively unchanged. In contrast, the ORP probes did not register this shift in potential or the ORP signal variability was so high that the signal shift was masked as illustrated in Fig. 5(b). Although this figure appears to suggest that there was a relatively good correlation between the ORP and MPS patterns, regression analysis showed that there was no correlation as indicated by $R^2 < 0.1510$ (Fig. SI-3). This lack of correlation between the MPS and ORP sensors became more evident as the system recovered from the "capping" and continued to stabilize. The ORP signals exhibited high fluctuations and variability during this period as illustrated by the 95% confidence intervals in Fig. 5(b). Furthermore, as the MPS signals were relatively stable, the ORP signals started drifting toward more positive values near the end of the experiment. The relative stability of the MPS signals after the system was capped is also illustrated in Video 2. This stability of MPS signals was not unexpected considering that oxygen diffusion was eliminated, and the system had to stabilize at the bio-electrochemical potential dictated by conditions in the sealed column. Beyond oxygen diffusion, this stability of the signals could probably be disturbed by the introduction of other environmental factors like temperature, other favorable electron acceptors like nitrates, or even the presence of photosynthetic organisms, which further increases the monitoring capabilities of the technology.

3.3. *Thermodynamic analysis and implications*

The trends illustrated in Figs. 4 and 5 are consistent with the predictions of thermodynamics for the processes exhibited by these two systems as illustrated in Fig. 6. This figure elucidates the same type of ΔE patterns when the systems were subjected to the same external influences. When high DOC water was added to the system, the total energy of the system increased ($\Delta H_{\text{System}} > 0$) because a "packaged" form of energy was introduced ($\text{d}H = T\text{d}S + V\text{d}P + \Sigma Y_i \text{d}X_i + \Sigma \mu_i \text{d}n_i$ in case of a nonhydrostatic open system, which

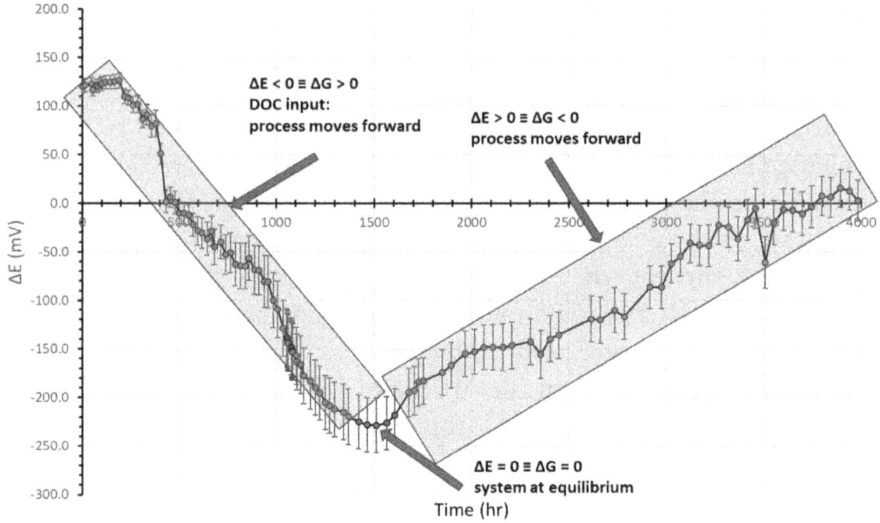

Fig. 6. Thermodynamic predictions for the processes exhibited by the two systems. The gray symbols represent the average OCP signals from the 48 MPS electrodes in chamber 1 for the first 4000 h of monitoring. The error bars represent 95% confidence intervals.

reduces to $\mathrm{d}H = T\mathrm{d}S + \Sigma\mu_i \mathrm{d}n_i$ under isobaric conditions when also all other relevant generalized coordinates remain constant[55]). The high DOC contains large quantities of reduced carbon forms (e.g., electrons in the high energy bonds), which represents an energy source for the microorganisms to utilize. Consequently, as DOC was added, the Gibbs free energy of the system was increased ($\mathrm{d}G = -S\mathrm{d}T + V\mathrm{d}P + \Sigma Y_i \mathrm{d}X_i + \Sigma\mu_i \mathrm{d}n_i$ in a general case of a nonhydrostatic open system, which reduces to $\mathrm{d}G = \Sigma\mu_i \mathrm{d}n_i$ under isobaric–isothermal conditions when also all other relevant generalized coordinates remain constant[54]). The chemical potentials of individual constituents are increased during this process ($\Delta\mu_i > 0$ when $\Delta a_i > 0$, as $a_i \sim c_i$, where a_i denotes the relative activity of species i in the system). Such chemical potential changes can be later utilized by the microorganisms to do work inside the system. The described change was registered through the drop in the electric potential of the system because $\Delta G = -nF\Delta E$. During the high DOC water injection, the $\Delta E_{\mathrm{system}}$ over time was decreased ($\Delta E_{\mathrm{system}}/\Delta t < 0$); and considering that $\Delta G = -nF\Delta E$, the change in the Gibbs free energy was also positive ($\Delta G > 0$). Although ΔG was increasing at this stage, the process moved forward because nonequilibrium conditions were induced by "priming" or "energizing" the system with DOC, which introduced new thermodynamic states ($\Delta S = k \ln \Omega$, where k is the Boltzmann constant and Ω is the number of thermodynamic states). The increase in number of new thermodynamic states was probably further facilitated by the biofilm "stripping" the electrons from the absorbed DOC, which resulted in the charging of the temporary electron acceptors (e.g., cytochromes and other similar functional proteins or nanostructures) within the biofilm and causing the MPS electrodes to exhibit drop in ΔE.

Once, however, the external input of high DOC water stopped, the system slowly moved to equilibrium where the change over time in $\Delta E = \Delta G = 0$ as illustrated in Fig. 6. Upon reaching the equilibrium, ΔE_{system} started increasing ($\Delta E > 0$; $\Delta G < 0$) due to the biochemical oxidation of the injected reduced carbon species (respiration), which were enzymatically facilitated by the microorganisms in the system. From open systems thermodynamics, it is known that a process can proceed spontaneously in the "forward" direction under isothermal–isobaric conditions when $\Delta G < 0$ (i.e., $\mathrm{d}G < 0$ considering infinitesimal progressions). Assuming a single biochemical reaction taking place in the system, the total differential of the Gibbs free energy is given by $\mathrm{d}G = -T\mathrm{d}S + V\mathrm{d}P + \Sigma Y_i \mathrm{d}X_i - A\mathrm{d}\xi$, where A denotes the thermodynamic affinity and $\mathrm{d}\xi$ is the change in the reaction extent.[54] As both A and $\mathrm{d}\xi$ are positive for the reaction in progress, under isobaric conditions, assuming also constant values of all relevant generalized coordinates, the expression for $\mathrm{d}G$ acquires the form $\mathrm{d}G = -T\mathrm{d}S - A\mathrm{d}\xi$. If the entropy change occurs solely due to the reaction progress, one can express the first term through $\mathrm{d}\xi$ as well ($\mathrm{d}S = \Delta_r S \mathrm{d}\xi$, where $\Delta_r S$ denotes the reaction entropy). So, the expression for $\mathrm{d}G$ reduces to $\mathrm{d}G = -(T\Delta_r S + A)\mathrm{d}x$. In brief, the essential driving force reduces to the fact that the energy introduced to the systems in the form of reduced carbon is released back into the universe, increasing its entropy.

When high DOC water was introduced at the bottom of the chamber, Video 2 illustrated a very interesting phenomenon. The sensors above the DOC induced ΔE gradient (around the 31st sensor — near the bottom), which were not exposed to high DOC concentrations, simultaneously dropped their OCPs once the pulse reached the gradient. This decrease in OCP appeared not to be induced by the local environment, but somehow was influenced by the sensors at the bottom of the chamber. Considering that the decrease in ΔE is proportional to the increasing entropy of the system, it may appear that the biofilm was trying to minimize the loss of usable energy by dispersing this entropy change across the chamber to the extent the conditions permit. It was also reasonable to postulate that the induced divergence from a stable baseline may be stemming from the same phenomenon; the discrete ΔE of each MPS was affected by the local abilities of a biofilm to disperse the changes in entropy that resulted from the metabolic processes across the entire biofilm network.

Interestingly, however, the changes in Gibbs free energy were not detected by the ORP sensors, except for rapid fluctuations in the ORP signal when the systems were shocked or exited the equilibrium conditions. This finding implied that the ORP electrodes were not capable of monitoring the "packaged" forms of energy introduced into a system unless the redox pairs were in bulk. Considering that the ORP may be considered as the gold standard in monitoring of aquatic environments, this deficiency severely limits their applicability.

4. Conclusions

The findings presented in this study extend beyond the postulated overarching hypothesis that spatial–temporal characterization of contaminant influence redox gradients in a quiescent system could be obtained by creating an MPS array system comprising multiple equidistant biofilm electrodes. The generated data show that the MPS arrays can detect and describe the spatial–temporal changes in an aquatic environment resulting from an influx of carbon rich water, which could not be detected by conventional ORP electrodes.

Interestingly, however, the experiments conducted over a long period of time revealed unusual behaviors. These observed behaviors suggested that biofilms may have an ability to create a large network through which they communicate by means of inducing changes in electric potentials like a sophisticated electronic device. The complex structure of biofilms may be parallel to one of the complex integrated circuits, which comprise transistors, resistors and capacitors. These "biological" circuits within the biofilm could be responsible for the shifts and fluctuations in the electric potentials, resulting from the metabolic processes, in order to create communication mechanisms. Unlike the vessel or other chemical-induced form of communications however, these communication mechanisms appear to be electrical in nature and raise questions on whether biofilms have the ability to disperse changes in entropy or energy. Considering that biofilms exhibit a level of intelligence by the sheer fact that they could chemically or electrically communicate at nano or microdistances, it is rational to postulate that biofilms have evolved the ability to rapidly communicate over long distances (>0.6 m) and distribute energy across their networks like, or potentially better than, more complex multicellular organisms.

Acknowledgment

The authors would like to extend their gratitude to Ms. Michell Peppers for helping with the illustrations and animations.

Conflict of interest

The corresponding author (K.H.) declares that, as an associate editor of Nano LIFE, there is a conflict of interest regarding this manuscript. However, K.H. confirms that he was not involved in the peer review process of the manuscript, and therefore he has not had any influence on the editorial decision-making process. The conflict of interest was disclosed to the editorial team, and appropriate steps were taken to ensure that the peer review and decision-making process for this manuscript were handled impartially and transparently.

References

1. Z. Lewandowski and H. Beyenal, *Fundamentals of Biofilm Research* (CRC Press, Boca Raton, FL, 2007).
2. K. Sauer, P. Stoodley, D. M. Goeres, L. Hall-Stoodley, M. Burmølle, P. S. Steward and T. Bjarnsholt, *Nat. Rev. Microbiol.* **20**, 608 (2022).
3. H.-C. Flemming, E. D. van Hullebuch, T. R. Neu, P. H. Nielsen, T. Seviour, P. Stoodley, J. Wingender and S. Wuertz, *Nat. Rev. Microbiol.* **21**, 70 (2022).
4. A. Penesyan, I. T. Paulsen, S. Kjelleberg and M. R. Gillings, *NPJ Biofilms Microbiomes* **7**, 80 (2021).
5. R. M. Donlan, *EID J.* **8**, 881 (2002).
6. A. Prindle, J. Liu, M. Asally, S. Ly, J. Garcia-Ojalvo and G. M. Süel, *Nature* **527**, 59 (2015).
7. R. Martinez-Corral, J. Liu, A. Prindle, G. M. Süel and J. Garcia-Ojalvo, *Philos. Trans. R. Soc. Lond. B Biol. Sci.* **374**, 1774 (2019).
8. S. Manna, C. Ghanty, P. Baindara, T. Kr. Barik and S. M. Mandal, *J. Basic Microbiol.* **60**, 819 (2020).
9. K. Rabbaey, N. Boon, S. D. Siciliano, M. Verhaege and W. Verstraete, *Appl. Environ. Microb.* **70**, 5373 (2004).
10. I. S. Chang, H. Moon, O. Bretschger, J. K. Jang, H. I. Park, K. H. Nealson and B. H. Kim, *J. Microbiol. Biotechnol.* **16**, 163 (2006).
11. A. Dewan, H. Beyenal and Z. Lewandowski, *Environ. Sci. Technol.* **42**, 7643 (2008).
12. A. E. Franks, K. P. Nevin, H. F. Jia, M. Izallalen, T. L. Woodard and D. R. Lovley, *Energ. Environ. Sci.* **2**, 113 (2009).
13. N. S. Malvankar, M. Vargas, K. P. Nevin, A. E. Franks, C. Leang, B. C. Kim, K. Inoue, T. Mester, S. F. Covalla, J. P. Johnson, V. M. Rotello, M. T. Tuominen and D. R. Lovley, *Nat. Nanotechnol.* **6**, 573 (2011).
14. J. Babauta, R. Renslow, Z. Lewandowski and H. Beyenal, *Biofouling* **28**, 789 (2012).
15. E. Marsili, D. B. Baron, I. D. Shikhare, D. Coursolle, J. A. Gralnick and D. R. Bond, *Proc. Natl. Acad. Sci. USA* **105**, 3968 (2008).
16. B. Erable, D. Feron and A. Bergel, *ChemSusChem* **5**, 975 (2012).
17. D. R. Bond and D. R. Lovley, *Appl. Environ. Microb.* **69**, 1548 (2003).
18. F. Mansfeld, *Electrochim. Acta* **52**, 7670 (2007).
19. H. Richter, K. McCarthy, K. P. Nevin, J. P. Johnson, V. M. Rotello and R. D. Lovley, *Langmuir* **24**, 4376 (2008).
20. Y. Liu, H. Kim, R. R. Franklin and D. R. Bond, *Chem. Phys. Chem.* **12**, 2235 (2011).
21. J. P. Busalmen, A. Esteve-Nunez, A. Berna and J. M. Feliu, *Bioelectrochemistry* **78**, 25 (2010).
22. J. T. Babauta, Electron Transfer mechanisms in electrochemically active biofilms, Ph.D. Thesis, Washington State University (2012).
23. X. Zhang, Extracellular electron transport of electroactive biofilm, *Bioelectrosynthesis: Principles and Technologies for Value-Added Products*, eds. A. Wang, W. Liu, B. Zhang and W. Cai (Wiley, 2020), pp. 295–305.

24. L. Zou, F. Zhu, Z. Long and Y. Huang, *J. Nanobiotechnol.* **19**, 120 (2021).
25. E. M. Conners, K. Rengasamy and A. Bose, *J. Ind. Microbiol. Biotechnol.* **49**, 1 (2022).
26. G. S. Jadhav and M. M. Ghangrekar, *Bioresource Technol.* **100**, 717 (2009).
27. K. P. Katuri, P. Kavanagh, S. Rengaraj and D. Leech, *Chem. Commun.* **46**, 4758 (2010).
28. T. Yu and L. P. Bishop, *Water Sci. Technol.* **37**, 195 (1998).
29. J. S. McLean, G. Wanger, Y. A. Gorby, M. Wainstein, J. McQuaid, S. I. Ishii, O. Bretschger, H. Beyenal and K. H. Nealson, *Environ. Sci. Technol.* **44**, 2721 (2010).
30. J. S. McLean, P. D. Majors, C. L. Reardon, C. L. Bilskis, S. B. Reed, M. F. Romine and J. K. Fredrickson, *J. Microbiol. Methods* **74**, 47 (2008).
31. J. T. Babauta, H. D. Nguyen and H. Beyenal, *Environ. Sci. Technol.* **45**, 6654 (2011).
32. A. P. Borole, D. Aaron, C. Y. Hamilton and C. Tsouris, *Environ. Sci. Technol.* **44**, 2740 (2010).
33. A. K. Manohar, O. Bretschger, K. H. Nealson and F. Mansfeld, *Bioelectrochemistry* **72**, 149 (2008).
34. K. B. Oldham and J. C. Myland, *Fundamentals of Electrochemical Science* (Academic Press, San Diego, 1994).
35. S. Srikanth, S. V. Mohan and P. N. Sarma, *Bioresource Technol.* **101**, 5337 (2010).
36. A. Larossa-Guerrero, K. Scott, K. P. Katuri, C. Godinez, I. M. Head and T. Curtis, *Appl. Microbiol. Biot.* **87**, 1699 (2010).
37. D. N. Myers, Water-quality sensors with case studies on floods, hurricanes, and harmful algal blooms, *Evaluating Water Quality to Prevent Future Disasters*, ed. S. Ahuja (Elsevier Inc., 2019), pp. 219–283.
38. S. A. Burge, K. D. Hristovski, R. S. Burge, D. A. Hoffman, D. Saboe, P. Chao, E. Taylor and S. S. Koenigsberg, *Sci. Total Environ.* **742**, 140528 (2020).
39. T. Sale, S. Gallo, K. K. Askarani, M. Irianni-Renno, M. Lyverse, H. Hopkins, J. Blotevogel and S. Burge, *J. Hazard. Mater.* **408**, 124403 (2021).
40. R. N. Glud, N. B. Ramsing and N. P. Revsbech, *J. Phycol.* **28**, 51 (1992).
41. T. C. Zhang and P. L. Bishop, *Water Sci. Technol.* **30**, 47 (1994).
42. R. Renslow, C. Donovan, M. Shim, J. Babauta, S. Nannapaneni, J. Schenk and H. Beyenal, *Phys. Chem. Chem. Phys.* **13**, 21573 (2011).
43. S. R. Burge, K. D. Hristovski, R. G. Burge, D. Saboe, D. A. Hoffman and S. S. Koenigsberg, *Sci. Total Environ.* **751**, 142342 (2021).
44. F. C. Brown, S. R. Burge, K. D. Hristovski, R. G. Burge, E. Taylor and D. A. Hoffman, *Maced. J. Chem. Chem. Eng.* **39**, 119 (2020).
45. D. Saboe, H. Ghasemi, M. M. Gao, M. Samardzic, K. D. Hristovski, D. Boscovic, S. R. Burge, R. G. Burge and D. A. Hoffman, *Sci. Total Environ.* **764**, 142876 (2021).
46. D. Saboe, K. D. Hristovski, S. R. Burge, R. G. Burge, E. Taylor and D. A. Hoffman, *Sci. Total Environ.* **766**, 144424 (2021).
47. K. D. Hristovski, S. R. Burge, D. Boscovic, R. G. Burge and F. Babanovska-Milenkovska, *J. Environ. Chem. Eng.* **10**, 107491 (2022).

48. S. N. Yang and Z. Lewandowski, *Biotechnol. Bioeng.* **48**, 737 (1995).
49. F. H. Xia, H. Beyenal and Z. Lewandowski, *Water Res.* **32**, 3631 (1998).
50. H. Beyenal and Z. Lewandowski, *Water Res.* **34**, 528 (2000).
51. C. C. H. Cronenberg and J. C. Vandenheuvel, *Biosens. Bioelectron.* **6**, 255 (1991).
52. H. Beyenal and Z. Lewandowski, *Biotechnol. Progr.* **18**, 55 (2002).
53. H. Beyenal and Z. Lewandowski, *Aiche J.* **47**, 1689 (2001).
54. H. Beyenal, A. Tanyolac and Z. Lewandowski, *Water Sci. Technol.* **38**, 171 (1998).
55. E. Keszei, *Chemical Thermodynamics* (Springer-Verlag, Berlin Heidelberg, 2012).

www.ingramcontent.com/pod-product-compliance
Lightning Source LLC
Chambersburg PA
CBHW051243060325
22889CB00004BA/29
9789819809011